D1264737

ALSO BY AMERICA'S TEST KITCHEN

FOR A FULL LISTING OF ALL OUR BOOKS

CooksIllustrated.com

AmericasTestKitchen.com

PRAISE FOR AMERICA'S TEST KITCHEN TITLES

"The book's depth, breadth, and practicality makes it a must-have for seafood lovers."
PUBLISHERS WEEKLY (STARRED REVIEW) ON FOOLPROOF FISH

"Another flawless entry in the America's Test Kitchen canon, *Bowls* guides readers of all culinary skill levels in composing one-bowl meals from a variety of cuisines."
BUZZFEED BOOKS ON BOWLS

Selected as the Cookbook Award Winner of 2019 in the Health and Special Diet Category
INTERNATIONAL ASSOCIATION OF CULINARY PROFESSIONALS (IACP) ON THE COMPLETE DIABETES COOKBOOK

"This is a wonderful, useful guide to healthy eating."
PUBLISHERS WEEKLY ON NUTRITIOUS DELICIOUS

"The sum total of exhaustive experimentation . . . anyone interested in gluten-free cookery simply shouldn't be without it."
NIGELLA LAWSON ON THE HOW CAN IT BE GLUTEN-FREE COOKBOOK

"*The Perfect Cookie* . . . is, in a word, perfect. This is an important and substantial cookbook. . . . If you love cookies, but have been a tad shy to bake on your own, all your fears will be dissipated. This is one book you can use for years with magnificently happy results."
THE HUFFINGTON POST ON THE PERFECT COOKIE

"The book offers an impressive education for curious cake makers, new and experienced alike. A summation of 25 years of cake making at ATK, there are cakes for every taste."
THE WALL STREET JOURNAL ON THE PERFECT CAKE

"True to its name, this smart and endlessly enlightening cookbook is about as definitive as it's possible to get in the modern vegetarian realm."
MEN'S JOURNAL ON THE COMPLETE VEGETARIAN COOKBOOK

"The America's Test Kitchen team elevates the humble side dish to center stage in this excellent collection of 1,001 recipes."
PUBLISHERS WEEKLY ON THE SIDE DISH BIBLE

"Offers a real option for a cook who just wants to learn some new ways to encourage family and friends to explore today's sometimes-daunting vegetable universe. This is one of the most valuable cooking resources for the home chef since Marian Morash's beloved classic *The Victory Garden Cookbook* (1982)."
BOOKLIST (STARRED REVIEW) ON VEGETABLES ILLUSTRATED

"A one-volume kitchen seminar, addressing in one smart chapter after another the sometimes surprising whys behind a cook's best practices. . . . You get the myth, the theory, the science, and the proof, all rigorously interrogated as only America's Test Kitchen can do."
NPR ON THE SCIENCE OF GOOD COOKING

"The 21st-century *Fannie Farmer Cookbook* or *The Joy of Cooking*. If you had to have one cookbook and that's all you could have, this one would do it."
CBS SAN FRANCISCO ON THE NEW FAMILY COOKBOOK

"The go-to gift book for newlyweds, small families, or empty nesters."
ORLANDO SENTINEL ON THE COMPLETE COOKING FOR TWO COOKBOOK

"The book's depth, breadth, and practicality makes it a must-have for seafood lovers."
PUBLISHERS WEEKLY ON FOOLPROOF FISH

"Some books impress by the sheer audacity of their ambition. Backed by the magazine's famed mission to test every recipe relentlessly until it is the best it can be, this nearly 900-page volume lands with an authoritative wallop."
CHICAGO TRIBUNE ON THE COOK'S ILLUSTRATED COOKBOOK

"It might become your 'cooking school,' the only book you'll need to make you a proficient cook, recipes included. . . . You can master the 100 techniques with the easy-to-understand instructions, then apply the skill with the recipes that follow."
THE LITCHFIELD COUNTY TIMES ON 100 TECHNIQUES

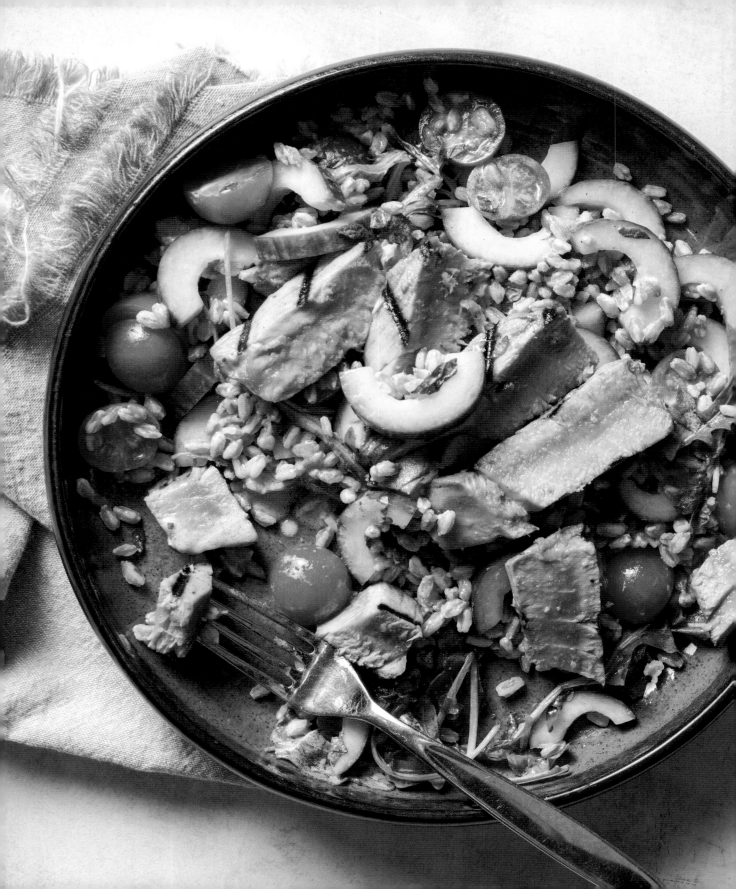

COOK FOR YOUR
GUT HEALTH

Quiet Your Gut, Boost Fiber, and Reduce Inflammation

with **ALICIA A. ROMANO**, MS, RD, LDN, CNSC

AMERICA'S TEST KITCHEN

Library of Congress Cataloging-in-Publication Data

Names: America's Test Kitchen (Firm), author.
Title: Cook for your gut health : quiet your gut, boost fiber, and reduce
    inflammation / America's Test Kitchen.
Description: Boston, MA : America's Test Kitchen, [2021] | Includes index.
Identifiers: LCCN 2020053201 (print) | LCCN 2020053202 (ebook) | ISBN
    9781948703529 (paperback) | ISBN 9781948703536 (ebook)
Subjects: LCSH: Gastrointestinal system--Diseases--Diet therapy--Recipes. |
    LCGFT: Cookbooks.
Classification: LCC RC819.D5 C66 2021 (print) | LCC RC819.D5 (ebook) |
    DDC 641.5/638--dc23
LC record available at https://lccn.loc.gov/2020053201
LC ebook record available at https://lccn.loc.gov/2020053202

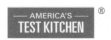

AMERICA'S TEST KITCHEN
21 Drydock Avenue, Boston, MA 02210

Printed in Canada
10 9 8 7 6 5 4 3 2

Distributed by
Penguin Random House Publisher Services
Tel: 800.733.3000

Pictured on front cover One-Pot Chicken with Braised Spring Vegetables (page 110)

Pictured on back cover Ratatouille with Poached Eggs (page 42); Seared Shrimp with Fresh Tomato Sauce and Cilantro-Lime Quinoa (page 218); Beef and Oat Berry Soup (page 76); Roasted Kabocha Squash with Maple and Sage (page 280); Roasted Halibut, Broccolini, and Potatoes with Mustard Sauce (page 208); Lentil Salad with Pomegranate and Walnuts (page 296)

Editorial Director, Books **Adam Kowit**

Executive Food Editor **Dan Zuccarello**

Executive Managing Editor **Debra Hudak**

Senior Editors **Camila Chaparro, Joseph Gitter, Lawman Johnson, Nicole Konstantinakos, Sacha Madadian, and Sara Mayer**

Test Cook **Sarah Ewald**

Editorial Assistant **Emily Rahravan**

Consulting Nutritionist **Alicia A. Romano, MS, RD, LDN, CNSC**

Design Director **Lindsey Timko Chandler**

Deputy Art Director **Janet Taylor**

Graphic Designer **Molly Gillespie**

Photography Director **Julie Bozzo Cote**

Photography Producer **Meredith Mulcahy**

Senior Staff Photographers **Steve Klise and Daniel J. van Ackere**

Staff Photographer **Kevin White**

Additional Photography **Joseph Keller and Carl Tremblay**

Food Styling **Joy Howard, Catrine Kelty, Steve Klise, Chantal Lambeth, Kendra McKnight, Ashley Moore, Christie Morrison, Marie Piraino, Elle Simone Scott, Kendra Smith, and Sally Staub**

PHOTOSHOOT KITCHEN TEAM

Photo Team and Special Events Manager **Alli Berkey**

Lead Test Cook **Eric Haessler**

Test Cooks **Hannah Fenton and Jacqueline Gochenouer**

Assistant Test Cooks **Gina McCreadie and Christa West**

Illustrations **Jay Layman**

Senior Manager, Publishing Operations **Taylor Argenzio**

Imaging Manager **Lauren Robbins**

Production and Imaging Specialists **Tricia Neumyer, Dennis Noble, and Amanda Yong**

Copy Editor **Deri Reed**

Proofreader **Vicki Rowland**

Indexer **Elizabeth Parson**

Chief Creative Officer **Jack Bishop**

Executive Editorial Directors **Julia Collin Davison and Bridget Lancaster**

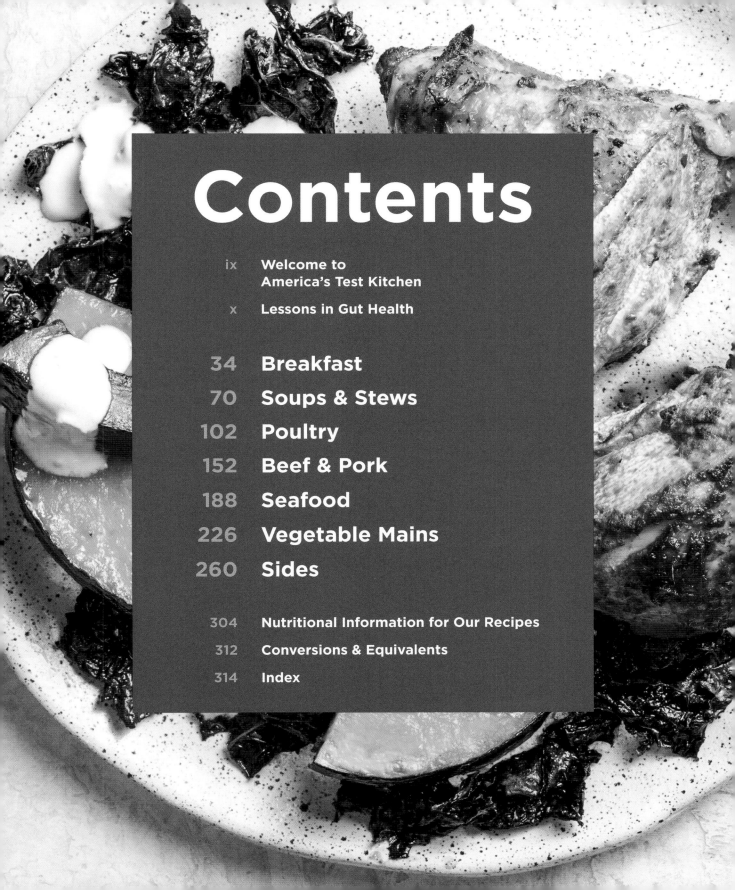

Contents

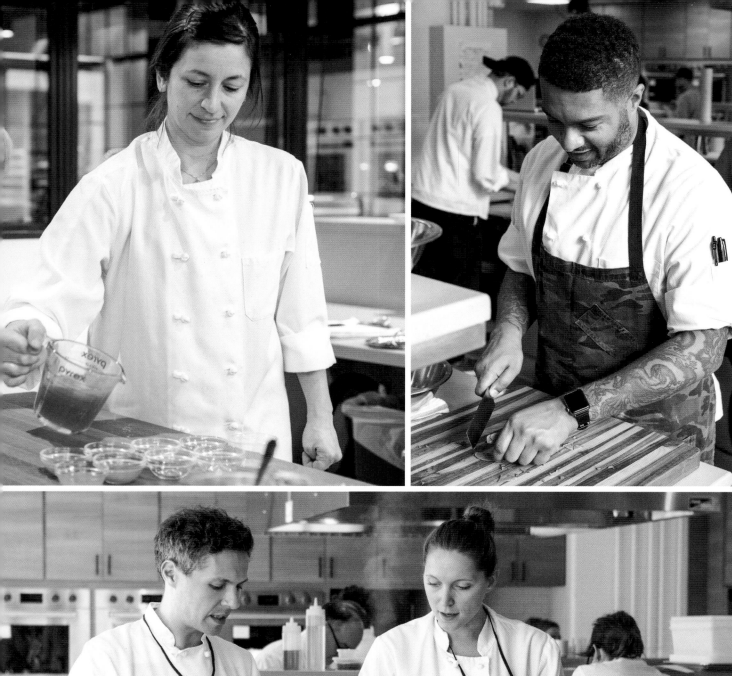

WELCOME TO AMERICA'S TEST KITCHEN

This book has been tested, written, and edited by the folks at America's Test Kitchen, where curious cooks become confident cooks. Located in Boston's Seaport District in the historic Innovation and Design Building, it features 15,000 square feet of kitchen space including multiple photography and video studios. It is the home of *Cook's Illustrated* magazine and *Cook's Country* magazine and is the workday destination for more than 60 test cooks, editors, and cookware specialists. Our mission is to empower and inspire confidence, community, and creativity in the kitchen.

We start the process of testing a recipe with a complete lack of preconceptions, which means that we accept no claim, no technique, and no recipe at face value. We simply assemble as many variations as possible, test a half-dozen of the most promising, and taste the results blind. We then construct our own recipe and continue to test it, varying ingredients, techniques, and cooking times until we reach a consensus. As we like to say in the test kitchen, "We make the mistakes so you don't have to." The result, we hope, is the best version of a particular recipe, but we realize that only you can be the final judge of our success (or failure). We use the same rigorous approach when we test equipment and taste ingredients.

All of this would not be possible without a belief that good cooking, much like good music, is based on a foundation of objective technique. Some people like spicy foods and others don't, but there is a right way to sauté, there is a best way to cook a pot roast, and there are measurable scientific principles involved in producing perfectly beaten, stable egg whites. Our ultimate goal is to investigate the fundamental principles of cooking to give you the techniques, tools, and ingredients you need to become a better cook. It is as simple as that.

To see what goes on behind the scenes at America's Test Kitchen, check out our social media channels for kitchen snapshots, exclusive content, video tips, and much more. You can watch us work (in our actual test kitchen) by tuning in to *America's Test Kitchen* or *Cook's Country* on public television or on our websites. Download our award-winning podcast *Proof*, which goes beyond recipes to solve food mysteries (AmericasTestKitchen.com/proof), or listen to test kitchen experts on public radio (SplendidTable.org) to hear insights that illuminate the truth about real home cooking. Want to hone your cooking skills or finally learn how to bake—with an America's Test Kitchen test cook? Enroll in one of our online cooking classes. And you can engage the next generation of home cooks with kid-tested recipes from America's Test Kitchen Kids.

Our community of home recipe testers provides valuable feedback on recipes under development by ensuring that they are foolproof. You can help us investigate the how and why behind successful recipes from your home kitchen. (Sign up at AmericasTestKitchen.com/recipe_testing.)

However you choose to visit us, we welcome you into our kitchen, where you can stand by our side as we test our way to the best recipes in America.

---

f facebook.com/AmericasTestKitchen
🐦 twitter.com/TestKitchen
▶ youtube.com/AmericasTestKitchen
📷 instagram.com/TestKitchen
📌 pinterest.com/TestKitchen

AmericasTestKitchen.com
CooksIllustrated.com
CooksCountry.com
OnlineCookingSchool.com
AmericasTestKitchen.com/kids

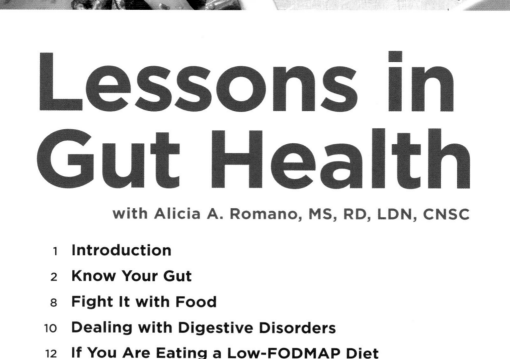

Lessons in Gut Health

with Alicia A. Romano, MS, RD, LDN, CNSC

INTRODUCTION

Whether because of lack of accessible research or unnecessary taboo, gut health, despite how important it is, only became of high public interest in recent years. But luckily it has quickly become part of the general health vernacular, an increasingly common consideration in and out of the doctor's office. Acute digestive discomfort, experienced by pretty much everyone once in a while (does every slice of pizza sit well with you?), and sometimes debilitating chronic GI disorders are gut issues on opposite ends of a spectrum. But no matter where you sit on that spectrum—maybe you're blissfully not on it at all—science shows that your gut is a set of organs (yes, a set) vital to your health and longevity, the reach of which goes far beyond your digestive system, influencing immunity, emotions, and how you absorb nutrients.

Your cooking is the easiest, most concrete way to promote a good gut, and therefore, general health; every time you feed yourself, you feed your gut. As trusted recipe developers, we're pleased to bring you a cookbook that, with whole foods, supports and promotes good gut health for most everyone—after all, everyone has a gut. At the same time, you can use this book if you're looking to calm occasional gastrointestinal symptoms or are among the 1 in 5 Americans who suffer from IBS.

What does cooking for your gut health look like? It's vibrant and satisfying. First and foremost, we emphasize fiber, as it's the number-one factor in promoting gut health in most people. It keeps you regular, it often carries prebiotics that feed good bacteria in your gut, and it can help prevent chronic inflammation of the GI tract. We call out the fiber content for every recipe, developing them to help you meet daily fiber goals. That means you can expect a rainbow of fruits and vegetables prepared with flair and hearty whole grains that satisfy you, plus supporting items, like healthful fats and lean proteins.

Eating for your gut shouldn't be restrictive; it should be abundant.

Start the day on a fiberful foot with breakfast dishes like Chickpea Shakshuka (page 40; adding chickpeas to the tomato sauce makes a filling egg-poaching medium). Pair sides—like Skillet-Roasted Broccoli with Smoky Sunflower Seed Topping (page 270) and Lentil Salad with Pomegranate and Walnuts (page 296)—from the side dish chapter with protein options as you like: We have chapters for lean but flavorful poultry, beef and pork, and seafood. Or take the guesswork out of rounding out the plate with one-dish meals like Chicken Mole with Cilantro-Lime Rice and Beans (page 122) and Soba Noodles with Roasted Eggplant and Sesame (page 252).

Eating for your gut shouldn't be restrictive; it should be abundant. A diverse diet is best for balancing good gut bacteria. But we also assist you if you've identified personal triggers (lactose and wheat are both common) or if you live gluten, dairy, or allium free. In fact, none of the recipes in this book use commonly irritating garlic or onion, instead getting foundational flavor through garlic-infused oil, aromatics like fresh ginger and fennel, or OK-to-eat allium like chives and scallion greens. These recipes showcase a variety of grains, many of them gluten free, and offer wheat-free variations if you need them. Likewise, our recipes show how to enjoy a bit of cheese while staying low in lactose, and most can be made dairy free.

If you've been diagnosed by your doctor with a gut disorder and are following The Low FODMAP Diet (universally backed for common gut disorders like IBS that we'll cover in detail) with a dietitian, you'll feel supported during and after the phased elimination of foods with our many naturally low-FODMAP recipes. And most others can simply be customized to be low FODMAP. Every recipe has an answer for the way your gut tells you to eat.

We make foolproof healthful recipes, but we couldn't go this alone. We consulted with nutritionist and dietitian Alicia A. Romano to guide us in the creation of these recipes and to give you an in-depth education on the evolving science of gut health, how to eat for it, and The Low FODMAP Diet. Dig in.

KNOW YOUR GUT

Before we focus on our favorite topic, food, it's important that we put your dietary choices into perspective: So what do we actually mean when we talk about the gut?

Hint: It's more than just your stomach. The gut is a concise way of talking about our digestive tract, also referred to as the gastrointestinal tract or GI tract. The gut, therefore, is a group of organs that starts with your mouth, extends to your esophagus, stomach, and small and large intestines, plus includes your organs that support digestive processes: your pancreas, liver, and gallbladder.

That's a lot of organs working in concert, but what makes keeping them healthy—keeping your gut healthy with foods outlined in the following pages—so important?

The gut is a bit of an overachiever; it's a boss tasked with several important jobs and it needs support, dietary and otherwise. Chiefly, there's digestion (breaking down your dinner) and absorption (receiving the nutrients from that dinner to keep your body going), and they are the building blocks for the health and proper function of our bodies. But the gut has more roles on its résumé than that. The gut influences the workings of the rest of your body: It's tightly connected to and communicates with your brain (see information on the gut-brain axis on page 4) and also plays a key role in your body's immunity.

Let's start with the most immediate concern for the gut, digestion, as well as cover the resources the gut can use to help complete its jobs smoothly.

Job #1: Digestion

Put simply, digestion is the process of breaking down the food we eat and turning it into nutrients essential for energy, growth and development, and cell repair within the body. As mentioned, our gut consists of a number of organs that play specific roles in the digestion process and we detail each in The Role of Digestive Organs (opposite).

We can support the gut in the digestive process with a healthy diet. Many common digestive complaints, like gas, bloating, and acid reflux—all unpleasant results of disruptions to the digestive process—may be related and responsive to modifications to your diet and eating habits. Here are some examples of nutritionally related digestive factors. (All of our recipes bear these in mind.)

The portion size of food you eat in a sitting
Large portions of high-fat food may contribute to reflux symptoms due to delayed emptying of the stomach and weakening of the gateway between the stomach and esophagus. If you're used to a heavy standard American diet, you'll find the recipes in this book to be moderately portioned.

The content of the food you eat in a sitting
The makeup of your meal, in protein, fat, carbohydrates, and fiber, can determine how difficult food will be to break down and how quickly it will move through your digestive tract. A low-fiber diet, for example, limited in produce and whole grains, may result in irregular bowel movements, so we focus on incorporating fiber into the full meals and side dishes in this book.

Whether the food you eat is liquid or solid
Liquefied food requires less effort for the gut to break down. How well you chew your food is a similar factor.

How fast you eat
The speed at which you eat can impact how well your food is digested.

Meal frequency
Eating with regularity, according to hunger throughout the day, can also promote regularity.

The Role of Digestive Organs

1 Mouth & Salivary Glands
- Teeth and tongue break up food particles.
- Saliva moistens and lubricates food; the enzyme amylase digests carbohydrates.

2 Pharynx & Esophagus
- Swallowing of food occurs.
- Food is transported to the stomach via peristalsis (muscle contractions); food passes through gastroesophageal sphincter, which acts as a gateway to the stomach.

3 Stomach
- Stomach acid (HCl) sterilizes food, killing most harmful bacteria, and food is broken down; HCl activates enzymes for digestion; pepsin breaks down proteins.
- Stomach uses churning motion to further break down food into a liquid material called chyme—this is what passes through the remainder of GI tract.
- Stores and churns food.

4 Small Intestine
- Digestion ends here.
- Nutrients are absorbed and packaged to be used by the rest of the body.

5 Large Intestine: Colon, Rectum & Anus
- Carbohydrates are fermented.
- Water and irons are reabsorbed.
- Feces form and are stored.
- Feces are eliminated through opening.

6 Pancreas, Liver & Gallbladder
- These additional organs store and release digestive enzymes that move the process along: The pancreas stores and releases enzymes for breaking down carbohydrates, fat, and protein; the liver produces bile, which is stored in the gallbladder and released to help emulsify fat.

ILLUSTRATION BY JAY LAYMAN

Job #2:
Working with the Brain

A diet that supports proper digestion (think: moderate portions, balanced macronutrients, plentiful fiber) can also ease your mind. The gut and brain are in constant communication, playing a game of telephone between the nervous system of the gut, called the enteric nervous system, and the central nervous system run by the brain. This link between the cognitive centers of the brain and intestinal function is known as the gut-brain axis. It means the brain plays a key role in digestion, telling us what, when, how much, and how fast to eat and drink. Reciprocally, the gut impacts mood and stress levels. In fact, bacteria in the gut actually make neuroactive compounds like serotonin, which regulates our emotions—if your stomach is well nourished, you can feel happier. In turn, the brain sends signals to the GI tract; that's why you might get that feeling in the "pit of your stomach" in times of stress or emotional hardship. Messages from the brain to the gut tune immune activity, muscle contractions (like peristalsis), and fluid secretion. When there is disruption to the brain for prolonged periods, such as in times of stress, or due to inadequate sleep or inflammation, the brain may perceive discomfort from the gut as stronger than usual.

Subdue the Stress

Lifestyle can have an impact on the quality of our health, and that extends to the gut. Stress can affect the smoothness of communications between the brain and gut and may trigger or heighten the perception of pain, bloating, and GI discomfort. Additionally, when we're stressed we may eat more or less than usual, and we may make poor dietary choices, which can influence digestion. Research continues to point to the role stress can play on the gut microbiome, influencing the type of gut bacteria we have available.

A priority in the health of our guts, then, lies in managing stress such as through maintaining a healthy social support network, engaging in regular physical exercise, and getting adequate sleep each night. If you are having a hard time managing stress in your life, it may be best to seek professional guidance.

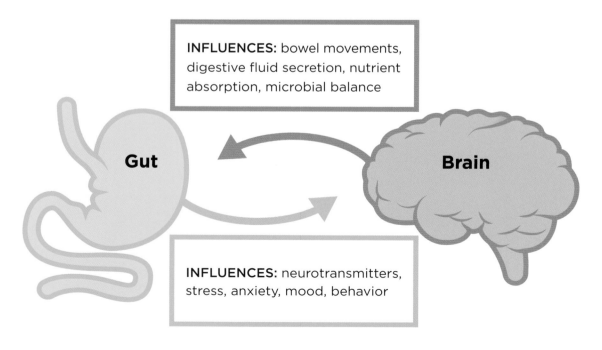

INFLUENCES: bowel movements, digestive fluid secretion, nutrient absorption, microbial balance

Gut

Brain

INFLUENCES: neurotransmitters, stress, anxiety, mood, behavior

Supporting Player:
The Gut Microbiome

No boss can work alone. It's important to acknowledge a supporting organ that lies within the gut: the gut microbiome.

The gut microbiome is an ecosystem of trillions of bacteria and microorganisms (including fungi, parasites, and viruses), collectively known as microbes, that coexist peacefully in a healthy person, with the largest community found in the small and large intestine. These microbes play a role in maintaining homeostasis—stability among body systems—by stimulating the immune system to go to work. Additionally, they go to work on the food you eat: Complex carbohydrates (fiber and starch) that are not easily digested will eventually encounter the microbes in the large intestine. Here, the microbes break down these carbohydrates through fermentation, producing short-chain fatty acids (SCFAs), essential food for intestinal cells and bacteria that helps them do their digestive job.

And what about probiotic supplements and their role? By definition, probiotics are live microorganisms (bacteria, yeast) that are among the same as the friendly ones that take up residence in your gut. (Our GI tracts have more than 100 trillion microorganisms representing more than 500 different species.) The idea is that if you add them to your diet, you can increase good bacteria and therefore gut function. So you can eat your friendly bacteria in foods in which they naturally occur: yogurt and kefir and fermented foods like kimchi, sauerkraut, pickles, miso, natto, and kombucha (see recipes on page 31). And dietary probiotic supplements make up a large portion of probiotic products. (Note: Like all US dietary supplements, they lack regulation and standardization, meaning there is no guarantee you are getting what you pay for.) Since we can't predict the population of bacteria unique to the individual and because a portion of what you ingest won't make it to the gut (due to sterilization in the stomach), your best bet is to first add probiotics through food sources so that you can also reap the benefits of the nutrients found naturally in those whole foods. Supplement with probiotics as advised by your doctor.

We don't yet know exactly what a healthy microbiome looks like and what its role in disease is. Plus, every individual has an entirely unique microbiome, shaped by both genetic and environmental factors. Currently, however, we can use what we do know about diet and lifestyle to potentially optimize the individual microbiome for better digestion and brain activity; a great way to do that is through the recipes in this book.

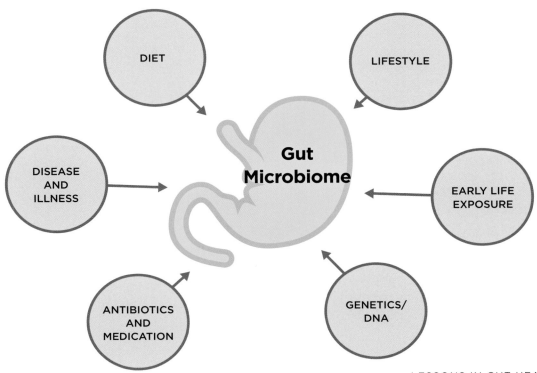

Job #3: Bolstering Immunity

The gut is a key player in the body's immune system. Think of the gut as a protective organ: It plays a role in blocking as many invasive organisms as it can, whether from the food you eat or even viruses in droplets in the air you breathe, preventing the spread of bacteria, toxins, and illnesses to other organs. In fact, 70 percent of your immune cells reside in the gut. (Yes, that means eating for your gut could mean fewer colds in the winter.)

First, the gut mechanically serves as a physical barrier to infections, starting at a mucous gel layer that's present throughout the gut and prevents bacteria from adhering. Further, movement of food through the GI tract (peristalsis) prevents bacteria from food from lingering, while stomach acid acts to sterilize food once it reaches the stomach. In a healthy gut, there is a tight barrier along its surface that controls what is absorbed into the bloodstream, further preventing harmful foodborne substances from entering the body and causing illness.

... the more fiber we eat, the better fueled our gut's good bacteria is.

But the reach goes beyond food invaders. Healthy digestion means you can absorb the nutrients from the good food you eat, which go on to support a number of bodily functions that bolster immunity.

Additionally, recall what we said about a healthy gut microbiome. Bacteria that are part of the normal intestinal tract act as good keepers of the gut, inhibiting colonization of invading bad bacteria (pathogens) simply by limiting space for them to exist and food for them to survive. These good bacteria put the immune system to work by stimulating the development of immune cells, chiefly T-cells. These are particularly important for the immune system, as they distinguish between good cells that your body should protect and bad ones (like cold viruses).

Again, that food for good gut bacteria is the aforementioned short-chain fatty acids created through the fermentation of complex carbohydrates in the gut. That means the more fiber we eat, the better fueled our gut's good bacteria is and the better able they are to protect our bodies when pathogens invade.

Cracks In the System

In some individuals, for a variety of reasons, the structure and integrity of the aforementioned gut lining may be compromised. The tight juncture or barrier that acts as the bodyguard for the gut doesn't work properly, leading to cracks or holes throughout the lining and opportunity for partially digested foods and viruses to penetrate the tissue beneath it. Some refer to this as "leaky gut syndrome." To be clear, we all have some degree of "cracks or holes" in our gut lining—this barrier is not completely impenetrable, and that's normal. However, current research shows that many aspects of the standard American diet (high amounts of processed foods, concentrated sugars, and saturated fats), lifestyle (high stress), and high intake of bowel damaging substances (alcohol, aspirin) may disrupt this balance and initiate this process, potentially driving prolonged inflammation.

Inflammation and the Gut

Inflammation is a buzz word in the world of gut health. How does diet combat harmful inflammation?

There are two types of inflammation. Acute inflammation refers to a short-term process occurring with your white blood cells in response to tissue injury or outside bacteria and viruses. It comes on rapidly and is usually short lived. This is the helpful kind of inflammation, an essential survival mechanism that helps the body fight potential infection and repair damaged tissue. In the gut, a little bit of acute inflammation isn't a bad thing: This may be the result of the food you eat, or it may be the gut's immune response to invading pathogens.

Chronic inflammation is problematic; it's when this usually short-term process lingers over months or years. Either the immune system response fails to eliminate the problem and inflammation stays active even after the initial threat (injury, illness, disease) has been eliminated, or the immune system acts in response to invaders that aren't, in fact, harmful. This chronic inflammatory process plays a role in challenging chronic diseases such as cardiovascular disease, diabetes, arthritis, asthma, and direct gut disorders, including chronic inflammatory diseases of the GI tract. A number of factors can influence chronic inflammation, including, for our purposes: poor diet, as well as environmental conditions, stressful lifestyle, infections, and some diseases.

Eating real foods that are nutrient dense supports your body's natural anti-inflammatory pathway while boosting your immunity.

There are no quick-fix solutions (even dietary ones) for any inflammation in the body. There are a number of suspicious treatments for "gut inflammation" on the market, from untested and heavily marketed supplements and herbs to cleanses and juicing and restrictive elimination diets, typically those that remove can-be nutritious foods like gluten and dairy. Many of these are not backed by science and can cause more harm.

It takes work, but the way to fight chronic inflammatory disorders through your gut isn't complicated: Eating real foods that are nutrient-dense supports your body's natural anti-inflammatory pathway—the pathway that helps prevent lingering, chronic inflammation—while boosting your immunity. We recommend eating as this book advises, with tons of recipes for a diet rich in plant-based foods that provide the fiber that we need to feed our gut bacteria and vital vitamins, minerals, phytonutrients, and antioxidants that collectively meet what our bodies' anti-inflammatory molecules need.

Some heavy-hitting anti-inflammatory plants you'll find in this book: blueberries, pomegranates, Swiss chard, and ginger. Also important: omega-3 fatty acids and other healthful unsaturated fats. The recipes in this book emphasize moderate fat from olive oil, fatty fish, avocado, and nuts and seeds. Research shows that these eating patterns may actually improve the diversity of our gut microbe community.

FIGHT IT WITH FOOD

Fiber for Everyone

So what should you eat to boost gut health? At the most basic level, the message is one you may have already heard (including so far in this introduction): Eat a varied and nutrient-dense diet that emphasizes plants. Incorporate healthful fats to enable the absorption of vitamins and minerals. Incorporate probiotic foods to help balance gut microflora. Limit highly processed foods. In this book you'll find real, uncomplicated food for all: no supplements, no gimmicks.

But the biggest focus of this book and a gut-healthy diet is fiber. Americans eat, on average, only 50 percent of the recommended dietary intake of fiber per day, and yet adequate fiber intake is an essential driver in promoting and maintaining our digestion. Plus, it plays an important role in prevention and management of a number of chronic diseases outside of the GI tract. What exactly is fiber? It's the part of plant foods—grains, fruits, vegetables, beans, nuts—that isn't entirely broken down in the small intestine during digestion. It moves to the colon to create the bulk and form of the stool. The key to serving you fiber in this book was simple and supplement-free: No matter the ingredients in our recipes—whether eggy breakfast dish or seafood dinner—we cooked them to accommodate plentiful vegetables and whole grains and legumes that have star status.

Fiber is categorized as insoluble or soluble, and both are present in fiber foods in different proportions. Insoluble fiber doesn't dissolve in water, so it passes through your digestive tract largely intact and helps to provide bulk to stool. Insoluble fiber makes food pass more quickly through the intestines, thus promoting regular bowel movements. It can be found in larger amounts in whole grains, fruit and vegetable skins, and nuts.

Soluble fiber dissolves in water to form a gel, creating the form of stool. It is fermented in the lower gut (insoluble fiber is not fermented) by bacteria there. One of the by-products of fiber fermentation is SCFAs (see page 5) that feed our gut bacteria. Soluble fiber's been shown to lower both LDL ("bad") cholesterol levels as well as total cholesterol levels and to slow the absorption of glucose, helping to maintain stable blood glucose levels. Soluble fiber is found in the fleshy parts of produce, in oats, barley, and dried beans.

A specific type of soluble fiber, prebiotics, not only ferments and produces SCFAs but is selectively targeted by just the good bacteria in your gut for this feast and therefore promotes the creation of more good bacteria. Prebiotics' benefits, then, extend to regulating the immune system, bowels, and cholesterol. Prebiotic foods include asparagus, jícama, oats, bananas, apples, beans, and onions and garlic. They're great to incorporate if they're tolerated. (If they aren't, there are plenty of other sources of fiber to focus on.)

Men age 50 or younger should take in 38 grams of fiber per day; women should take in 25 grams. Men age 51 or older should take in 30 grams per day; women, 21 grams. Increase your fiber slowly to aid in tolerance, as you may experience temporary bloating, gas, diarrhea, or constipation as you acclimate.

Simple Fiber Solutions

Try these ways to add fiber to your day.

- *Sprinkle it:* Add chia or flax seeds and berries to your yogurt or oatmeal.
- *Vary with vegetables:* Add wilted spinach or leftover cooked veggies to eggs.
- *Love legumes:* Try legume-based pastas made from chickpeas and lentils; add beans to sauces, pasta dishes, or salads.
- *Spiralize it:* Add shredded or spiralized vegetables to any pasta or soup.
- *Get garnishing:* Sprinkle sides or salads with nuts, seeds, or pickled vegetables.
- *Snack smart:* Crunch on popcorn, whole-wheat crackers, and steamed edamame.
- *Go bowling:* A bowl of berries or other fresh fruit will fill you up between meals.

Ranking Fiber

Find the fiber content of your favorite plant-based foods and those in our recipes to help you build and supplement your meals.

Food	Portion	Grams of Fiber	Food	Portion	Grams of Fiber
Lentils	1 cup (cooked)	15.5	Green beans	1 cup	3.5
Black beans	1 cup (cooked)	15	Sweet corn	1 cup (boiled)	3.5
Lima beans	1 cup (cooked)	13	Brown rice	1 cup (cooked)	3.5
Chickpeas	1 cup (cooked)	12.5	Almonds	¼ cup (1 ounce)	3.5
Chia seeds	2 tablespoons	10	Canned pumpkin	½ cup	3.5
Artichoke hearts	1 cup	10.5	Kabocha squash	1 cup	3
Green peas	1 cup (cooked)	9	Fennel	1 cup sliced	3
Raspberries	1 cup	8	Potatoes	1 small (with skin)	3
Bulgur	1 cup (cooked)	8	Banana	1 medium	3
Freekeh	1 cup (cooked)	8	Orange	1 medium	3
Oat berries	1 cup (cooked)	8	Strawberries	1 cup	3
Whole-wheat pasta	1 cup (cooked)	6	Asparagus	1 cup	3
Pearled barley	1 cup (cooked)	6	Kale	1 cup (cooked)	3
Parsnips	1 cup sliced	6	Okra	1 cup	3
Jícama	1 cup sliced	6	Celery	1 cup chopped	2.5
Broccoli	1 cup (cooked)	5	Bell pepper	1 medium	2.5
Avocado	½ avocado	5	Pineapple	1 cup pieces	2.5
Quinoa	1 cup (cooked)	5	Eggplant	1 cup cubed	2.5
Edamame	1 cup shelled	6	Cauliflower	1 cup chopped	2
Apple (with skin)	1 medium	4.5	Tomato	1 cup chopped	2
Spinach	1 cup (cooked)	4	Escarole	1 cup chopped	2
Swiss Chard	1 cup (cooked)	4	Millet	1 cup (cooked)	2
Cabbage	1 cup (cooked)	4	Snap Peas	1 cup	2
Brussels sprouts	1 cup (cooked)	4	Radishes	½ cup sliced	1
Potato (with skin)	1 cup (cooked)	4	Zucchini	1 cup sliced	1
Sweet potato (no skin)	1 medium (cooked)	4			
Carrots	1 cup chopped	4			

DEALING WITH DIGESTIVE DISORDERS

For many, getting adequate fiber—through nutritious dishes like the recipes in this book make—can do wonders for overall and digestive health. These recipes can support the functional GI disorders (most notably IBS and constipation) detailed below. Note that there are also GI disorders that are outside the scope of this book when it comes to diet. We want to give a brief description of other disorders as well so you know when diet may not be the answer. In any case, this book cannot replace medical advice.

Functional GI Disorders

Stomach aches and pains. Bloating. Abdominal cramping. Frequent trips to the bathroom. Going too long before "going." These are just a few of the symptoms and complaints that go hand in hand with functional GI disorders (FGIDs), the most common GI disorders in the general population and that affect nearly 2 in 4 persons worldwide. They often lead to side effects that can impair quality of life. These are conditions such as IBS and constipation (but also include functional dyspepsia, functional vomiting, and functional abdominal pain), in which the GI tract looks normal and structures are intact, but they don't, yes, *function* properly or feel normal. Diagnosis requires a workup with your medical team and may include tests to view your GI tract.

There are dietary and lifestyle factors that may play a role in creating FGIDs or making them worse, including eating a diet low in fiber (that's where we help), stress, certain medications, inadequate exercise, changes in routine or traveling, resisting the urge to have a bowel movement, and overusing laxatives that may weaken the bowel muscles. Any impairment to the gut-brain interaction rather than to gut structures can be functional (there are more than 30 recognized FGIDs!), but two common diagnoses are IBS and constipation.

Irritable Bowel Syndrome (IBS)

IBS is the most prevalent FGID worldwide, affecting about 1 in 5 Americans annually and 1 in 8 persons worldwide. This diagnosis usually comes after other conditions are ruled out, including inflammatory bowel disease (IBD), celiac disease, ulcers, food allergies, and colitis. Symptoms of IBS can include abdominal pain and cramps, excess gas, bloating, change in bowel habits, and alternating constipation and diarrhea.

IBS can be quite debilitating for patients, with a cascade of symptoms. The scientific and medical communities are still learning about what contributes to IBS, from how our brain and gut talk to how we digest and absorb food and what our gut has been exposed to (infection, previous antibiotic therapy). Only a small number of people with IBS have very severe symptoms, and in some cases, people can control symptoms by managing diet, lifestyle, and stress (these again!).

Constipation

The technical definition of being constipated is having fewer than three bowel movements per week; however, how often we go can vary considerably. Regardless, the longer we go between regular bowel movements, the more difficult it becomes to pass stool. As a result, stools can be dry and hard, bowel movements can be painful, and we can have a feeling of incomplete bowel emptying. We shouldn't be shy talking about our bowels: Studies show that constipation accounts for almost 8 million health care visits in the US annually. Constipation can either be idiopathic in nature (of an unknown cause) or due to a

Note that the recommendations in this book do not take precedence over medical advice. If you are experiencing prolonged GI symptoms that are not responsive to common dietary therapy, you should seek medical attention. Additionally, if you have a known GI diagnosis, you should speak with your physician and dietitian about appropriate dietary practices, as their recommendations may vary.

slow-moving intestine or related to IBS (known as IBS-C); additional medical causes of constipation exist and are diagnosed by your gastrointestinal physician.

Turning back to our lesson on digestion (see page 2), the colon is responsible for absorbing water from waste to create stool. In the case of constipation, the colon absorbs too much water from the stool, often due to food passing too slowly through the digestive tract. This dries out the stool, making it hard in consistency and difficult to pass. Eating high-fiber foods and drinking adequate fluid (see page 26 for flavorful sippers) are major parts of a healthful diet to manage constipation: Water is necessary to keep our stool soft and bulky rather than dry and hard. We suggest drinking about half your body weight in ounces of water per day.

In addition to *what* you eat, it's important to eat with regularity to achieve regularity. When we eat, we stimulate digestion that makes the intestines move and groove.

So rather than skipping meals or eating erratically, aim for three or four discrete meals. Consult your doctor for other tips on becoming more regular if this is a concern. And note that if you experience persistent constipation that does not respond to modifications in lifestyle and diet or is associated with significant abdominal pain, major bloating, or blood in the stool, you should swiftly seek medical attention.

When basic diet, even increasing fiber adequately, and lifestyle adjustments are not enough to relieve IBS or constipation, a more tailored dietary approach, known as The Low FODMAP Diet (see page 12) may be advised by your medical team. The Low FODMAP Diet is a science-backed dietary approach for the management of IBS developed by Monash University in Melbourne, Australia. It offers a great deal of symptom management for those suffering with IBS. We discuss The Low FODMAP Diet in detail in the following pages and provide you with clearly labeled low-FODMAP recipes throughout the book.

Autoimmune Disorders

Outside of FGIDs, there are autoimmune GI disorders to mention that this book, or any diet, is not enough to treat; these conditions are medically diagnosed and treated, and their nutritional management is highly individualized.

Inflammatory Bowel Disease (IBD)

IBD covers autoimmune disorders that involve chronic inflammation of the lining of the gut, including ulcerative colitis (UC) (inflammation and sores in the innermost lining of the large intestine, often accompanied by bloody diarrhea) and Crohn's disease (inflammation of the lining of the digestive tract that can extend entirely through the intestinal wall and may result in diarrhea, narrowing of the GI tract, abnormal openings in the GI tract, and malabsorption). These conditions usually involve debilitating symptoms and in some cases may lead to serious or life-threatening complications, and thus appropriate medical management is paramount.

The nutritional management of IBD isn't one-size-fits-all and is modified based on the state of IBD—whether the condition is "active" (a flare) or "at rest" (remission). Although no specific diet has been shown to prevent or treat IBD, specific diet strategies may help, including actually limiting fiber during a flare.

Celiac Disease

Celiac disease is another serious autoimmune disease in which the body mounts an immune response to eating gluten, a protein found in wheat, barley, and rye. The immune system creates inflammation that damages the lining of the small intestine, creating a cascade of symptoms of varying severity including diarrhea, bloating, gas, fatigue, dizziness, flu-like symptoms, and poor absorption. Other effects may include anemia (low blood counts) and bone thinning (osteoporosis). Treatment involves a strict gluten-free diet to help manage symptoms, heal the gut, and prevent long-term and serious complications.

IF YOU ARE EATING A LOW-FODMAP DIET

In some cases, simply upping your fiber and changing lifestyle habits may not be enough to combat FGIBs like IBS, so your primary care or gastrointestinal physician may recommend trialling a diet therapy known as The Low FODMAP Diet. This medically tailored diet is highly researched in the realm of IBS and is typically advised under the guidance of a registered dietitian. The Low FODMAP Diet consists of eliminating commonly bothersome fermentable carbohydrates for a spell, with a structured reintroduction of different types. The end goal: symptom reduction and the most liberal diet possible. Three in four individuals with a diagnosis of IBS will benefit from a dietary restriction of FODMAPs. A large portion of the recipes in this book satisfy the requirements of the complete elimination phase of this diet to support you if you need it—while still getting adequate fiber. (Achieving adequate fiber while eating low FODMAP is an area where patients often need help.)

What Are FODMAPs?

Most food we eat is broken down and absorbed in the small intestine. The portion of food that makes it past the small intestine (mostly sugars and fibers) arrives to the large intestine mostly undigested and, in the case of sugars, soluble fibers, and prebiotic soluble fibers (see page 8), ready to be feasted on by gut bacteria. The end result: fermentation and gas production. The process of fermentation—feeding our gut bacteria—is necessary for a healthy gut. In the case of IBS and other FGIBs however, the result can be a chain reaction resulting in the aforementioned uncomfortable GI symptoms. Scientists have come to understand that in the case of IBS, certain types of fermentable short-chain carbohydrates are particularly poorly absorbed by the small intestine, and during digestion they pull water into the GI tract and create a fast food source—a feeding frenzy, essentially—for bacteria in the gut, which for some people can cause bloating, abdominal pain, constipation, and diarrhea. This understanding led to the development of The Low FODMAP Diet by Monash University. This therapy aims at cutting off these fast-food supplies and improving overall symptom tolerance for IBS sufferers. FODMAP is an acronym for the different types of potentially offending carbohydrates (see High & Low-Fodmap Food List on page 14).

The diet has continued to evolve since its development. It is impossible to guess the FODMAP content of food; researchers at Monash University continue to use careful lab analyses to measure FODMAP contents and update guidelines for practitioners and consumers. Many common foods are considered high FODMAP, including wheat, barley, rye, garlic, onion, apples, watermelon, pears, cauliflower, mushrooms, honey, cow's milk, and sugar-free candies and gum—to name a few big ones that bother a lot of people. These foods are categorized by different FODMAP groups, as we can see in the chart. (Note: Some foods have multiple FODMAPs.)

As you might suspect, you shouldn't simply eliminate foods from your diet willy-nilly. For example, we've discussed the importance of certain foods, like prebiotic ones, which may be limited on this diet. The Low FODMAP Diet is a phased dietary approach to IBS management and includes three steps that allow one to reduce the overall load of FODMAP foods and reintroduce them in a systematic way as triggers are identified: 1. Elimination (eliminating all FODMAP categories for two to six weeks to identify if they're a bother); 2. Reintroduction (methodically determining which FODMAP foods you can eat freely, which ones might need to be portion controlled or enjoyed only on occasion, and which you need to limit most often); and 3. Individualization (finding long-term, successful, nutritionally varied eating solutions). The goal: the most liberal diet possible with minimized GI symptoms. And that will look different for everyone. It's recommended that you follow it under the guidance of a registered dietitian; you can use our recipes to support you in doing so and in the future when you know what FODMAPs are your no-nos.

Lactose versus Dairy

Dairy products from cow's, sheep's, and goat's milk contain a type of natural sugar called lactose—one of the small-chain carbohydrates that can be hard to digest. In many cases, this is due to lactose intolerance, the most common food intolerance globally. Lactose intolerance occurs due to a decreased production of the digestive enzyme lactase that is needed to break down lactose. The result of intolerance: gas, bloating, and diarrhea.

Now, there's a big misconception that *all* dairy products need to be avoided in order to follow both a low-FODMAP diet and a generally healthful diet for the gut. However, even if you suffer from lactose intolerance, studies show that you may still be able to tolerate small amounts of dairy in your diet—we call this a low-lactose diet. What's more, not all dairy products are created equal. For example, the amount of lactose in a cup of milk (11 grams) is much higher than the amount of lactose in an ounce of hard cheese (often just 1 gram). So even on a low-lactose diet, you can likely enjoy small amounts of dairy throughout the day, a sprinkle of goat cheese on Chickpea Shakshuka (page 40) or a dollop of yogurt on Curried Millet with Almonds and Raisins (page 290).

Since there are so many individuals who suffer from diagnosed lactose intolerance, we chose to adapt all the recipes in this book to have the option to be low in lactose by developing recipes to work with lactose-free and dairy-free milk alternatives and featuring naturally low-lactose cheese. For completely dairy-free recipes, look for the round blue tag next to recipes and variations. If you do not suffer from a lactose intolerance or a dairy allergy, feel free to use your favorite cow's, sheep's, or goat's milk products.

F	**Fermentable**	Fermentable is a modifier for all of the following carbohydrates in the chart: They're fibers and sugars that act as fast food for bacteria in the lower gut during digestion; those with functional GI disorders experience heightened discomfort from these.
O	**Oligosaccharides** (fructans and galacto-oligosaccharides (GOS))	Fructans: wheat, garlic, onions, leeks, shallots, green peas, snow peas, snap peas, sun-dried tomatoes, artichokes GOS: kidney, pinto, white, great Northern, black beans; large amounts of chickpeas and lentils
D	**Disaccharides** (lactose)	Milk (cow's, sheep's, goat's), soft cheese (cottage, ricotta, cream cheese), ice cream, yogurt
M	**Monosaccharides** (fructose)	Mangoes, apples, pears, cherries, figs, dried fruit, honey, agave, high-fructose corn syrup Note: All fruits naturally contain fructose. These listed contain a great excess of fructose.
A	**[and]**	
P	**Polyols** (sorbitol and mannitol)	Sorbitol: apples, blackberries, peaches, plums, some candy and gum Mannitol: cauliflower, snow peas, some candy and gum

High- & Low-FODMAP Food List

A diet low in FODMAPs isn't meant to be limiting; take a look at a snapshot of foods you should limit next to those you can eat more abundantly.

Food Category	High-FODMAP Foods	Low-FODMAP Foods
Vegetables	Artichokes, asparagus, cauliflower, garlic, green peas, mushrooms, onions, sugar snap peas	Arugula, collard greens, kale, spinach, carrots, parsnips, bell pepper, cucumber, potato, tomato, kabocha squash
Fruits	Apples, ripe bananas, pears, nectarines, peaches, watermelon, grapefruit, dried fruit, figs, raspberries, cherries, plums, prunes, persimmons, mangoes	Blueberries, strawberries, raspberries, cantaloupe, honeydew, kiwi, pineapple, grapes, oranges, lemons, limes, papaya
Dairy/Dairy Alternatives	Soft cheese, condensed or evaporated milk, milk, ice cream, yogurt, soy milk made from whole soybeans	Lactose-free milk, lactose-free yogurt, plant-based milks (see page 19), canned coconut milk; feta, goat, cheddar, Parmesan, mozzarella cheeses
Grains	Wheat, barley, rye	Rice, quinoa, corn, millet, oats, polenta, slow-leavened sourdough bread (see page 27), soba noodles (100 percent buckwheat), gluten-free pasta and bread (see page 19)
Legumes	Black beans, pinto beans, great Northern beans, lima beans, navy beans, soybeans, split peas	Small amounts of canned chickpeas (¼ cup) and lentils (½ cup)
Nuts/Seeds	Pistachios, cashews	Measured amounts of almonds, pecans, hazelnuts, walnuts, Brazil nuts, peanuts, and pine nuts; sunflower, pumpkin, chia, flax, hemp, and poppy seeds; peanut butter (2 tablespoons), almond butter (1 tablespoon)
Baking Items	Flours made from wheat, barley, rye or beans; agave syrup, honey, molasses; chicory root, high-fructose corn syrup, sugar alcohols; garlic/onion powder, seasoning blends with garlic/onion	Wheat-free/bean-free flour blends (corn, quinoa, rice, etc.); maple syrup, dark chocolate, table sugar, confectioners' sugar, brown sugar, garlic oil

Allium and Wheat: Limiting or Eliminating Fructans

Fructans, short-chain carbohydrates that are part of the "O" in FODMAPs, are abundant in our diets, with wheat accounting for nearly 70 percent of our fructan intake, followed by onion. Intolerance to fructan foods occurs in a great number of patients with IBS. However, strict avoidance of fructans long term is unnecessary and counterproductive for those patients who are not bothered by them since many fructans act as prebiotics (see page 8).

We wanted to make sure our recipes could be universally enjoyed among readers struggling with functional GI conditions, so we made two decisions regarding these fructans: 1. We omitted fructan-containing allium (garlic and onions): We didn't need them with our workarounds. 2. We limited wheat, always offering a wheat-free substitution when we used it.

So rather than cooking with an abundance of allium, we created easy ways for the home cook to savor the flavor of these ingredients without the fructans. For those without a fructan intolerance, feel free to feed yourself and your gut by adding chopped prebiotic garlic and onion where you like. For those going through a low-FODMAP elimination or who have found that large amounts of allium are a trigger for symptoms, find that our flavorful recipes avoid them by calling for garlic oil where one might use allium. Cooking in garlic-infused oil, for which we provide a recipe (page 20), adds all of the aroma of garlic with none of the fructans, as these carbohydrates are water- but not oil-soluble. You can also make dishes deeply flavored from the start by sautéing other aromatic vegetables like sweet, anise-y fennel or finish by garnishing with low-FODMAP allium—chives and the green parts of scallions (see Allium to Eat and Not Eat).

Although we have chosen to reduce the amount of wheat in our recipes in this book, we are not encouraging a wheat-free diet for everyone, nor are we suggesting that a gluten-free diet is necessary to quiet your gut. In fact, there are a number of benefits to 100 percent whole-wheat products: prebiotic fiber, vitamins, and minerals. Unfortunately, we know the carbohydrates in wheat contain fructans, which cause many to experience GI symptoms after eating. Aside from fructans, gluten, the protein found in wheat, barley, and rye, should be

Allium to Eat and Not Eat

If you need to avoid fructans, eat allium from the right, not from the left.

NO

- Garlic cloves
- Onions
- Shallots
- White parts of scallions and leeks

YES

- Green parts of scallions and leeks
- Chives
- Garlic oil

strictly avoided when adhering to a diet for celiac disease. Our recipes that keep the wheat have the flexibility to fit your needs: If you're avoiding wheat because it contains fructans and is high FODMAP, look for recipes with the low-FODMAP icon; if you are avoiding gluten altogether, look for the gluten-free icon. You can also look to our substitutions—every recipe that includes wheat or gluten has instructions on how to make it wheat and gluten free. In order to ensure you meet your dietary needs, you'll find a vast array of recipes highlighting nutritious wheat-free ancient grains like quinoa and millet that pack a similar nutritional punch.

Serving Sizes and the Monash App

Monash University's Low FODMAP Diet isn't exactly intuitive; there are intricacies to doing it right. One is that it's important to understand that some foods that are considered low FODMAP are considered so only at certain portion sizes—eat large amounts and you could be pushing the FODMAP limit. Luckily, researchers and scientists at Monash University meticulously investigate foods and their FODMAP content. We highly recommend downloading their app, the Monash University FODMAP Diet. It uses a traffic-light system, indicating which foods contain FODMAPs and whether the FODMAP categories in the food are found in no-to-low amounts (green), moderate amounts (yellow), or high amounts (red). Also indicated are what serving sizes contain what levels of FODMAPs. Here's a summary of some things to know when navigating the diet and app.

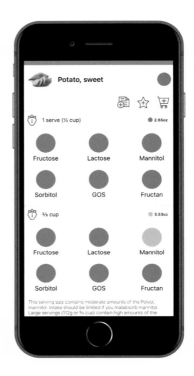

- *Green light, go:* Some foods have virtually no FODMAPs. These are green-light foods in all FODMAP categories; you can go ahead and enjoy them. Typically, the portion you'd need to eat for these be considered high FODMAP would be much larger than you could consume.

- *Green light, but go slow:* There are also portion-based low-FODMAP foods; these are the foods that are a go at certain portions, and the app will provide an acceptable ounce amount. Unfortunately, if you go beyond that portion you'll overfill your FODMAP cup.

- *Yellow light, eat with caution:* If a food is given a yellow circle, it is moderate in the FODMAP at hand and should be eaten extremely infrequently.

- *Red light, don't eat:* If you have an intolerance to the carbohydrate category that a food item is high (red) in, you should avoid it.

- *Stop FODMAP stacking:* When you eat two or more servings of foods from the same FODMAP group in one sitting, even if the foods are in a proper serving size, FODMAPs can stack, and your cup can overfill. (It is important to note that FODMAP stacking is not an issue for all and can typically be identified under the guidance of your dietitian.)

Low-FODMAP, High-Fiber Foods

If you're following a low-FODMAP diet, the message about eating more fiber might feel like a contradiction. Yes, adequate fiber intake can be a challenge if you're eliminating beans, whole-wheat products, and/or high-FODMAP vegetables and fruits (we're looking at you, asparagus, artichokes, cauliflower, and apples). But there are still plenty of ways to find fiber that won't interfere with digestion. Our recipes will help. Additionally, the easiest way to look at getting fiber is to think in terms of simple swaps. If you have to cut out A, what is the B you can replace it with? For example, if you have to cut out high-fiber Brussels sprouts and cauliflower, you can replace them with kale or collard greens. Below find high-fiber items (generally 3 or more grams per serving) you can eat to satiety without worrying about FODMAPs.

Food	Fiber / Serving
Parsnips	6 grams/1 cup sliced
Collard greens	6 grams/1 cup cooked
Carrots	3 grams/1 cup sliced
Kabocha squash	3 grams/1 cup
Potatoes	3 grams/1 small with skin
Wild rice	3 grams/1 cup
Quinoa	5 grams/1 cup
Canned lentils	4.5 grams/½ cup
Strawberries	3 grams/1 cup

What to Forget About

Eating for your gut might seem daunting. We want to ease your mind (and gut) and remind you there is plenty to eat.

Some Fat Is Fine

Although we know that fatty, greasy foods can be a GI irritant, incorporating healthful unsaturated fats (such as fatty fish and the oils from nuts, seeds, and plants) is encouraged (and may provide further anti-inflammatory benefit). Choose these and limit fried foods and large amounts of saturated fats from fatty marbled cuts of meat, lard, butter, and the like.

Animal Protein Is OK

For the most part, high-protein foods such as poultry, fish, meat, and eggs are fine, as the low-FODMAP diet is about carbohydrates. Fatty cuts of meat and processed meat tend to be high in saturated fat and should be limited. Also be aware of the use of high-FODMAP seasonings.

Don't Follow Fad Eliminations

As outlined on page 13, you can eat dairy and gluten—unless you have an allergy or celiac disease. Many dairy products work quite well on a low-FODMAP diet.

Sugar Isn't the Enemy

Following general guidelines minimizing added sugar and maximizing nutritious foods is key for health. This does not mean we have to avoid sugar overall to achieve a healthy gut. We like to encourage quality and moderation over quantity.

Skip Quick Fixes

If it sounds too good to be true, it is. There are so many diet trends not backed by science. Our guts crave a diverse diet, not gimmicks or unnecessary restrictions.

Choose Ingredients with Care

If you are following a low-FODMAP diet or specialized plan, you should be careful when purchasing certain items that might include hidden irritants, like those listed below. Of course, this list isn't exhaustive, and you should always check ingredient labels, watching for allium flavorings and celery powder; lactose and dairy (milk powder sneaks into items for protein and browning properties); and wheat (wheat or gluten-based thickeners).

Oat Products

Oats are a gift for those who are fructan or gluten free and might be missing wheat flour products; you can happily enjoy granola, chewy oat berry salads, and baked goods made with oat flour that satisfy like wheat. Just be aware that suitable-to-eat oats are commonly cross-contaminated with wheat, because of how they grow and are processed. Look for oat products—oats of all types (quick, old-fashioned, steel-cut), oat berries (groats), oat flour, and snack bars and other items made with oats—that are certified gluten free if gluten is a concern.

Tomato Products

Tomato and garlic or tomato and onion are common pairs. Make sure to buy canned tomato products and jarred sauces without the addition of allium or allium powders. (We take care of the aromatic quality of the dish in each recipe.)

Broths

We call for chicken, beef, and vegetable broths in this book. As you probably know from experience, broth often is infused with allium, and the same is true for store-bought varieties. We love our allium-free recipes for all of these broths (see page 24), but if you're purchasing broth, check the label. Fructan-free vegetable broths can be difficult to find, but Imagine, Zoup!, and Gourmend brands are good choices for chicken and beef broths.

Soy Sauce and Oyster Sauce

Soy sauce points up the flavor of gut-friendly dishes. Be sure to buy gluten-free soy sauce or tamari if you're cooking gluten free. And check your oyster sauce bottle before purchasing as many brands use wheat-based thickener.

Customization: The Key to Our Gut-Healthy Recipes

  MAKE IT LOW FODMAP

  MAKE IT DAIRY FREE

  MAKE IT GLUTEN FREE

We cannot stress it enough: Gut health is highly individualized. Yes, everyone has a gut that needs caring for, but some could have a condition that requires a doctor's and dietitian's assistance and, after all, everyone has a different microbiome and microbial makeup. That's why we've developed recipes that can meet your unique needs, whomever you are. Use them every day to support a healthful, holistic way of eating with varied nutrition or use them on occasion, when the recipes are appropriate for your condition.

You can be sure you'll get adequate fiber if you cook from this book. Round icons tag recipes for their low-FODMAP, dairy-free, or gluten-free status. And at the bottom of the page, find your dietary customizations. These methods for making dishes low FODMAP never restrict or reduce the amount you can eat—you'll never find a serving-size reduction without a replacement ingredient of some kind, and you'll never find an omission of an ingredient necessary for flavor.

STOCKING UP

While it's true that the gut-friendly pantry might look different for everyone, there are some staples we recommend having on hand to make cooking easier. Some are high in fiber for helping to make hearty meals; others are helpful for adding flavor to gut-friendly foods.

Produce

Vegetables and fruit are always on the menu and should always be in the kitchen. In-season produce tastes best, but there are some items we recommend buying regularly.

Storage Vegetables

Having long-storing vegetables on hand makes it easy to produce a gut-friendly meal, even when you haven't planned ahead. As a bonus, many of these recipes are packed with nutrients, and they're often low FODMAP. Consider keeping winter squash (try kabocha found on pages 114 and 280), carrots and potatoes (free from FODMAPs), and sweet potatoes (low FODMAP at 2.65 ounces).

Leaves of Green

Dark, leafy greens like kale, collard greens, and Swiss chard are nutritious and great for getting your fiber, whether they star in dishes like Kale and Black Bean Breakfast Burritos (page 46) or get stirred into recipes for robust flavor and heft like Smoky Chicken and Lentil Soup with Swiss Chard (page 74). All of these greens are low FODMAP at any portion size. Lighter salad greens often are too, so you can feel good buying greens like escarole, arugula, and spinach for a main or side salad.

The Herb Garden

We recommend continually restocking scallions (using only green parts) and chives since they're both approved allium that can add oniony bite to a dish. Herbs of all kinds are great for adding fresh, pleasantly grassy flavor to foods.

The FODMAP-Free Fruit Bowl

You want to eat nutritious fresh fruits, but those high in fructose can be bothersome. Some fruits are safe when eaten to appetite and make a great snack: strawberries, raspberries (2 ounces), grapes, kiwi, oranges, papaya, and pineapple.

Lactose and Dairy Alternatives

Since many people eating for their gut health don't in fact need to avoid dairy or the proteins in dairy but rather the sugars (lactose), there are high-flavor dairy products you can use in moderation in low-lactose recipes. Think hard cheese for grating over dishes, cooking in butter, dolloping a bit of yogurt. If you want to make a dish lactose free, you can use lactose-free milks and yogurts; if you want to make a dish dairy free, you can use dairy-free milks and yogurts. We like Silk Unsweetened Almond Milk as an all-purpose choice and a number of plant-based yogurts can make a good sauce.

Grains and Grain Alternatives

If you need to avoid wheat or gluten, there are plenty of grains to enjoy that your diet will benefit from, like rice of all varieties, oat berries, quinoa, millet, and buckwheat soba noodles. You can use gluten-free breads and flours (find our recipes on pages 30–31) in recipes; be sure to look out for high-FODMAP ingredients like milk powder or bean flours. Beware also of white flour in some corn tortilla brands. And there are a host of gluten-free pastas made from everything from corn to beans. If you eat low FODMAP, choose those made from rice, corn, or quinoa. We like Jovial brand.

Flavor Boosters

With most allium and some umami-rich ingredients missing from low-FODMAP recipes, you should know how to finesse the flavor of dishes. A full spice rack comes in handy. Spices for rubbing onto meat or blooming before cooking, or for sprinkling over dishes are a sure way to, well, spice things up. (Make sure to check for allium powders in store-bought spice blends. Chili powder is a common example so we call for chipotle chile powder.) Miso and soy sauce provide umami depth. Nuts and seeds add richness when you omit cheese or avocado. And we've provided a reliable arsenal of low-FODMAP sauces and condiment recipes (see pages 21–25).

GUT-FRIENDLY MEAL BUILDERS

Sometimes it's in the sauce. Gut-friendly dishes, like any, can benefit from a foundational or finishing flavor booster, but those can come from the very ingredients and condiments that commonly carry FODMAPs—most often fructans for flavoring, or thickeners that are sometimes hidden. So why not make them at home? Here are our recipes that will allow you to add aromatic qualities to dishes with quick condiments you make; along with homemade, gut-friendly versions of ingredients (broths and dressings) that traditionally include FODMAPs; and supplements to your meals in the form of breads and beverages that promote a healthy gut.

Allium Alternatives

Whether you're eliminating fructans, the fermentable carbohydrates found in allium, through a low-FODMAP diet or have simply found that garlic and onions don't sit well with you (as is common), you can solve almost all flavor fears with our all-purpose garlic oil. Fructans are water-, not fat-, soluble so infusing garlic cloves into neutral-tasting canola oil creates a fructan-free aromatic cooking staple. And an "infusion" doesn't mean a time commitment; we simmer garlic cloves in oil for just 3 to 5 minutes for the flavor we want. That makes your garlic oil jar easy to replenish. (It is not safe to store homemade garlic oil for more than 3 days.) Start sautéing vegetables for a stew or finish dishes with a drizzle and you'll think you've incorporated allium in your cooking. (You can also use store-bought garlic oil, but it will taste less fresh.)

GARLIC OIL
Makes about ½ cup

Extra-virgin olive oil can be substituted for the canola oil. This recipe can be doubled or tripled.

- ½ **cup canola oil**
- 4 **garlic cloves, smashed and peeled**

Heat oil and garlic in small saucepan over medium-low heat until fragrant and starting to bubble, 3 to 5 minutes. Let cool completely. Strain oil through fine-mesh strainer into airtight container; discard solids. (Garlic oil can be refrigerated for up to 3 days.)

Garlic Oil Infusions

For an aromatic twist, add any one of the following ingredients along with the garlic and let the mixture sit at room temperature for 4 hours before straining. Match these oils with complementary flavor profiles in our recipes, or introduce new profiles to basic sides.

- 1 tablespoon dried rosemary or thyme

- 2 tablespoons chopped dried porcini or shiitake mushrooms

- 1 tablespoon cracked fennel, caraway, mustard, coriander, dill, or cumin seeds

- 2 (3-inch) strips lemon, lime, or orange zest

- 1 lemongrass stalk, trimmed to bottom 6 inches, halved lengthwise, and sliced thin

- 1 (2-inch) piece ginger, sliced into ¼-inch-thick rounds

Suitable Sauces

Some of cooking's most foundational sauces—vinaigrettes that start with a minced shallot, herb condiments chopped up with garlic, lactose-heavy accompaniments—include FODMAPs for flavor. And buying them at the store can mean fruitless time wasted scanning packages for allium seasonings, milk powders, or wheat-based thickeners in unexpected places. Here are homemade sauces to drizzle vibrant flavor on lean meats, salad greens, vegetable dishes, and more—while keeping them gut-friendly.

MAKE-AHEAD VINAIGRETTE
Makes about 1 cup

Regular or light mayonnaise can be used in this recipe. Do not use blackstrap molasses. You can substitute garlic oil for the extra-virgin olive oil.

- 1 tablespoon mayonnaise
- 1 tablespoon molasses
- 1 tablespoon Dijon mustard
- ½ teaspoon table salt
- ¼ cup wine vinegar
- ½ cup extra-virgin olive oil, divided
- ¼ cup canola oil

1 Combine mayonnaise, molasses, mustard, and salt in 2-cup jar with tight-fitting lid. Stir with fork until mixture is milky in appearance and no lumps of mayonnaise or molasses remain. Add vinegar, seal jar, and shake until smooth, about 10 seconds.

2 Add ¼ cup olive oil, seal jar, and shake vigorously until thoroughly combined, about 10 seconds. Repeat, adding remaining ¼ cup olive oil and canola oil in 2 additions, shaking vigorously until thoroughly combined after each addition. (Dressing can be refrigerated for up to 1 week. Shake before serving.)

BASIL PESTO
Makes about 1 cup

- ¼ cup pine nuts, toasted and cooled
- 2 cups fresh basil leaves
- 1 ounce Parmesan cheese, grated (½ cup)
- ¼ cup extra-virgin olive oil
- 2 tablespoons garlic oil (see page 20)
- ½ teaspoon table salt

Process pine nuts, basil, Parmesan, olive oil, garlic oil, and salt in food processor until smooth, about 1 minute, scraping down sides of bowl as needed. (Pesto can be refrigerated for up to 3 days or frozen for up to 1 month. To prevent browning, press plastic wrap flush to surface or top with thin layer of olive oil. Serve at room temperature.)

CHIMICHURRI
Makes about 1 cup

For a milder sauce, omit or use the lesser amount of pepper flakes.

- 3 tablespoons hot water
- 2 teaspoons dried oregano
- ½ teaspoon table salt
- 1 cup fresh parsley leaves
- ½ cup fresh cilantro leaves
- ⅛–¼ teaspoon red pepper flakes
- ½ cup garlic oil (see page 20)
- 2 tablespoons red wine vinegar

1 Combine hot water, oregano, and salt in small bowl; let sit for 5 minutes to soften oregano.

2 Pulse parsley, cilantro, and pepper flakes in food processor until coarsely chopped, about 10 pulses. Transfer mixture to medium bowl and stir in oil, vinegar, and water mixture. Cover and let sit at room temperature for at least 1 hour. Season with salt and pepper to taste. (Chimichurri can be refrigerated for up to 2 days. Whisk before serving at room temperature.)

CHERMOULA
Makes about 1 cup

- 1½ cups fresh cilantro leaves
- ½ cup garlic oil (see page 20)
- ¼ cup lemon juice (2 lemons)
- 1 teaspoon ground cumin
- 1 teaspoon paprika
- ¼ teaspoon table salt
- ⅛ teaspoon cayenne pepper (optional)

Process all ingredients in food processor until smooth, about 1 minute, scraping down sides of bowl as needed. (Chermoula can be refrigerated for up to 2 days. Whisk before serving at room temperature.)

FRESH TOMATO SALSA
Makes about 3 cups

For a milder salsa, omit the jalapeño or use the lesser amount. For a spicier salsa, reserve and add jalapeño seeds.

- 1½ pounds tomatoes, cored and cut into ½-inch pieces
- ¼ cup chopped fresh cilantro
- 4 scallions, green parts only, sliced thin
- ½-1 jalapeño chile, stemmed, seeded, and minced
- 1 tablespoon garlic oil (see page 20)
- 2 teaspoons lime juice, plus extra for seasoning

Place tomatoes in colander and let drain for 30 minutes. As tomatoes drain, layer cilantro, scallions, and jalapeño on top of tomatoes. Shake colander to drain excess juice, then transfer vegetables to bowl. Stir in oil and lime juice. Season with salt, pepper, and extra lime juice to taste. (Salsa can be refrigerated for up to 24 hours.)

ORANGE-BASIL RELISH
Makes about 1 cup

We enjoy using basil here, but any fresh herb will work.

- 3 oranges
- 2 scallions, green parts only, minced
- 2 tablespoons chopped fresh basil
- 2 teaspoons lemon juice
- 2 teaspoons extra-virgin olive oil

1 Cut away peel and pith from oranges. Cut oranges into 8 wedges, then slice crosswise into ½-inch-thick pieces. Place orange pieces in strainer set over bowl and let drain for 15 minutes; measure out and reserve 1 tablespoon drained juice.

2 Combine orange juice, scallions, basil, lemon juice, and oil in bowl. Stir in orange pieces and let sit for 15 minutes. Season with salt and pepper to taste. (Relish can be refrigerated for up to 2 days.)

HERBED YOGURT SAUCE
Makes 1 cup

You can substitute lactose-free or dairy-free yogurt (see page 19) for plain yogurt.

- 1 cup plain yogurt
- 2 tablespoons minced fresh cilantro
- 2 tablespoons minced fresh mint
- 1 tablespoon garlic oil (see page 20)

Whisk all ingredients in bowl until smooth and season with salt and pepper to taste. Cover and refrigerate for at least 30 minutes. (Sauce can be refrigerated for up to 4 days. Whisk before serving.)

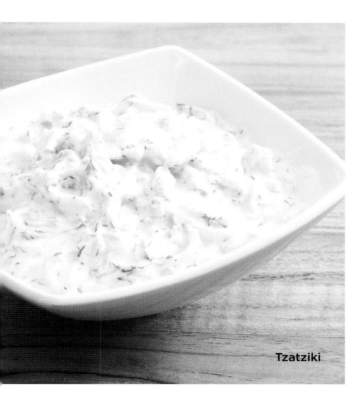

Tzatziki

PEANUT DIPPING SAUCE
Makes about 1 cup

You can use smooth or chunky peanut or almond butter. For a milder sauce, omit the chili oil or use the lesser amount.

- 6 tablespoons peanut or almond butter
- 6 tablespoons water
- 2 tablespoons rice vinegar
- 2 tablespoons soy sauce
- 4 teaspoons grated fresh ginger
- ¼–1 teaspoon chili oil

Whisk all ingredients together in bowl until smooth. (Peanut sauce can be refrigerated for up to 3 days. Serve at room temperature.)

FRESH TOMATO SAUCE
Makes 4 cups (enough for 1 pound of pasta)

Be sure to choose the ripest tomatoes you can find. If you plan to freeze the sauce, hold off on adding the basil until right before serving.

- 3 tablespoons garlic oil (see page 20)
- 2 pounds plum tomatoes, cored and cut into ½-inch pieces
- ¾ teaspoon table salt
- ½ teaspoon pepper
- 2 tablespoons chopped fresh basil

Heat oil in large saucepan over medium heat until shimmering. Stir in tomatoes, salt, and pepper. Increase heat to medium-high and cook until tomatoes are broken down and sauce is slightly thickened, about 10 minutes. Stir in basil and season with salt and pepper to taste. (Sauce can be refrigerated for up to 4 days or frozen for up to 1 month.)

TZATZIKI
Makes about 1 cup

You can substitute lactose-free or dairy-free Greek yogurt (see page 19) for plain Greek yogurt.

- ½ cucumber, peeled, halved lengthwise, seeded, and shredded
- ¼ teaspoon table salt
- ½ cup plain Greek yogurt
- 1 tablespoon garlic oil (see page 20)
- 1 tablespoon minced fresh dill

Toss cucumber with salt in colander and let drain for 15 minutes. Whisk yogurt, oil, and dill together in bowl, then stir in cucumber. Cover and refrigerate for at least 30 minutes. Season with salt and pepper to taste. (Tzatziki can be refrigerated for up to 2 days.)

Low-FODMAP Broths

In addition to being the warming base for soulful soups and stews, broth is a common pantry ingredient for adding to savory recipes—bubbling braises or steaming vegetables. Traditionally, long-simmered homemade broth includes not only the main ingredient for the flavor profile (chicken, beef, or vegetables) but aromatic vegetables—definitely including onion, often including garlic. If the broth is store bought, extracts or powders from these ingredients are often used for this purpose (see page 18). But do they have to? We successfully developed chicken, beef, and even vegetable broth without offending ingredients, turning instead to garlic oil for sautéing, safe-to-eat dark green parts of leeks, and complementary aromatic vegetables.

CHICKEN BROTH
Makes about 8 cups

If you have a large pot (at least 12 quarts), you can easily double this recipe to make 1 gallon.

- 1 tablespoon garlic oil (see page 20)
- 3 pounds whole chicken legs, backs, and/or wings, hacked into 2-inch pieces
- 1 leek, dark green parts only, chopped coarse and washed thoroughly
- 8 cups water
- 3 bay leaves
- ½ teaspoon table salt

1 Heat oil in Dutch oven over medium-high heat until just smoking. Pat chicken dry with paper towels. Brown chicken in 2 batches, about 5 minutes per batch; transfer to bowl. Add leek to fat left in pot and cook over medium heat until softened, about 5 minutes.

2 Return browned chicken and any accumulated juices to pot, cover, and reduce heat to low. Cook, stirring occasionally, until chicken has released its juices, about 20 minutes.

3 Stir in water, bay leaves, and salt, scraping up any browned bits, and bring to simmer. Reduce heat to low, cover, and simmer until broth is rich and flavorful, about 1 hour. Strain broth through fine-mesh strainer into large container; discard solids. Let broth settle for 5 to 10 minutes, then defat using wide, shallow spoon or fat separator. (Cooled broth can be refrigerated for up to 4 days or frozen for up to 1 month.)

BEEF BROTH
Makes about 8 cups

You can substitute 4 pounds of beef chuck, cut into 3-inch chunks, plus 2 pounds of small marrow bones for the beef shanks. If you have a large pot (at least 12 quarts), you can easily double this recipe to make 1 gallon.

- 1 tablespoon garlic oil (see page 20), plus extra as needed
- 6 pounds beef shanks, meat cut from bone in large chunks
- 1 leek, dark green parts only, chopped coarse and washed thoroughly
- ½ cup dry red wine
- 8 cups water
- 2 bay leaves
- ½ teaspoon table salt

1 Heat oil in Dutch oven over medium-high heat until just smoking. Pat beef and bones dry with paper towels. Brown beef and bones in 3 or 4 batches, about 5 minutes per batch, adding extra oil as needed, up to 1 tablespoon. Transfer beef and bones to bowl. Add leek to fat left in pot and cook over medium heat until softened, about 5 minutes.

2 Stir in wine, scraping up any browned bits, and cook until reduced by about half, about 2 minutes. Return browned beef and bones and any accumulated juices to pot, cover, and reduce heat to low. Cook, stirring occasionally, until beef has released its juices, about 20 minutes.

3 Stir in water, bay leaves, and salt, scraping up any browned bits, and bring to simmer. Reduce heat to low, cover, and simmer until meat is tender and broth is rich and flavorful, 1½ to 2 hours. Strain broth through fine-mesh strainer into large container; reserve beef for another use and discard remaining solids. Let broth settle for 5 to 10 minutes, then defat using wide, shallow spoon or fat separator. (Cooled broth can be refrigerated for up to 4 days or frozen for up to 1 month.)

VEGETABLE BROTH
Makes 1¾ cups base (enough for 7 quarts broth)

Kosher salt aids in grinding the vegetables. The broth base contains enough salt to keep it from freezing solid, making it easy to remove 1 tablespoon at a time. For gluten-free broth, use gluten-free soy sauce or tamari.

- 1 **pound leeks, dark green parts only, chopped and washed thoroughly (4 cups)**
- ¾ **cup chopped celery root**
- 2 **carrots, peeled and chopped (⅔ cup)**
- ½ **cup fresh parsley leaves and thin stems**
- 2 **tablespoons kosher salt**
- 1½ **tablespoons tomato paste**
- 3 **tablespoons soy sauce**

1 Process leeks, celery root, carrots, parsley, and salt in food processor to fine paste, about 4 minutes, scraping down sides of bowl as needed. Add tomato paste and process for 1 minute, scraping down sides of bowl every 20 seconds. Add soy sauce and process for 1 minute.

2 Transfer mixture to airtight container and tap firmly on counter to remove air bubbles. Press small piece of parchment paper flush against surface of mixture and cover. (Paste can be refrigerated for up to 1 week or frozen for up to 6 months.)

3 To make 1 cup of broth, stir 1 tablespoon fresh or frozen broth base into 1 cup boiling water. If particle-free broth is desired, let broth steep for 5 minutes, then strain through fine-mesh strainer.

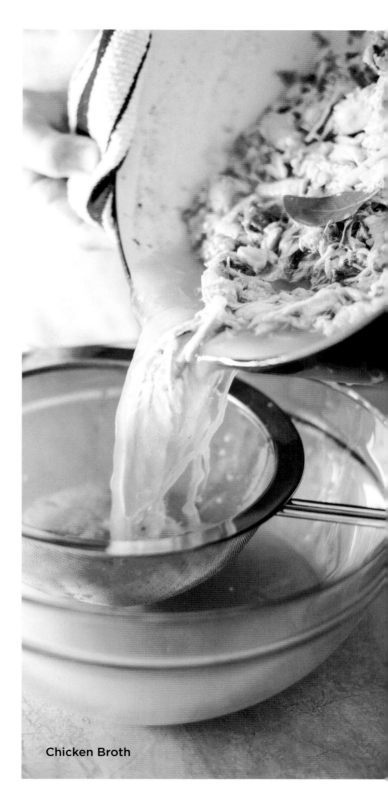

Chicken Broth

Healthful Hydration

Getting adequate fluids goes hand-in-hand with healthful food and fiber; you can't benefit from one without the other. And sugary beverages won't do it. If you want to drink more than water all day, turn to these refreshing flavorful drinks, all of which limit sugar and instead find flavor from infused produce and teas. You won't want to stop sipping.

CUCUMBER-LEMON WATER
Makes about 4 cups

- 1 cucumber, peeled, halved lengthwise, and seeded
- 4 cups water
- 2 teaspoons grated lemon zest plus 1 tablespoon juice

Shred cucumber on large holes of box grater to yield 1 cup pulp; transfer to bowl. Stir in water and lemon zest and juice and let steep for 1 hour. Strain through fine-mesh strainer into pitcher (or strain into second bowl and transfer to pitcher); discard solids. Serve at room temperature, chilled, or over ice. (Infused water can be refrigerated for up to 3 days.)

CANTALOUPE-MINT ICED GREEN TEA
Makes about 4 cups

Chinese green tea will produce a grassy, floral tea, whereas Japanese green tea will be more savory. Three tea bags can be substituted for the loose-leaf tea. This recipe can be easily doubled.

- ½ small ripe cantaloupe, seeded
- 2 tablespoons loose-leaf decaffeinated green tea
- 3 cups hot water (175 degrees)
- 1 cup ice water
- 3 tablespoons chopped fresh mint
- 2 tablespoons sugar (optional)
- 1 tablespoon lemon juice

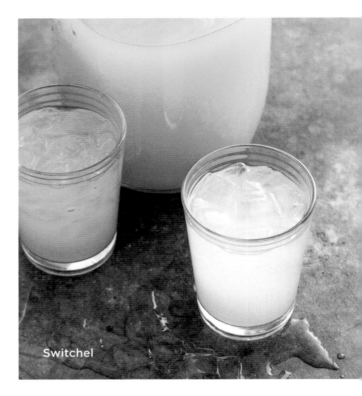

Switchel

1 Cut cantaloupe into 4 quarters, but do not peel. Grasping peel, shred flesh on large holes of box grater to yield 1 cup pulp; set aside. Place tea in bowl. Add hot water and steep for 4 minutes. Add ice water, mint, sugar, if using, lemon juice, and reserved cantaloupe. Stir tea with wooden spoon until sugar is dissolved. Let steep for 1 hour.

2 Strain tea through fine-mesh strainer into pitcher (or strain into second bowl and transfer to pitcher); discard solids. Refrigerate for at least 1 hour before serving over ice. (Strained tea can be refrigerated for up to 3 days.)

RASPBERRY-BASIL ICED BLACK TEA
Makes about 4 cups

We prefer frozen raspberries here since they are generally less expensive, but you can use fresh, ripe raspberries. Two tea bags can be substituted for the loose-leaf tea. This recipe can be easily doubled.

7½ ounces (1½ cups) frozen raspberries, thawed

3 tablespoons chopped fresh basil

2 tablespoons sugar (optional)

2 teaspoons lemon juice

1½ teaspoons loose-leaf decaffeinated black tea

3 cups boiling water

1 cup ice water

1 Place raspberries, basil, sugar, if using, and lemon juice in bowl. Using wooden spoon, mash until no whole berries remain. Place tea in second bowl. Add boiling water and steep for 4 minutes. Add ice water and raspberry mixture. Stir tea with wooden spoon until sugar is dissolved. Let steep for 1 hour.

2 Strain tea through fine-mesh strainer into pitcher (or strain into third bowl and transfer to pitcher); discard solids. Refrigerate for at least 1 hour before serving over ice. (Strained tea can be refrigerated for up to 3 days.)

SWITCHEL
Makes 8 cups

This sharp, gingery drink will get more potent with ginger flavor the longer it remains unstrained.

6 cups water

¾ cup cider vinegar

½ cup pure maple syrup

¼ cup old-fashioned rolled oats

2 tablespoons grated fresh ginger

1 teaspoon grated lemon zest

¼ teaspoon table salt

Bring all ingredients to simmer in large saucepan over medium-high heat. Remove from heat and let cool completely. Transfer switchel to bowl, cover, and refrigerate for at least 6 hours or up to 24 hours. Strain switchel through fine-mesh strainer into pitcher (or strain into second bowl and transfer to pitcher); discard solids. Serve chilled or over ice. (Strained switchel can be refrigerated for up to 3 days.)

Low-FODMAP Breads and Gluten-Free Flour Blends

Bread shouldn't be demonized, and while many can eat it, there are some who cannot tolerate the fructans in wheat and cannot eat bread. Or can they? In the case of low-FODMAP bread (beyond gluten-free bread), there's another option: slow-rise sourdough. It's a fascinating phenomenon: The slow fermentation process of a sourdough starter–leavened bread kills the fructans in wheat so those suffering from IBS do not experience unpleasant effects. It doesn't hurt that a loaf of chewy, flavorful sourdough bread is among the most delicious you can have. And of course, the test kitchen has tackled the tall order of creating a gluten-free loaf of bread, a whole-grain one at that, plus gluten-free flour blends for those with celiac disease or who avoid gluten. This bread is also suitable for those following a low-FODMAP diet, and the blends can be used for flour in the recipes in this book.

SOURDOUGH BREAD
Makes 1 large round loaf

For the best results, weigh your ingredients. Because step 2 of this recipe takes between 12 and 18 hours to complete, it's best to start it early in the morning or in the evening. It's important to move on to step 3 as soon as the dough is domed and bubbly. If ambient temperatures are above 80 degrees, use ice-cold water in the dough; if ambient temperatures are below 70 degrees, rising times will be closer to the end of the time ranges. This recipe requires a heavy-bottomed Dutch oven of at least 5 quarts in volume.

LEVAIN
3 tablespoons (1 ounce) bread flour

2 tablespoons (1 ounce) cool water (70 degrees)

2 teaspoons (½ ounce) mature Sourdough Starter (recipe follows)

DOUGH
3⅓ cups (18⅓ ounces) bread flour

1¾ teaspoons table salt

1¼ cups plus 2 tablespoons (11 ounces) cool water (70 degrees)

1 For the levain: Combine flour, water, and starter in small bowl and stir with wooden spoon until uniform. Cover with plastic wrap and let sit until doubled in volume, 3 to 5 hours. Transfer to refrigerator and use within 7 days.

2 For the dough: Whisk flour and salt together in bowl. Combine water and 3 tablespoons (2 ounces) levain (discard remainder) in large bowl and whisk until smooth. Add flour mixture to water mixture and stir using wooden spoon, scraping up dry flour from bottom of bowl until dough comes together, then knead by hand in bowl until shaggy ball forms and no dry flour remains. Cover bowl with plastic wrap and let sit at room temperature until subtly domed, lightly bubbly, and just doubled in volume, 12 to 18 hours.

3 Transfer dough to lightly floured counter. Gently press dough into 8- to 10-inch disk, then fold edges toward middle to form round. Cover loosely with plastic and let rest for 15 minutes. Meanwhile, line colander or banneton with large linen or cotton dish towel and dust liberally with flour. Repeat pressing and folding of dough to form round, then place dough seam side down on counter and form into tight round. (To round, set dough on unfloured counter. Loosely cup your hands around dough and, without applying pressure to dough, move your hands in small circular motions. Tackiness of dough against counter and circular motion should work dough into smooth, even ball, but if dough sticks to your hands, lightly dust your fingers with flour.) Place dough seam side up on floured towel in colander and loosely fold edges of towel over dough to enclose. Cover top of dough loosely with plastic wrap. Let sit at room temperature 1 hour, then refrigerate for 12 to 24 hours (whatever is most convenient).

4 One hour before baking bread, adjust oven rack to middle position, set covered heavy-bottomed Dutch oven on rack, and heat oven to 475 degrees.

5 Lay 12- by 12-inch sheet of parchment paper on counter and spray generously with vegetable oil spray. Uncover colander and unfold edges of towel. Lay parchment sprayed side down over loaf, then invert colander onto counter. Remove colander and towel.

6 Carefully remove Dutch oven from oven, place on stovetop, and set lid aside. Using razor blade or sharp knife, make one 7-inch-long, ½-inch-deep slit along top of dough. Pick up dough by lifting parchment edges and lower into Dutch oven. Carefully cover pot and transfer to oven. Bake for 20 minutes.

7 Remove lid, reduce oven temperature to 425 degrees, and continue to bake until loaf is deep brown and registers 210 degrees, 15 to 25 minutes longer. Carefully remove bread from pot; transfer to wire rack, and let cool completely before slicing, 2 to 3 hours. (Store uneaten bread cut side down on cutting board for up to 3 days.)

SOURDOUGH STARTER
Makes 1 starter

For the best results, weigh your ingredients and use organic flour (which is richer in micro-organisms than conventional flour) and bottled or filtered water (which is free of the chlorine in tap water that can kill those essential micro-organisms). Be sure to include white and either whole-wheat or rye flour in the bulk flour mixture; whole-grain flours are more nutritious than white flour and are more likely to contain the needed bacteria and yeast, making them ideal nourishment for the nascent culture. (Once the starter is mature, you maintain it with just white flour; non-organic is fine.) Once the starter is ready for use, it can easily be scaled up to the necessary proportions. Note that the time frame of each step is approximate: How quickly your starter moves from one step to the next will depend on the flour you're using to refresh it and how hospitable the environment is for yeast and bacteria activity. Let visual cues be your guide and use the day count as a reference. You'll need 2 small lidded containers, such as 4-ounce canning jars, and 1 larger lidded container, such as a 16-ounce canning jar.

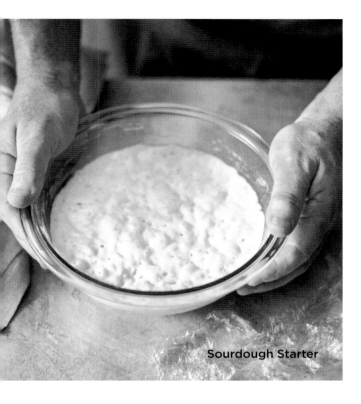

Sourdough Starter

1½ **cups organic bread flour or King Arthur All-Purpose Flour**

1½ **cups organic whole-wheat or rye flour**

Warm room-temperature (70- to 80-degree) bottled or filtered water

1 Create bulk batch of flour mixture by combining bread or all-purpose flour with whole-wheat or rye flour in sealable container (weighing ingredients will become vital later, but volume is fine here). Using spoon, mix 4 teaspoons (⅓ ounce; 10 grams) flour mixture and 2½ teaspoons (⅓ ounce; 10 grams) water in small jar. Cover with plastic wrap or loosely with lid and let sit at warm room temperature (70 to 80 degrees) for 1 to 3 days. Visual cue to move to the next step: Starter is bubbly, wet-looking (there might even be liquid pooled on top), and fragrant—even pungent.

2 Stir starter well and transfer 2 teaspoons (⅓ ounce; 10 grams) to clean jar; reserve remaining starter as backup in original jar and store in refrigerator. Stir 4 teaspoons (⅓ ounce; 10 grams) flour mixture and 2½ teaspoons (⅓ ounce; 10 grams) water into starter mixture until no dry flour remains. Cover with plastic wrap or loosely with lid and let sit at warm room temperature for 24 hours. Repeat every 24 hours for 4 to 10 days. Visual cue to move to next step: Starter is bubbly and fragrant less than 12 hours after previous refreshment.

3 Refresh starter as before every 12 hours. At this stage, in addition to saving leftover starter as backup, you can collect generations of backup starter in a larger sealed jar; store it in the refrigerator to keep on hand for use in other nonbread applications such as pancakes, biscuits, and crackers. If at any point the starter activity slows down or stops altogether, return to refreshing the culture once daily.

4 Cues that starter is mature and ready for baking: Starter doubles or triples in volume within 12 hours of being refreshed and smells yeasty/bready/yogurty. Conduct a "float test": Place a blob of starter in a jar with water. If starter floats, it's producing and retaining ample amounts of carbon dioxide, meaning the yeast population has increased sufficiently.

5 If your starter exhibits the signs of maturity and passes the float test, you can move it to the refrigerator. Measure out 1½ tablespoons (1 ounce; 28 grams) starter and transfer to clean bowl (save any leftover starter in refrigerator as backup culture). Stir 7 tablespoons (2 ounces; 57 grams) all-purpose flour and ¼ cup (2 ounces; 57 grams) room-temperature (70 degrees) water into starter until no dry flour remains. Place mixture in jar, seal it well but loosely, and let sit at room temperature until it has about doubled in volume, 3 to 6 hours (use rubber band around container to mark the mixture's starting volume). Once mixture has doubled, transfer jar to refrigerator. Repeat process every 7 to 14 days.

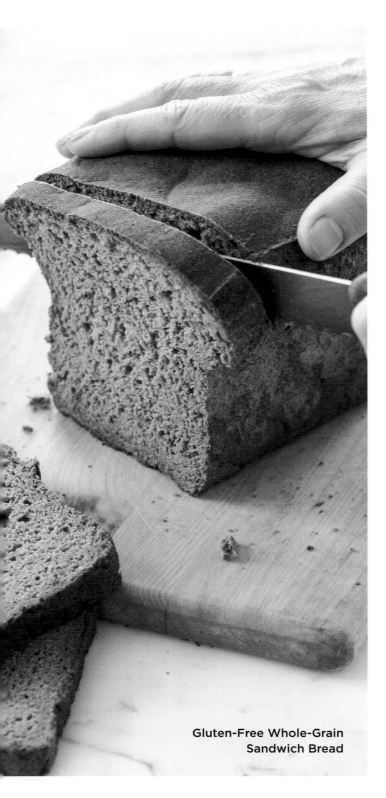

**Gluten-Free Whole-Grain
Sandwich Bread**

GLUTEN-FREE WHOLE-GRAIN SANDWICH BREAD
Makes 1 loaf

Do not substitute other whole-grain blends for the ATK Whole-Grain Gluten-Free Flour Blend; they will not work. Psyllium is crucial to the structure of the bread; do not omit. For a dairy-free version, substitute vegetable oil for butter. Note that not all brands of baking powder are gluten free. This recipe calls for an 8½ by 4½-inch loaf pan; if using a 9 by 5-inch loaf pan, the dough will not rise as high and the bread will not be quite as tall.

17	ounces (2 cups plus 2 tablespoons) warm water (110 degrees)
2¼	teaspoons instant or rapid-rise yeast
3	tablespoons plus 1 teaspoon sugar, divided
2	large eggs plus 1 large yolk
2	tablespoons unsalted butter, melted and cooled
19½	ounces (4⅓ cups) ATK Whole-Grain Gluten-Free Flour Blend (recipe follows)
3	tablespoons powdered psyllium husk
2	teaspoons baking powder
1½	teaspoons table salt

1 Adjust oven rack to middle position and heat oven to 200 degrees. As soon as oven reaches 200 degrees, turn it off. (This will be warm proofing box for dough. Do not begin step 2 until oven has been turned off.) Spray 8½ by 4½-inch loaf pan with canola oil spray.

2 Combine warm water, yeast, and 1 teaspoon sugar in bowl and let sit until bubbly, about 5 minutes. Whisk in eggs and yolk and melted butter. Using stand mixer fitted with paddle, mix flour blend, psyllium, baking powder, salt, and remaining 3 tablespoons sugar together on low speed until combined, about 1 minute. Slowly add yeast mixture and mix until combined, scraping down bowl as needed, about 1 minute. Increase speed to medium and beat until dough is sticky and uniform, about 6 minutes. (Dough will resemble cookie dough.)

3 Using rubber spatula, scrape dough into prepared pan. Using wet hands, press dough gently into corners and smooth top. Run finger around entire edge of loaf, pressing down slightly, so that sides are about ½ inch shorter than center. Cover loosely with plastic wrap, place in warmed oven, and let rise for 10 minutes; do not let plastic touch oven rack.

4 Remove pan from oven and let sit on counter until loaf has risen ½ inch above rim of pan, about 20 minutes. Meanwhile, heat oven to 350 degrees.

5 Remove plastic and spray loaf with water. Bake until top is browned, crust is firm, and loaf sounds hollow when tapped, about 1½ hours, rotating pan halfway through baking. Turn off oven and leave bread in oven for 15 minutes longer.

6 Remove bread from oven and let cool in pan for 10 minutes. Unmold bread onto wire rack and let cool completely, about 3 hours. Serve. (Cooled bread can be wrapped in double layer of plastic wrap and stored at room temperature for up to 3 days. Alternatively, cooled bread can be sliced, wrapped in double layer of plastic wrap, and frozen for up to 1 month.)

ATK ALL-PURPOSE GLUTEN-FREE FLOUR BLEND
Makes 42 ounces (about 9⅓ cups)

If you don't bring the flour to room temperature before using, the recipe may not work as expected. You can use this flour as a low-FODMAP and gluten-free all-purpose flour substitute in our recipes.

24 ounces (4½ cups plus ⅓ cup) white rice flour

7½ ounces (1⅔ cups) brown rice flour

7 ounces (1⅓ cups) potato starch

3 ounces (¾ cup) tapioca starch

Whisk all ingredients together in large bowl until well combined. (Flour blend can be refrigerated for up to 3 months or frozen for up to 6 months. Bring to room temperature before using.)

ATK WHOLE-GRAIN GLUTEN-FREE FLOUR BLEND
Makes 45 ounces (about 10 cups)

We had good results with Bob's Red Mill ground golden flaxseeds. Do not substitute ground brown flaxseeds because the flavor will be too strong. Do not attempt to grind flaxseeds yourself because you will not be able to grind them fine enough. If you don't bring the flour to room temperature before using, the recipe may not work as expected.

24 ounces (5¼ cups) teff flour

8 ounces (1¾ cups) brown rice flour

8 ounces (2⅓ cups) ground golden flaxseeds

5 ounces (1 cup) sweet white rice flour

Whisk all ingredients together in large bowl until well combined. (Flour blend can be refrigerated for up to 3 months or frozen for up to 6 months. Bring to room temperature before using.)

Probiotic Partners

On page 5, we discuss the role of probiotics in maintaining a balanced, healthy gut microbiome. Here we've included probiotic foods (including making a low-FODMAP version of kimchi) that not only give you a bacterial boost but that can accompany gut-healthy foods as condiments to create great-tasting meals. You can use the homemade yogurts in any recipe in the book that calls for yogurt, or simply enjoy them for breakfast or snacking.

SAUERKRAUT
Makes about 1½ quarts

This recipe requires at least 6 days of fermenting time. You will need a ½-gallon widemouthed jar for this recipe.

2½ pounds green cabbage (1 head), quartered, cored, and sliced ⅛ inch thick (7 cups)

2 tablespoons kosher salt, divided

1½ teaspoons juniper berries

2 cups water

1 Cut out parchment paper round to match diameter of ½-gallon widemouthed jar. Toss cabbage with 4 teaspoons salt in large bowl. Using your hands, forcefully knead salt into cabbage until cabbage has softened and begins to release moisture, about 3 minutes. Stir in juniper berries.

2 Tightly pack cabbage mixture and any accumulated liquid into jar, pressing down firmly with your fist to eliminate air pockets as you pack. Press parchment round flush against surface of cabbage.

3 Dissolve remaining 2 teaspoons salt in water and transfer to 1-quart zipper-lock plastic bag; squeeze out air and seal bag well. Place inside second zipper-lock bag, press out air, and seal well. Place bag of brine on top of parchment and gently press down. Cover top of jar with triple layer of cheesecloth and secure with rubber band.

4 Place jar in 50- to 70-degree location away from direct sunlight and let ferment for 6 days; check jar daily, skimming residue from surface and pressing to keep cabbage submerged. After 6 days, taste sauerkraut daily until it has reached desired flavor (this may take up to 7 days longer; sauerkraut should be pale and translucent, with a tart and floral flavor).

5 When sauerkraut has reached desired flavor, discard cheesecloth, bag of brine, and parchment; skim off any residue. Serve. (Sauerkraut and accumulated juices can be transferred to clean jar, covered, and refrigerated for up to 6 weeks; once refrigerated, flavor of sauerkraut will continue to mature).

KIMCHI
Makes about 2 quarts

If gochugaru is unavailable, you can substitute ⅓ cup red pepper flakes. For the most balanced flavor, we prefer a fermentation temperature of 65 degrees. This recipe requires at least 9 days of fermenting time. You will need a ½-gallon widemouthed jar for this recipe.

- **1 head napa cabbage (2½ pounds), cored and cut into 2-inch pieces**
- **4½ teaspoons kosher salt, divided**
- **½ cup gochugaru**
- **⅓ cup sugar**
- **¼ cup low-sodium soy sauce (see page 18)**
- **3 tablespoons fish sauce**
- **1 (2-inch) piece fresh ginger, peeled and chopped coarse**
- **20 scallions, green parts only, cut into 2-inch pieces**
- **1 carrot, peeled and cut into 2-inch matchsticks**

1 Toss cabbage with 2½ teaspoons salt in bowl, cover, and let sit at room temperature for 1 hour. Transfer cabbage to colander, squeeze to drain excess liquid, and return to now-empty bowl. Cut out parchment paper round to match diameter of ½-gallon widemouthed glass jar.

2 Process gochugaru, sugar, soy sauce, fish sauce, and ginger in food processor until no large pieces of ginger remain, about 20 seconds. Add gochugaru mixture, scallions, and carrot to cabbage and toss to combine. Tightly pack vegetable mixture into jar, pressing down firmly with your fist to eliminate air pockets as you pack. Press parchment round flush against surface of vegetables.

3 Dissolve remaining 2 teaspoons salt in water and transfer to 1-quart zipper-lock plastic bag; squeeze out air and seal bag well. Place inside second zipper-lock bag, press out air, and seal well. Place bag of brine on top of parchment and gently press down. Cover jar with triple layer of cheesecloth and secure cheesecloth with rubber band.

4 Place jar in 50- to 70-degree location away from direct sunlight and let ferment for 9 days; check jar daily, skimming residue and mold from surface and pressing to keep mixture submerged. After 9 days, taste kimchi daily until it has reached desired flavor. (This may take up to 11 days longer; cabbage should be soft and translucent with a pleasant cheesy, fishy flavor.)

5 When kimchi has reached desired flavor, remove cheesecloth, bag of water, and parchment, and skim off any residue or mold. Serve. (Kimchi and accumulated juice can be transferred to clean jar, covered, and refrigerated for up to 3 months; while refrigerated, kimchi will continue to soften and develop flavor.)

HOMEMADE YOGURT
Makes about 4 cups

The success of this recipe hinges on using yogurt that contains live and active cultures. The longer the yogurt cooks, the tangier it will be. You will need two 16-ounce Mason jars with lids for this recipe.

3½ cups whole milk

¼ cup nonfat dry milk powder

¼ cup plain yogurt with live and active cultures

1 Adjust oven rack to middle position. Heat milk in large saucepan over medium-low heat (do not stir while heating), until milk registers 185 degrees. Remove pot from heat, gently stir in milk powder, and let cool to 160 degrees, 7 to 10 minutes. Strain milk mixture into bowl and let cool until it registers 110 degrees, stirring occasionally to prevent skin from forming, about 30 minutes.

2 Combine yogurt and ½ cup cooled milk in small bowl, then gently stir into remaining cooled milk. Cover tightly with plastic wrap and poke several holes in plastic. Place bowl in oven and turn on oven light, creating a warm environment of 100 to 110 degrees. Let yogurt sit undisturbed until thickened and set, 5 to 7 hours.

3 Transfer yogurt to refrigerator and let sit until completely chilled, about 3 hours. Stir yogurt to recombine before serving. (Yogurt can be refrigerated for up to 1 week; stir to recombine before serving.)

VARIATION
Homemade Greek-Style Yogurt
Set fine-mesh strainer over 8-cup liquid measuring cup and line with double layer of coffee filters. Transfer chilled yogurt to prepared strainer, cover with plastic, and refrigerate until about 2 cups of liquid have drained into measuring cup, 7 to 8 hours. Transfer drained yogurt to jar with tight fitting lid, discarding liquid.

HOMEMADE ALMOND MILK YOGURT
Makes about 3 cups

To promote the fermentation required in making low-FODMAP dairy-free yogurt, we used probiotic capsules, since typical yogurt starters are often sourced from dairy products. You can find agar-agar and probiotic capsules at your local natural food store. The flavor of the yogurt may vary depending on the brand of probiotic used; we developed this recipe using RenewLife Ultimate Flora Critical Care 50 Billion capsules. Do not substitute agar-agar flakes for the agar-agar powder.

1¾ teaspoons agar-agar powder

¼ cup water

3 cups almond milk

1 50-billion probiotic capsule

1 Adjust oven rack to middle position. Sprinkle agar-agar over water in small bowl and let sit until softened, about 10 minutes.

2 Heat milk in large saucepan over medium-low heat until just simmering. Add softened agar-agar and cook, whisking constantly, until fully dissolved. Strain milk mixture into bowl and let cool until it registers 110 degrees, stirring occasionally to prevent skin from forming, about 30 minutes.

3 Twist open probiotic capsule and whisk contents into cooled milk mixture; discard capsule's casing. Cover bowl tightly with plastic wrap and poke several holes in plastic. Place bowl in oven and turn on oven light, creating a warm environment of 100 to 110 degrees. Let yogurt sit undisturbed for at least 12 hours or up to 24 hours. (Yogurt will not thicken while sitting.)

4 Transfer yogurt to refrigerator and let sit until completely chilled and set, about 3 hours. Process yogurt in blender until smooth, about 30 seconds, before serving. (Yogurt can be refrigerated for up to 1 week; stir to recombine before serving.)

VARIATION
Homemade Greek-Style Almond Milk Yogurt
Increase agar-agar powder to 2 teaspoons. Using whisk, break up chilled yogurt into small pieces, then transfer to blender and process until smooth, about 30 seconds.

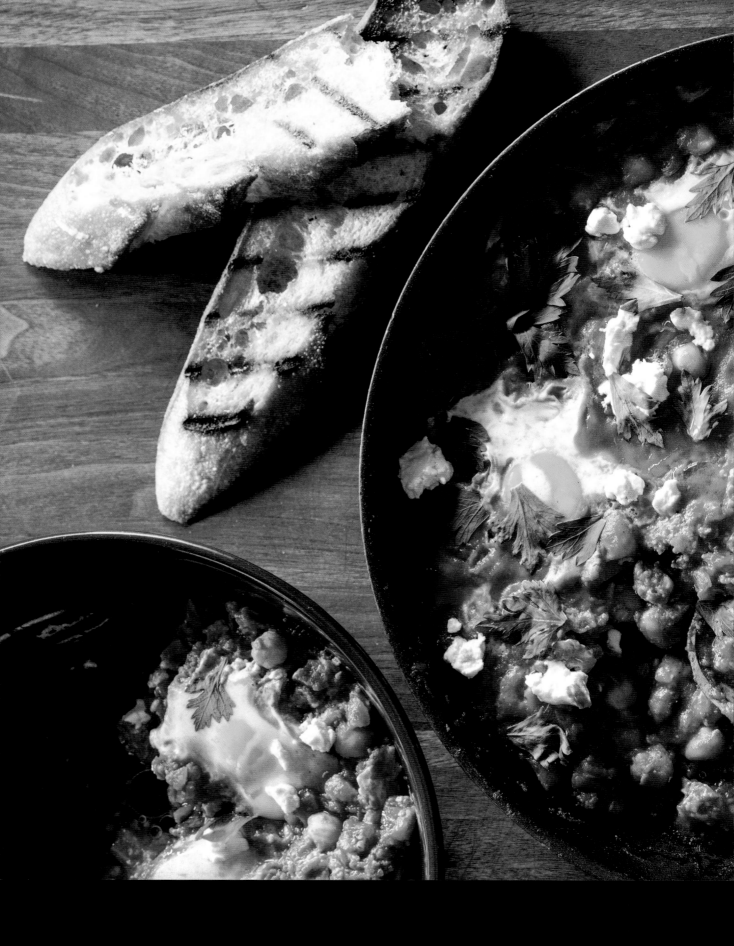

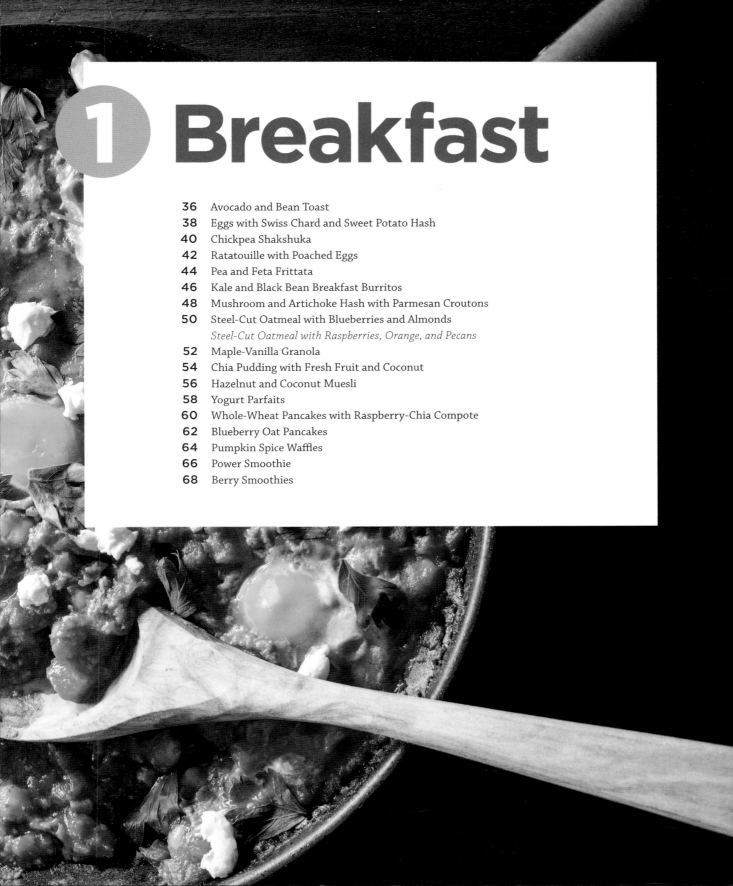

1 Breakfast

AVOCADO AND BEAN TOAST

SERVES 4

DAIRY FREE

WHY THIS RECIPE WORKS Avocado toast is one of our favorite healthful snacks, but we wanted a topped toast that was a bit more substantial and could stand alone as breakfast. That meant adding some fiber, and sustaining protein as well. Mashed black beans and shingled avocado slices on toast, brightened with citrus, marinated tomatoes, fresh cilantro, and quick-pickled radishes was our winning combination that boosted fiber in a flash. By simply mashing our beans with hot water, oil, and lime zest and juice, we were able to get a well-textured base. The pickled vegetables cut through the richness and really made this toast taste like a treat. A hearty slice of whole-grain rustic bread ably carried all of these contrasting flavors and textures. For an accurate measure of boiling water, bring a full kettle of water to a boil and then measure out the desired amount.

4 radishes, trimmed and sliced thin

½ teaspoon grated lime zest plus ¼ cup lime juice (2 limes), divided

1 teaspoon sugar

½ teaspoon plus ⅛ teaspoon table salt, divided

4 ounces grape or cherry tomatoes, quartered

4 teaspoons extra-virgin olive oil, divided

⅛ teaspoon pepper, divided

1 (15-ounce) can black beans, rinsed

¼ cup boiling water

4 (2-ounce) slices rustic 100-percent whole-grain bread, toasted

1 ripe avocado, halved, pitted, and sliced thin

¼ cup fresh cilantro leaves

1 Combine radishes, 3 tablespoons lime juice, sugar, and ½ teaspoon salt in bowl and let sit at room temperature for 15 minutes. Drain radishes and set aside.

2 Combine tomatoes, 1 teaspoon oil, pinch salt, and pinch pepper in bowl. Using potato masher, mash beans, boiling water, lime zest and remaining 1 tablespoon juice, remaining pinch salt, remaining pinch pepper, and remaining 1 tablespoon oil in second bowl to coarse paste, leaving some whole beans intact. Season with salt and pepper to taste.

3 Spread mashed bean mixture evenly on toasted bread slices and shingle avocado slices over beans. Top with tomatoes, cilantro, and pickled radishes. Serve.

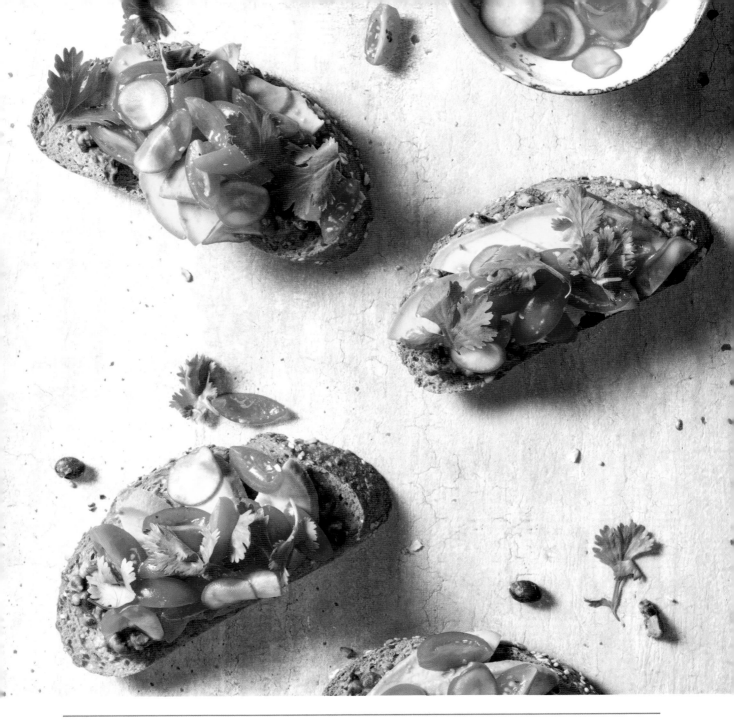

PER SERVING

Dietary Fiber 13g **Cal** 340;
Total Fat 14g, **Sat Fat** 2g;
Chol 0mg; **Sodium** 600mg;
Total Carb 48g, **Total Sugars** 6g,
Added Sugars 0g; **Protein** 11g

 MAKE IT GLUTEN FREE Substitute gluten-free bread for whole-grain bread.

EGGS WITH SWISS CHARD AND SWEET POTATO HASH

SERVES 4

WHY THIS RECIPE WORKS With two types of potatoes, garlicky (thank you, garlic oil) Swiss chard, and four fried eggs, this breakfast has what the standard eggs and potatoes are missing: varied flavors and textures and synchronized perfectly cooked eggs with runny yolks, plus fiber, nutrients, and low-FODMAP status. Microwaving the potato cubes before browning them in a pan keeps cooking quick and also ensures well cooked potatoes that brown in the time their centers are fluffy-creamy. Both potatoes contribute fiber, with the red potatoes helping to keep the dish low FODMAP and the sweet potatoes contributing their sweet flavor and abundant nutrients. The Swiss chard takes just 3 minutes to wilt in the skillet the potatoes brown in; the eggs fry in there next. A little lemon juice and paprika season the vegetable mixture and the runny yolks marry the elements on the plate with richness.

1¼ pounds red potatoes, unpeeled, cut into ½-inch pieces

12 ounces sweet potatoes, peeled and cut into ½-inch pieces

1 tablespoon garlic oil (see page 20), divided

12 ounces Swiss chard, stemmed and cut into 1-inch pieces

½ teaspoon table salt, divided

2 teaspoons lemon juice

3 tablespoons extra-virgin olive oil, divided

1 teaspoon paprika

8 large eggs, divided

1 Microwave red potatoes and sweet potatoes in large covered bowl until almost tender, about 10 minutes, stirring halfway through microwaving; drain away excess liquid and set aside.

2 Heat 1 teaspoon garlic oil in 12-inch nonstick skillet over medium heat until shimmering. Add chard and ¼ teaspoon salt and cook until tender, about 3 minutes. Using tongs, transfer chard to bowl and stir in lemon juice. Wipe skillet clean with paper towels.

3 Heat 2½ tablespoons olive oil in now-empty skillet over medium-high heat until just smoking. Add potato mixture and remaining ¼ teaspoon salt and cook, stirring occasionally, until golden brown, about 10 minutes. Off heat, push potatoes to sides of skillet. Add remaining 2 teaspoons garlic oil and paprika to center and cook until fragrant, about 15 seconds. Stir paprika mixture into potatoes and season with salt and pepper to taste. Divide hash evenly among 4 serving plates and top with chard mixture.

4 Crack 4 eggs into bowl. Crack remaining 4 eggs into second bowl. Heat remaining 1½ teaspoons olive oil in now-empty skillet over medium-high heat until shimmering. Working quickly, pour 1 bowl of eggs into one side of skillet and second bowl of eggs into other side of skillet. Cover and cook for 1 minute. Remove skillet from heat and let sit, covered, 15 to 45 seconds for runny yolks (white around edge of yolk will be barely opaque), 45 to 60 seconds for soft but set yolks, and about 2 minutes for medium-set yolks. Using rubber spatula, gently separate eggs into 4 portions and transfer to plates with Swiss chard mixture and hash. Serve.

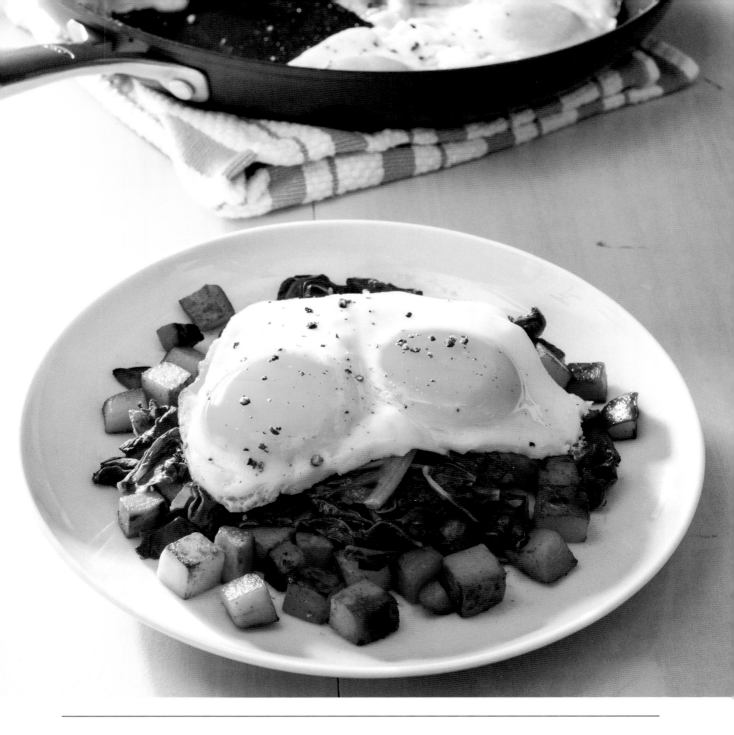

PER SERVING

Dietary Fiber 6g **Cal** 440;
Total Fat 24g, **Sat Fat** 5g;
Chol 370mg; **Sodium** 670mg;
Total Carb 39g, **Total Sugars** 6g,
Added Sugars 0g; **Protein** 18g

CHICKPEA SHAKSHUKA

SERVES 4

GLUTEN FREE

WHY THIS RECIPE WORKS The beloved dish of eggs poached in spicy tomato sauce enjoyed throughout the Mediterranean, Middle East, and North Africa gets a fiber boost with the untraditional addition of chickpeas. Incorporating canned chickpeas into the sauce maintains the ease that convenience products (canned tomatoes and jarred roasted red peppers) lend many versions of shakshuka. And in addition to substance, the chickpeas add nutty depth to the dish. Eggs poached in the tomato-chickpea sauce and a sprinkle of goat cheese on top finish the extra-hearty dish with richness. Spooning sauce over the whites of the eggs as they cook ensures the eggs cook evenly. We're serving this for breakfast but it's filling and robust enough to be a great eggs-for-dinner option. Serve the shakshuka with toasted bread (slow-leavened sourdough (see page 27) or gluten-free if needed) to scoop up the sauce.

- 1 tablespoon garlic oil (see page 20), plus extra for drizzling
- 1 (15-ounce) can chickpeas, rinsed
- 1½ teaspoons smoked paprika
- 1 teaspoon ground cumin
- 1 (28-ounce) can crushed tomatoes
- 1 cup jarred roasted red bell peppers, rinsed, patted dry, and chopped coarse
- ¼ teaspoon table salt
- ¼ teaspoon pepper
- 8 large eggs
- 2 ounces goat cheese, crumbled (½ cup)
- 2 tablespoons chopped fresh parsley

1 Heat oil in 12-inch nonstick skillet over medium-high heat until shimmering. Add chickpeas, paprika, and cumin and cook until fragrant, about 1 minute. Stir in tomatoes, red peppers, salt, and pepper and bring to simmer. Cover, reduce heat to medium-low, and cook until flavors meld, about 5 minutes. Season with salt and pepper to taste.

2 Off heat, using back of spoon, make 8 shallow 1½-inch indentations in sauce (7 around perimeter and 1 in center). Crack 1 egg into each indentation. Spoon sauce over edges of egg whites so whites are partially covered and yolks are exposed.

3 Bring to simmer over medium heat (there should be small bubbles across entire surface). Reduce heat to maintain simmer. Cover and cook until whites are just set and yolks are still runny, 4 to 7 minutes, rotating skillet occasionally for even cooking. Sprinkle with goat cheese and parsley and drizzle with extra oil. Serve.

PER SERVING
Dietary Fiber 7g **Cal** 350;
Total Fat 18g, **Sat Fat** 6g;
Chol 380mg; **Sodium** 720mg;
Total Carb 23g, **Total Sugars** 9g,
Added Sugars 0g; **Protein** 22g

 MAKE IT LOW FODMAP Reduce chickpeas to 1 cup.

 MAKE IT DAIRY FREE Omit goat cheese.

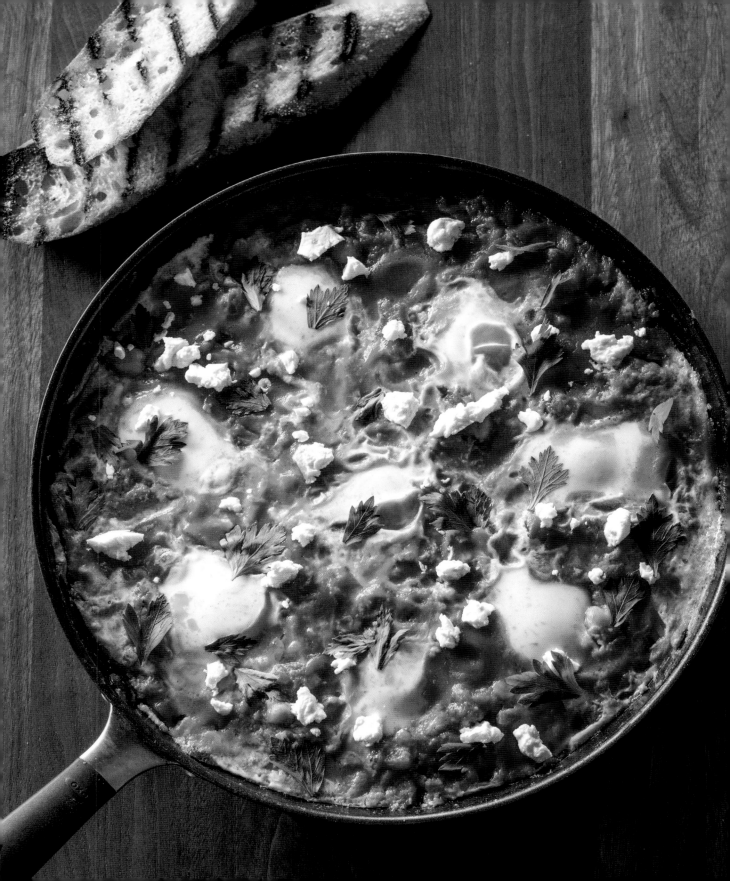

RATATOUILLE WITH POACHED EGGS

SERVES 4

WHY THIS RECIPE WORKS Ratatouille is all about summer vegetables—specifically, zucchini, eggplant, and tomatoes. The classic French dish showcases their taste and abundance by emphasizing simple ingredients cooked in a flavorful stew. The dish can serve as a side or a paired entrée, but here we make it a standout stand-alone breakfast option by cooking it in a skillet and poaching eggs directly in the stew. Browning the vegetables was critical to developing and deepening their flavor; otherwise the ratatouille tasted bland and soggy. Since zucchini and eggplant have very different cooking times, we browned the zucchini first and then removed it from the pan before cooking the eggplant to make sure we didn't get mush. Poaching the eggs right in the ratatouille worked like a charm. Leaving the skin on the eggplant helps keep the pieces intact during cooking.

3 tablespoons garlic oil (see page 20), divided, plus extra for drizzling

1¼ pounds zucchini, cut into ¾-inch pieces

1¼ pounds eggplant, cut into ¾-inch pieces

¾ teaspoon table salt, divided

¼ teaspoon pepper, divided

1 pound plum tomatoes, cored and cut into ½-inch pieces

¾ cup water

1 teaspoon herbes de Provence

1 teaspoon red wine vinegar

4 large eggs

1 ounce Parmesan cheese, grated (½ cup)

¼ cup chopped fresh basil

1 Heat 1 tablespoon oil in 12-inch nonstick skillet over medium-high heat until just smoking. Add zucchini and cook until well browned, 5 to 8 minutes; transfer to bowl.

2 Add eggplant, remaining 2 tablespoons oil, ½ teaspoon salt, and ⅛ teaspoon pepper to now-empty skillet and cook over medium-high heat until eggplant is well-browned, 6 to 9 minutes. Stir in tomatoes, water, herbes de Provence, remaining ¼ teaspoon salt, and remaining ⅛ teaspoon pepper. Simmer until eggplant and tomatoes are softened, 7 to 10 minutes. Stir in zucchini and any accumulated juices and the vinegar.

3 Off heat, using back of spoon, make 4 shallow 1½-inch indentations in ratatouille. Crack 1 egg into each indentation. Spoon sauce over edges of egg whites so whites are partially covered and yolks are exposed.

4 Bring to simmer over medium heat (there should be small bubbles across entire surface). Reduce heat to maintain simmer. Cover and cook until whites are just set and yolks are still runny, 4 to 7 minutes, rotating skillet occasionally for even cooking. Sprinkle with Parmesan and basil and drizzle with extra oil. Serve.

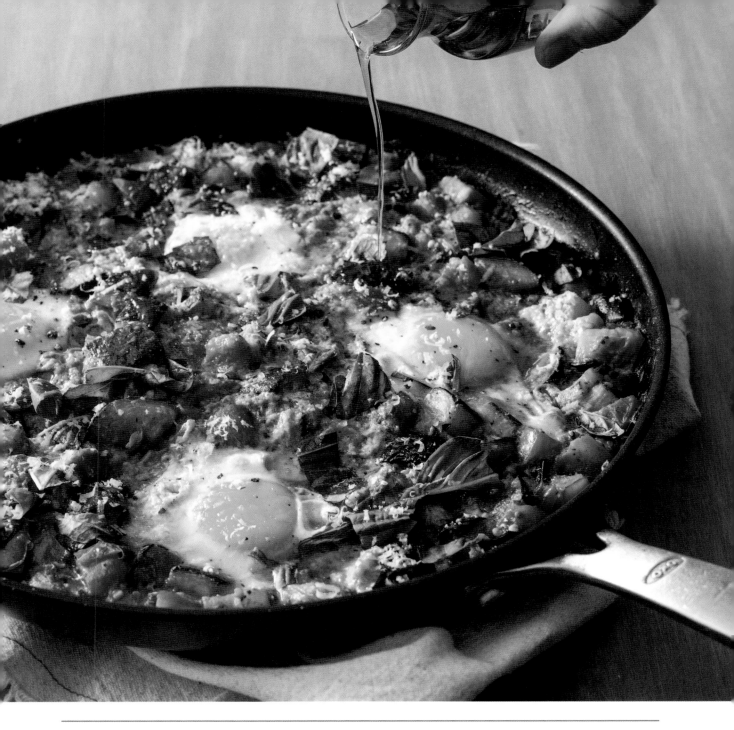

PER SERVING

Dietary Fiber 7g **Cal** 280;
Total Fat 18g, **Sat Fat** 4g;
Chol 190mg; **Sodium** 650mg;
Total Carb 18g, **Total Sugars** 11g,
Added Sugars 0g; **Protein** 14g

DF **MAKE IT DAIRY FREE** Omit Parmesan cheese.

PEA AND FETA FRITTATA

SERVES 4

GLUTEN FREE

WHY THIS RECIPE WORKS You really can't go wrong with a good-for-you frittata for breakfast; the extra-thick omelet is sturdy enough to hold plenty of vegetables among its creamy curds. Despite their diminutive size, peas really pack fiber and we thought they'd be a fun addition to a frittata, contributing pops of sweetness in every bite and an attractive polka-dotted presentation. Balancing them is salty-briny low-lactose feta cheese, fresh oregano, and bright lemon. To make it a meal (this frittata works well for lunch or dinner, too), we serve it with a fresh fennel and arugula salad that's quick to put together. Look for a trail that fills in slowly in step 3; if it fills in quickly, not enough egg has coagulated and the finished frittata will contain pockets of undercooked egg. Slice the fennel as thinly as possible. You will need a 12-inch ovensafe nonstick skillet for this recipe.

12 large eggs

⅓ cup whole milk

½ teaspoon plus pinch table salt, divided

2 ounces feta cheese, crumbled into ½-inch pieces (½ cup)

2 tablespoons minced fresh oregano

2 tablespoons extra-virgin olive oil, divided

2 cups frozen peas

Pinch red pepper flakes (optional)

½ teaspoon grated lemon zest plus 2½ teaspoons juice, divided

6 ounces (6 cups) baby arugula

1 fennel bulb, stalks discarded, bulb halved, cored, and sliced thin

1 Adjust oven rack to middle position and heat oven to 350 degrees. Whisk eggs, milk, and ½ teaspoon salt in bowl until well combined. Stir in feta and oregano.

2 Heat 1 teaspoon oil in 12-inch ovensafe nonstick skillet over medium-high heat until shimmering. Add peas, pepper flakes, and ¼ cup water. Cover and cook until peas are bright green and just tender, 3 to 5 minutes. Uncover, stir in lemon zest and ½ teaspoon juice and cook until skillet is dry, about 1 minute.

3 Add egg mixture and cook, using rubber spatula to stir and scrape bottom of skillet until large curds form and spatula leaves trail through eggs but eggs are still very wet, about 30 seconds. Smooth curds into even layer and cook, without stirring, for 30 seconds. Transfer skillet to oven and bake until frittata is slightly puffy and surface bounces back when lightly pressed, 6 to 9 minutes.

4 Using rubber spatula, loosen frittata from skillet and transfer to cutting board. Let sit for 5 minutes. Meanwhile, whisk remaining 5 teaspoons oil, remaining 2 teaspoons lemon juice, and remaining pinch salt together in large bowl. Add arugula and fennel and toss to coat. Season with salt and pepper to taste. Serve.

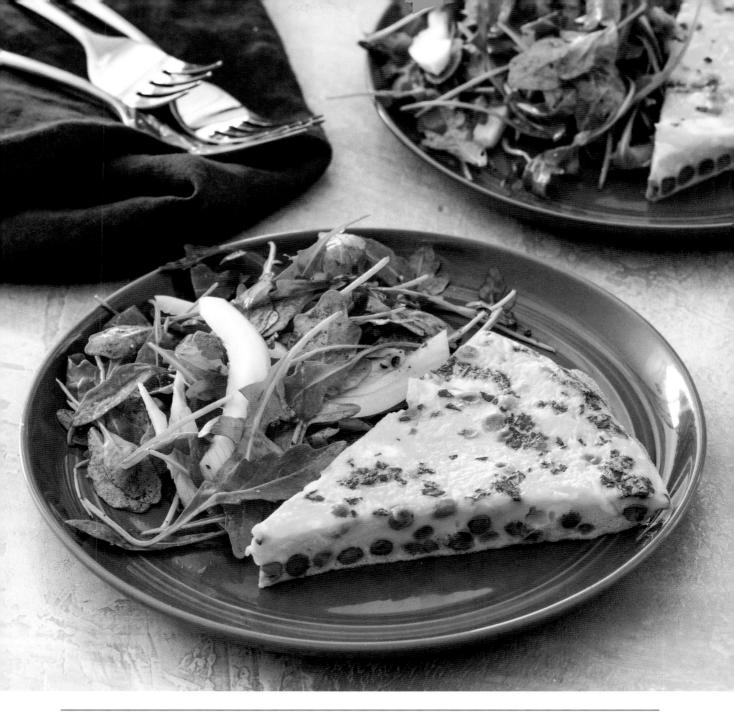

PER SERVING

Dietary Fiber 6g **Cal** 420;
Total Fat 25g, **Sat Fat** 8g;
Chol 575mg; **Sodium** 730mg;
Total Carb 19g, **Total Sugars** 9g,
Added Sugars 0g; **Protein** 28g

LF **MAKE IT LOW FODMAP** Substitute dairy-free or lactose-free milk (see page 19) for whole milk. Substitute 2 cups frozen broccoli florets, thawed and chopped, for peas. Increase arugula to 8 ounces and reduce fennel to ½ bulb.

DF **MAKE IT DAIRY FREE** Substitute dairy-free (see page 19) milk for the whole milk. Omit feta.

KALE AND BLACK BEAN BREAKFAST BURRITOS

SERVES 6

DAIRY FREE

WHY THIS RECIPE WORKS Burritos are a beloved meal anytime for their abundant delicious ingredients all wrapped up in a soft tortilla parcel. The addition of an egg scramble, which packs in protein, usually defines a breakfast burrito, but the rest is less defined—and usually not as nutritious. We start the morning right by including a usual suspect, fiberful black beans, and a stellar surprise, hearty kale, along with the fluffy scrambled eggs. We begin with a flavorful base of sautéed poblano and cumin to wake everything up, then add our beans, mashing half to create a cohesive mixture. Next, we quickly braise our kale until tender, then scramble the eggs before folding the kale back in. All of this happens in a single skillet. We spread the bean mixture onto whole-wheat tortillas, add the kale-egg scramble, and finish with tomato and a drizzle of garlic oil. Softening the tortillas in the microwave makes them easy to roll. Serve with hot sauce if desired.

2 tablespoons garlic oil (see page 20), divided, plus extra for drizzling

1 poblano chile, stemmed, seeded, and chopped fine

½ teaspoon table salt, divided

½ teaspoon ground cumin

1 (15-ounce) can black beans, rinsed

2 teaspoons lime juice

12 ounces kale, stemmed and chopped

8 large eggs

¼ teaspoon pepper

6 (10-inch) 100 percent whole-wheat flour tortillas

1 tomato, cored and chopped fine

1 Heat 1 tablespoon oil in 12-inch nonstick skillet over medium-high heat until shimmering. Add poblano and ⅛ teaspoon salt and cook until softened, about 3 minutes. Stir in cumin and cook until fragrant, about 15 seconds. Stir in beans and ½ cup water and cook until beans are heated through, about 4 minutes. Off heat, mash half of beans to chunky paste with potato masher. Stir in lime juice and season with salt and pepper to taste; transfer mixture to bowl and cover to keep warm. Wipe skillet clean with paper towels.

2 Heat 2 teaspoons oil in now-empty skillet over medium-high heat until shimmering. Add kale and ⅛ teaspoon salt, cover, and cook until kale begins to wilt, about 2 minutes. Stir in ¼ cup water, cover, and cook until kale is tender, 2 to 4 minutes. Using tongs, transfer kale to separate bowl. Wipe skillet clean with paper towels.

3 Whisk eggs, 2 tablespoons water, pepper, and remaining ¼ teaspoon salt in bowl until well combined. Heat remaining 1 teaspoon oil in now-empty skillet over medium-high heat until shimmering. Add egg mixture and cook, using rubber spatula to constantly and firmly scrape along bottom and sides of skillet, until eggs begin to clump and spatula leaves trail on bottom of skillet, 1½ to 2½ minutes. Off heat, add kale and constantly fold eggs and kale until eggs have finished cooking, 30 to 60 seconds. Cover to keep warm.

4 Wrap tortillas in damp dish towel and microwave until warm and pliable, about 1 minute. Lay warm tortillas on counter and spread bean mixture evenly across center of each tortilla, close to bottom edge. Top with kale-egg mixture then sprinkle with tomato and drizzle with extra oil to taste. Working with 1 tortilla at a time, fold sides then bottom of tortilla over filling, then continue to roll tightly into burrito. Serve immediately.

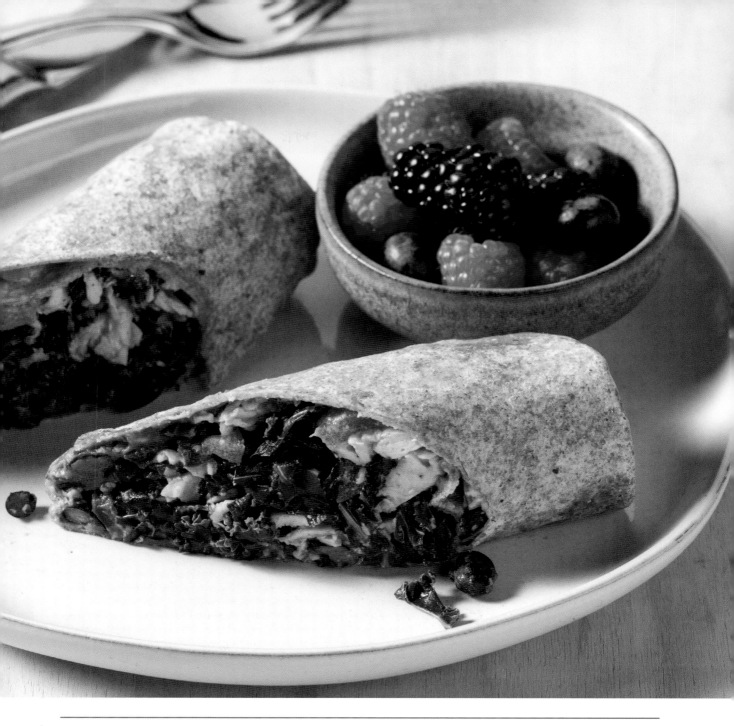

PER SERVING

Dietary Fiber 8g **Cal** 320;
Total Fat 15g, **Sat Fat** 4g;
Chol 250mg; **Sodium** 750mg;
Total Carb 31g, **Total Sugars** 2g,
Added Sugars 0g; **Protein** 16g

LF **MAKE IT LOW FODMAP** Substitute canned lentils for black beans and gluten-free wraps for whole-wheat tortillas.

GF **MAKE IT GLUTEN FREE** Substitute gluten-free wraps for whole-wheat tortillas.

MUSHROOM AND ARTICHOKE HASH WITH PARMESAN CROUTONS

SERVES 4

WHY THIS RECIPE WORKS Breakfast hash is a delicious savory skillet meal, but many of the classic versions, like corned beef hash, provide little nutrition. In addition to replacing meat with meaty vegetables (there's a pound and a half of mushrooms here), this hash forgoes the potatoes and calls for fiber-filled artichokes. But our hash still needed a starchy element for cohesiveness; we took the opportunity to incorporate a wholesome grain instead. Parmesan croutons made from rustic whole-grain bread was an inspiring departure. We pressed our mixture into the skillet with the back of a spatula, flipping and packing it a few times to achieve good browning and cohesion. A final dollop of brightly seasoned yogurt livened up all the flavors. Any mix of wild mushrooms can be used here. While we prefer the flavor and texture of jarred whole baby artichoke hearts in this recipe, you can substitute 18 ounces frozen artichoke hearts, thawed and patted dry, for the jarred.

6 tablespoons plus 1 teaspoon garlic oil (see page 20), divided

2 (2-ounce) slices rustic 100-percent whole-grain bread, cut into ½-inch pieces

¼ cup grated Parmesan cheese

1½ pounds chanterelle, cremini, oyster, and/or shiitake mushrooms, stemmed and cut into ½-inch pieces

¼ teaspoon table salt

3 cups jarred whole baby artichoke hearts packed in water, drained, quartered, and patted dry

2 teaspoons minced fresh sage

½ cup plain Greek yogurt

½ teaspoon grated lemon zest plus 1 tablespoon juice

1 Heat 2 tablespoons oil in 12-inch nonstick skillet over medium heat until shimmering. Add bread and cook, stirring constantly, until beginning to brown, 3 to 5 minutes. Add Parmesan and continue to cook, stirring constantly and breaking up clumps, until croutons are golden brown, about 2 minutes; transfer to bowl.

2 Heat 2 tablespoons oil in now-empty skillet over medium-high heat until shimmering. Add mushrooms and salt, cover, and cook, stirring occasionally, until mushrooms have released their liquid, 8 to 10 minutes.

3 Uncover and stir in 2 tablespoons oil, artichokes, sage, and reserved croutons. Using back of spatula, firmly pack hash into skillet and cook undisturbed for 2 minutes. Meanwhile, whisk yogurt, lemon zest and juice, and remaining 1 teaspoon oil together in small bowl and season with salt and pepper to taste; set aside.

4 Flip hash, one portion at a time, and repack into skillet. Repeat flipping process every few minutes until hash is well browned, about 6 minutes. Season with salt and pepper to taste. Top individual portions with 2 tablespoons yogurt mixture before serving.

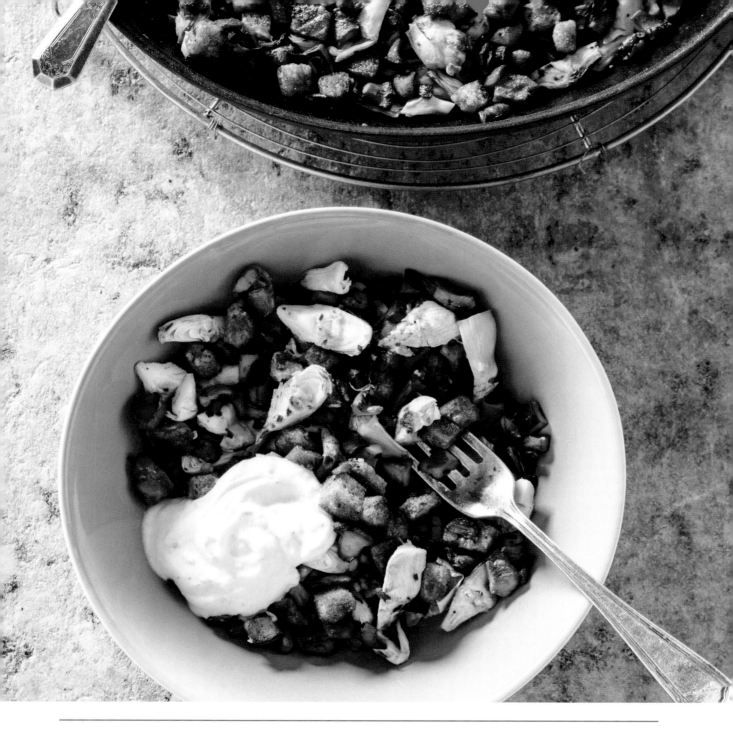

PER SERVING

Dietary Fiber 7g **Cal** 440;
Total Fat 29g, **Sat Fat** 7g;
Chol 10mg; **Sodium** 650mg;
Total Carb 33g, **Total Sugars** 6g,
Added Sugars 0g; **Protein** 13g

DF **MAKE IT DAIRY FREE** Omit Parmesan cheese and cook bread in step 1 until golden brown, 5 to 7 minutes. Substitute dairy-free yogurt (see page 19) for Greek yogurt.

GF **MAKE IT GLUTEN FREE** Substitute gluten-free bread for whole-grain bread.

STEEL-CUT OATMEAL WITH BLUEBERRIES AND ALMONDS

SERVES 4

WHY THIS RECIPE WORKS Steel-cut oats, which are dried oat kernels cut crosswise into coarse bits, create an oatmeal that is full of texture while still being luscious and creamy. Bonus: They're a low-FODMAP whole grain. With whole grains typically comes a longer cooking time, but we keep our breakfast speedy by soaking the oats in just-boiled water overnight and then heating them through in the morning, for getting up and going. We didn't need dairy to cook our oatmeal, as the oat mixture becomes creamy enough through the soaking and cooking in water. Cinnamon and nutmeg provide the classic, warm-spice flavor we like in oatmeal. A topping of blueberries adds sweetness and more fiber and nutrition, while chopped toasted almonds provide contrasting crunch to the creamy porridge. Do not substitute rolled oats for the steel-cut oats. This oatmeal reheats well, so you can quickly serve it up again later in the week.

4 cups water, divided

1 cup steel-cut oats (see page 18)

¼ teaspoon table salt

1 tablespoon packed brown sugar

¼ teaspoon ground cinnamon

Pinch ground nutmeg

2½ ounces (½ cup) blueberries, divided

3 tablespoons whole almonds, toasted and chopped

1 Bring 3 cups water to boil in large saucepan over high heat. Off heat, stir in oats and salt, cover, and let sit for at least 12 hours or up to 24 hours.

2 Stir remaining 1 cup water, sugar, cinnamon, and nutmeg into oats and bring to boil over medium-high heat. Reduce heat to medium and cook, stirring occasionally, until oats are softened but still retain some chew and mixture thickens and resembles warm pudding, 4 to 6 minutes.

3 Remove saucepan from heat and let sit for 5 minutes. Stir to recombine and serve, sprinkling individual portions evenly with blueberries and almonds.

VARIATION
Steel-Cut Oatmeal with Raspberries, Orange, and Pecans
Substitute 1 teaspoon grated orange zest for cinnamon and nutmeg, raspberries for blueberries, and pecans for almonds.

PER SERVING

Dietary Fiber 6g **Cal** 230;
Total Fat 5g, **Sat Fat** 0.5g;
Chol 0mg; **Sodium** 150mg;
Total Carb 39g, **Total Sugars** 6g,
Added Sugars 3g; **Protein** 7g

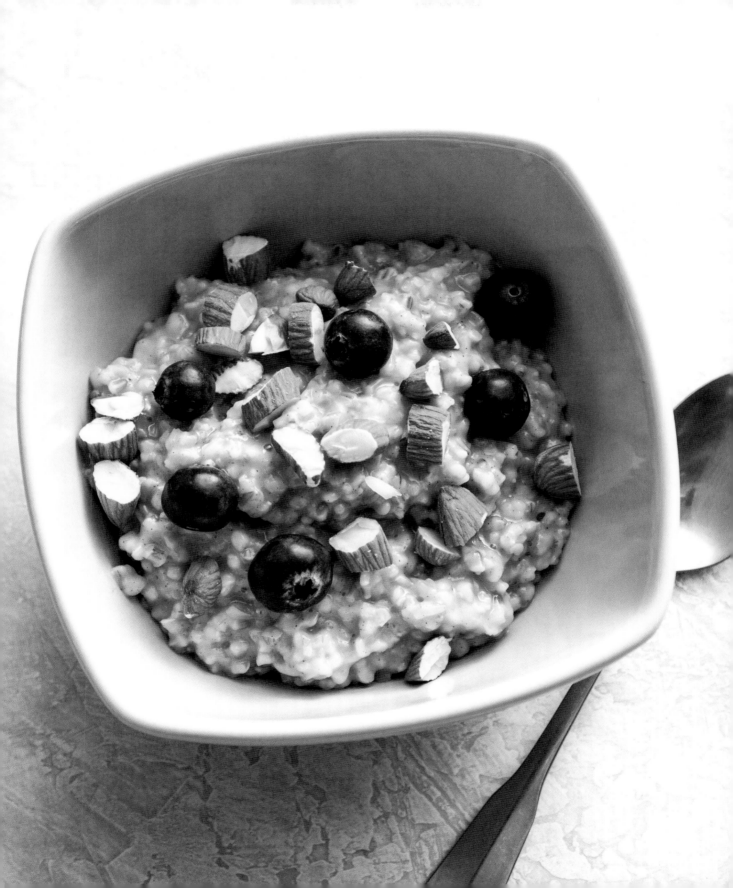

MAPLE-VANILLA GRANOLA

MAKES ABOUT 7 CUPS

WHY THIS RECIPE WORKS Granola should be a healthy, nutrient-dense breakfast or snack, but store-bought versions most often come up short. We wanted to bring granola back to where it began: a collection of toasted oats and nuts held together in generous clumps by a kiss of sweetness. We found that the secret to the perfect texture was to firmly pack the granola mixture into a rimmed baking sheet before baking. Once it was baked, we had a granola "bark" that we could break into crunchy clumps of any size. Coarsely chopped almonds, flaked coconut, and raisins added a welcome crunch and sweetness. Maple syrup and a hefty amount of vanilla rounded things out with rich, warm sweetness and, once baked, held everything together. Do not substitute quick oats, instant oats, or steel-cut oats for the rolled oats in this recipe.

⅓ cup extra-virgin olive oil

⅓ cup maple syrup

1 tablespoon vanilla extract

½ teaspoon table salt

3 cups (9 ounces) old-fashioned rolled oats (see page 18)

2 cups unsweetened flaked coconut

1 cup whole almonds, chopped coarse

½ cup raisins

1 Adjust oven rack to upper-middle position and heat oven to 325 degrees. Line rimmed baking sheet with parchment paper.

2 Whisk oil, maple syrup, vanilla, and salt together in large bowl. Fold in oats, coconut, and almonds until thoroughly coated.

3 Transfer mixture to prepared baking sheet and spread into thin, even layer. Using stiff metal spatula, press on mixture until very compact. Bake until golden brown, 25 to 30 minutes, rotating sheet halfway through baking.

4 Remove granola from oven and let cool on wire rack for 1 hour. Break cooled granola into pieces of desired size and stir in raisins. Serve. (Granola can be stored at room temperature for up to 2 weeks.)

PER ⅔-CUP SERVING

Dietary Fiber 6g **Cal** 380;
Total Fat 26g, **Sat Fat** 11g;
Chol 0mg; **Sodium** 120mg;
Total Carb 35g, **Total Sugars** 14g,
Added Sugars 6g; **Protein** 7g

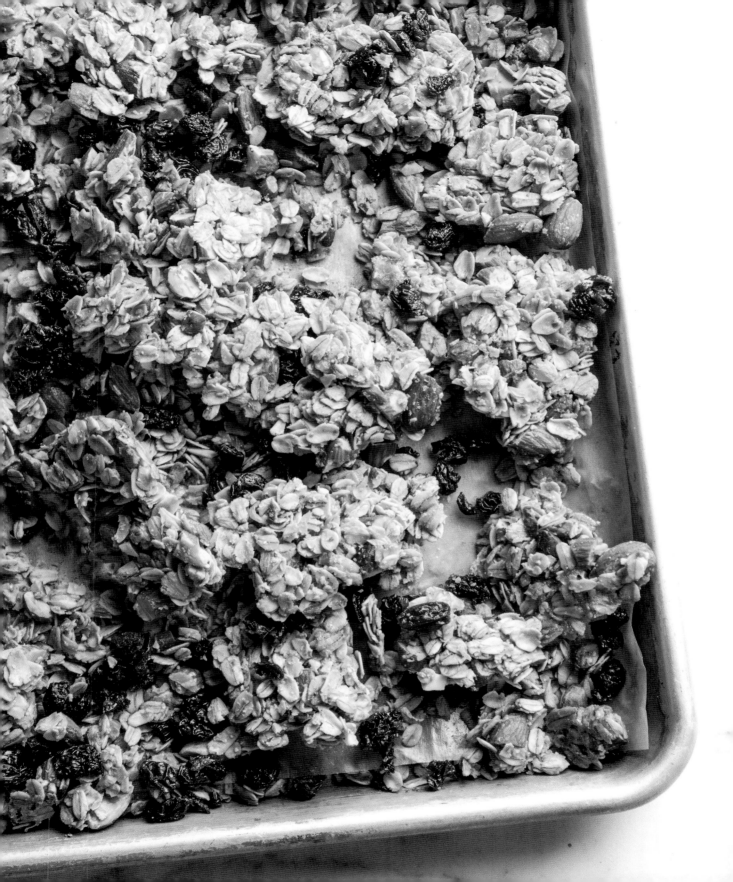

CHIA PUDDING WITH FRESH FRUIT AND COCONUT

SERVES 4

GLUTEN FREE

WHY THIS RECIPE WORKS Chia pudding comes together by what seems like Jack and the Beanstalk–level magic. When chia seeds are combined with liquid and left to soak overnight they create a gel, which thickens and produces a no-cook tapioca-like pudding—a spectacular alternative to the usual yogurt for breakfast. Pudding alchemy aside, chia is great because it's a nutritional powerhouse, packed with fiber (plus protein and omega-3 fatty acids) that will keep you full for hours. And with a neutral flavor, it's the perfect canvas for fruity toppings. This recipe takes little effort, just time. Soaking the seeds overnight is a hands-off way of making the pudding ready for morning. Before we put it to bed, we give the pudding a quick second whisk 15 minutes after its initial mixing to make sure all the chia is hydrated and to prevent clumping. To flavor the pudding, we keep things simple with vanilla extract and maple syrup, which pair nicely with almost any toppings you have at your breakfast table.

2 cups milk

½ cup chia seeds

2 tablespoons maple syrup, plus extra for serving

1½ teaspoons vanilla extract

¼ teaspoon table salt

5 ounces (1 cup) blueberries, raspberries, sliced strawberries, and/or sliced bananas

¼ cup unsweetened flaked coconut, toasted

1 Whisk milk, chia seeds, maple syrup, vanilla, and salt together in bowl. Let mixture sit for 15 minutes, then whisk again to break up any clumps. Cover bowl with plastic wrap and refrigerate for at least 8 hours or up to 1 week.

2 Adjust consistency of pudding with water as needed. Top individual portions with ¼ cup blueberries and 1 tablespoon coconut, and drizzle with extra maple syrup before serving.

PER SERVING

Dietary Fiber 10g **Cal** 260;
Total Fat 14g, **Sat Fat** 6g;
Chol 10mg; **Sodium** 200mg;
Total Carb 27g, **Total Sugars** 14g,
Added Sugars 6g; **Protein** 8g

 MAKE IT LOW FODMAP Substitute dairy-free or lactose-free milk (see page 19) for milk.

 MAKE IT DAIRY FREE Substitute dairy-free milk (see page 19) for milk.

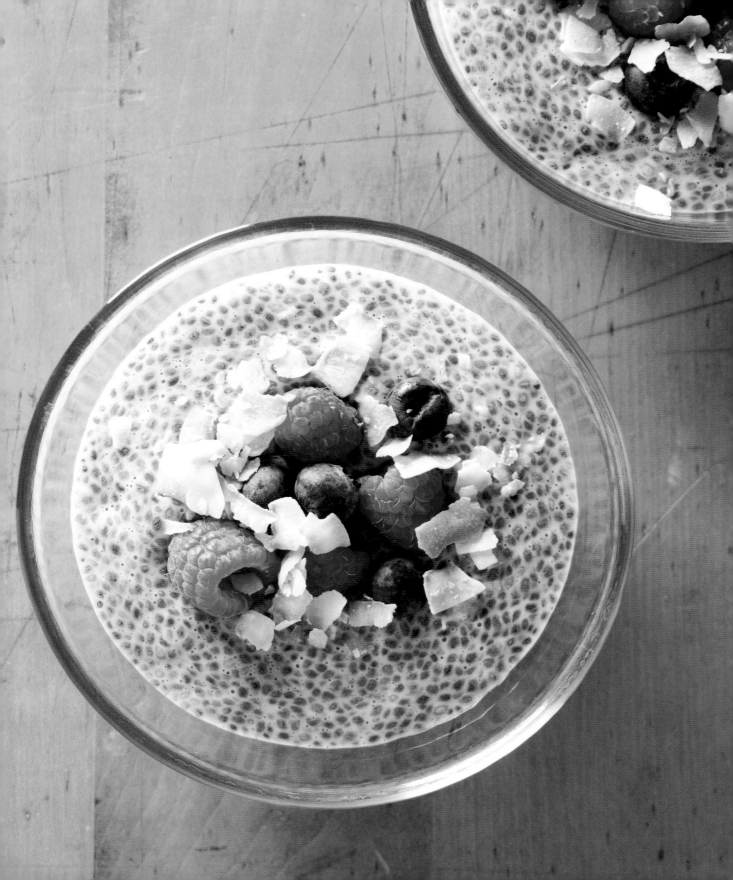

HAZELNUT AND COCONUT MUESLI

SERVES 4

GLUTEN FREE

WHY THIS RECIPE WORKS Starting your day right gives you the fuel and focus to conquer your tasks and can set the stage for your food choices for the rest of the day. We think every breakfast should fill you like a weekend brunch—even if it has to be ready fast. This muesli is a satisfying, nutrient-packed oat dish that's soaked overnight to soften the oats and improve digestibility; all you need to do in the morning is sprinkle your bowl with some berries. While traditional muesli uses all raw ingredients, we found that toasting the nuts brought depth and complexity to this simple dish. For our nut, chopped hazelnuts offered a pleasing aroma and crunch. Dried cranberries and shredded coconut, which soften during soaking, provided moderate pops of sweetness. To make a single serving, combine ½ cup muesli with ⅓ cup milk in bowl, cover, and refrigerate overnight. Muesli can also be served like cereal (no soaking overnight). Serve with maple syrup if desired.

1½ cups (4½ ounces) old-fashioned rolled oats (see page 18)

¼ cup dried cranberries or raisins

¼ cup hazelnuts, toasted, skinned, and chopped

¼ cup unsweetened shredded coconut

½ teaspoon cinnamon, optional

1⅓ cups milk

5 ounces (1 cup) blueberries or raspberries

1 Combine oats, cranberries, hazelnuts, coconut, and cinnamon, if using, in bowl. (Muesli can be stored at room temperature for up to 2 weeks.)

2 Stir milk into muesli until combined. Cover and refrigerate for at least 12 hours or up to 24 hours. Top individual portions with ¼ cup blueberries before serving.

PER SERVING
Dietary Fiber 6g **Cal** 300;
Total Fat 13g, **Sat Fat** 5g;
Chol 10mg; **Sodium** 40mg;
Total Carb 43g, **Total Sugars** 16g,
Added Sugars 0g; **Protein** 8g

 MAKE IT LOW FODMAP Substitute dairy-free milk or lactose-free milk (see page 19) for milk.

 MAKE IT DAIRY FREE Substitute dairy-free milk (see page 19) for milk.

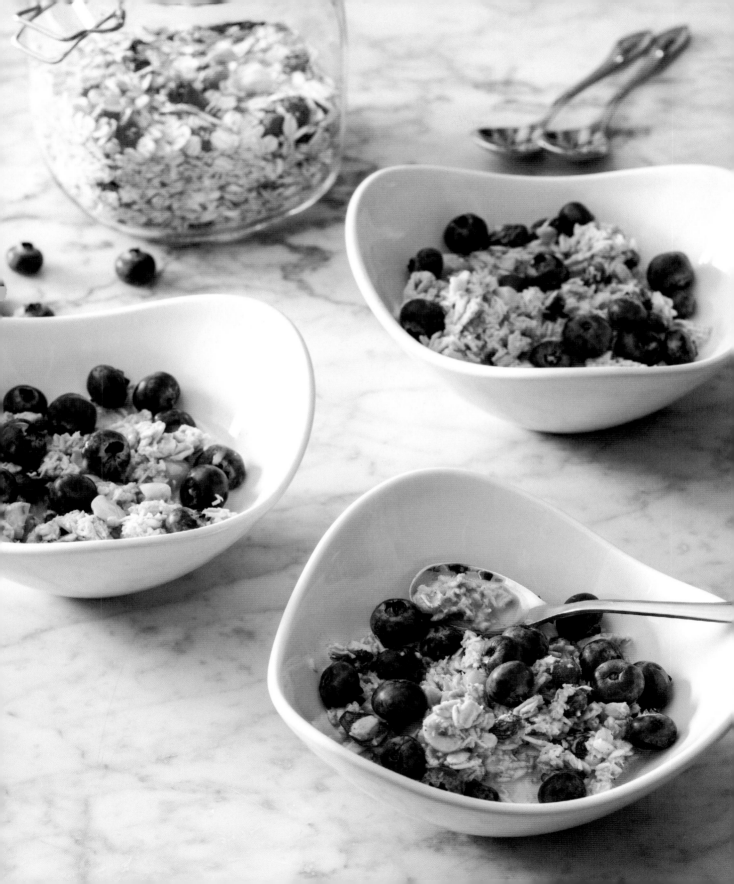

YOGURT PARFAITS

SERVES 4

WHY THIS RECIPE WORKS Creamy yogurt, fruit, and a topping are an easy and healthful start to the day—and layering them in a tall glass makes the simplest of breakfasts feel like a special occasion. Fiber-rich berries naturally sweeten the plain yogurt and add lots of freshness. Parfaits need crunch and we give ours plenty with toasted almonds and sunflower seeds. Do not substitute frozen fruit. Serve the parfaits within 15 minutes of assembling or the nuts and seeds will begin to turn soggy.

¾ cup whole almonds, toasted and chopped

½ cup raw sunflower seeds, toasted

2 cups plain yogurt, divided

20 ounces (4 cups) blackberries, blueberries, raspberries, and/or sliced strawberries, divided

Combine almonds and sunflower seeds in bowl. Using four 16-ounce glasses, spoon ¼ cup yogurt into each glass, then top with ½ cup berries, followed by 3 tablespoons nut mixture. Repeat layering process with remaining yogurt, berries, and nut mixture. Serve.

PER SERVING
Dietary Fiber 10g **Cal** 390;
Total Fat 26g, **Sat Fat** 4.5g;
Chol 15mg; **Sodium** 60mg;
Total Carb 30g, **Total Sugars** 16g,
Added Sugars 0g; **Protein** 14g

 MAKE IT LOW FODMAP Substitute walnuts or pecans for almonds. Use strawberries for the berries. Substitute dairy-free or lactose-free yogurt (see page 19) for plain yogurt.

 MAKE IT DAIRY FREE Substitute dairy-free yogurt (see page 19) for plain yogurt.

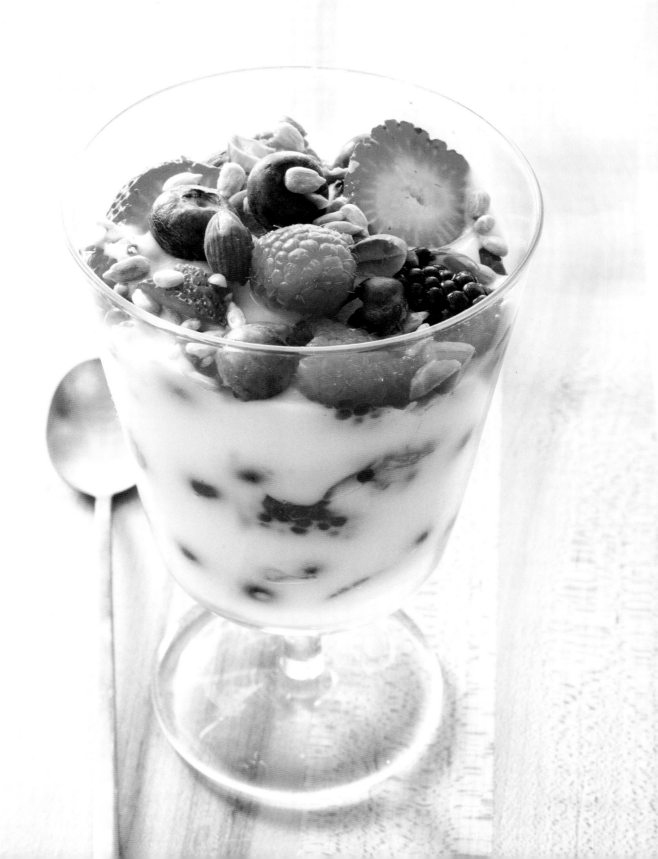

WHOLE-WHEAT PANCAKES WITH RASPBERRY-CHIA COMPOTE

MAKES 15 PANCAKES; SERVES 4 TO 6

WHY THIS RECIPE WORKS Pancakes seemed like the perfect opportunity to showcase more fiber-rich whole-wheat flour; the flour's earthy, robust flavor would pair well with a sweet fruit topping. But would the results be dense and heavy? Most whole-wheat pancake recipes shy away from using only whole-wheat flour, cutting the mix with white. But when we prepared a batch of 100 percent whole-wheat pancakes, rather than being leaden they turned out light, fluffy, and tender. The reason? The bran in the whole-wheat flour—the same stuff that contributes healthful fiber—cuts through any gluten strands that form, preventing the pancakes from becoming tough. In fact, while recipes for pancakes made with white flour advise undermixing to avoid tough pancakes, with whole-wheat flour we could whisk our batter until smooth. These pancakes aren't just the best for you; they're simply the best and so deserve the best topping: A quick and easy raspberry compote, sneakily thickened to a glossy consistency and made even more fiber-rich with chia seeds, is bright and sweet—elegant even. An electric griddle set at 350 degrees can be used in place of a skillet.

COMPOTE
- 5 ounces (1 cup) raspberries
- 1 tablespoon sugar
- 1 tablespoon water
- Pinch table salt
- 1 tablespoon chia seeds
- ¼ teaspoon vanilla extract

PANCAKES
- 2 cups (11 ounces) whole-wheat flour
- 2 tablespoons sugar
- 1½ teaspoons baking powder
- ½ teaspoon baking soda
- ½ teaspoon table salt
- 2¼ cups buttermilk
- 5 tablespoons plus 2 teaspoons canola oil, divided
- 2 large eggs

1 **For the compote:** Cook raspberries, sugar, water, and salt in small saucepan over medium-low heat, mashing occasionally with potato masher, until bubbling and raspberries have broken down, 4 to 6 minutes. Off heat, stir in chia seeds and vanilla and let sit until thickened, about 10 minutes. (Compote can be refrigerated for up to 3 days, bring to room temperature and stir to recombine before serving.)

2 **For the pancakes:** Adjust oven rack to middle position and heat oven to 200 degrees. Set wire rack in rimmed baking sheet and place in oven.

3 Whisk flour, sugar, baking powder, baking soda, and salt together in large bowl. Whisk buttermilk, 5 tablespoons oil, and eggs in second bowl until combined. Whisk buttermilk mixture into flour mixture until smooth. (Mixture will be thick; do not add more buttermilk.)

4 Heat 1 teaspoon oil in 12-inch nonstick skillet over medium heat until shimmering, 3 to 5 minutes. Using paper towels, wipe out oil, leaving thin film in pan. Using ¼-cup measure, portion batter into pan, spreading each into 4-inch round using back of spoon. Cook until edges are set, first side is golden, and bubbles on surface are just beginning to break, 2 to 3 minutes.

5 Flip pancakes and cook until second side is golden, 1 to 2 minutes. Transfer to wire rack in oven. Repeat with remaining batter, adding remaining oil to pan as necessary. Serve with compote.

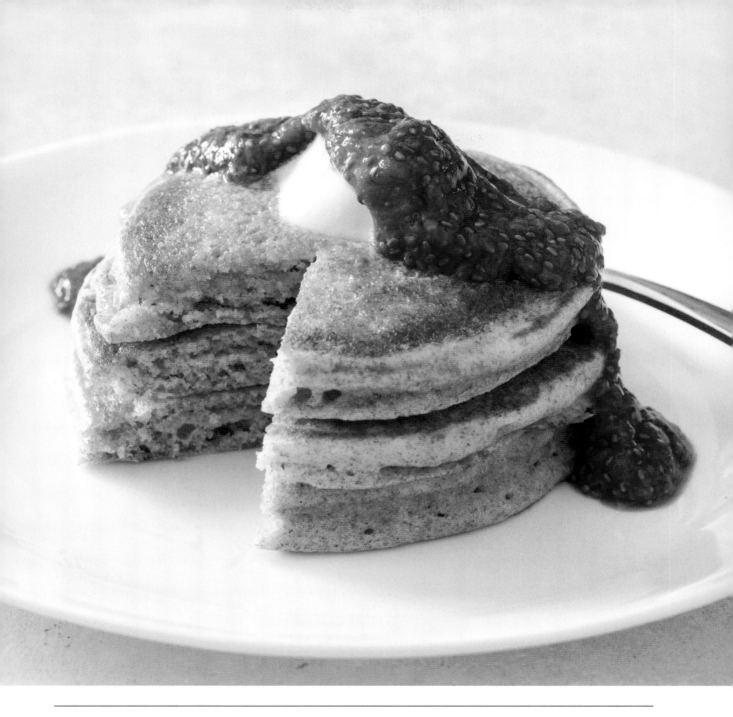

**PER 3-PANCAKE SERVING WITH
2 TABLESPOONS COMPOTE**

Dietary Fiber 9g **Cal** 470;
Total Fat 19g, **Sat Fat** 2.5g;
Chol 80mg; **Sodium** 670mg;
Total Carb 63g, **Total Sugars** 15g,
Added Sugars 8g; **Protein** 15g

 MAKE IT DAIRY FREE Substitute dairy-free milk (see page 19) for buttermilk and add 2 tablespoons lemon juice to milk mixture.

BLUEBERRY OAT PANCAKES

MAKES 18 PANCAKES; SERVES 6

WHY THIS RECIPE WORKS Not every food with the word "cake" in it is simple to make good alternative versions of if you're eating wheat- or gluten-free. But because pancakes don't require loads of structure—just enough to make them more fluffy than dense—they're a great candidate for remodeling. This breakfast classic gets a boost here from gluten-free whole grains; we zeroed in on oats for their nutty flavor, hearty texture, and high fiber content. We were able to create a smooth base for our batter using three-quarters oat flour with ½ cup whole-wheat, but the pancakes are also good with FODMAP-friendly gluten-free flour substituted for that mere ½ cup. Stirring some whole oats into our pancakes as well, presoaked to soften, gives them a satisfying texture. Fresh blueberries, cinnamon, and nutmeg pair nicely with the toasty oats. We prefer using store-bought oat flour as it has a very fine grind and creates the most fluffy pancakes, but you can make your own in a pinch: Grind 1½ cups (4½ ounces) old-fashioned rolled oats in a food processor to a fine meal, about 2 minutes; note pancakes will be denser if using ground oats. Do not use toasted oat flour, or quick, instant, or thick-cut oats in this recipe. An electric griddle set at 350 degrees can be used in place of a skillet. Serve with maple syrup, if desired.

2 cups buttermilk, divided, plus extra as needed

1 cup (3 ounces) old-fashioned rolled oats (see page 18)

1½ cups (4½ ounces) oat flour (see page 18)

½ cup (2¾ ounces) whole-wheat flour

2½ teaspoons baking powder

1 teaspoon ground cinnamon

¼ teaspoon table salt

⅛ teaspoon ground nutmeg

2 large eggs

3 tablespoons plus 2 teaspoons canola oil, divided

3 tablespoons sugar

2 teaspoons vanilla extract

7½ ounces (1½ cups) blueberries

1 Adjust oven rack to middle position and heat oven to 200 degrees. Set wire rack in rimmed baking sheet and place in oven. Combine 1 cup buttermilk and oats in bowl and let sit at room temperature until softened, about 15 minutes.

2 Whisk oat flour, whole-wheat flour, baking powder, cinnamon, salt, and nutmeg together in large bowl. Whisk remaining 1 cup buttermilk, eggs, 3 tablespoons oil, sugar, and vanilla in second bowl until frothy, about 1 minute. Make well in center of dry ingredients, add all of egg mixture to well, and gently stir until just combined. Using rubber spatula, fold in oat-buttermilk mixture until just combined.

3 Heat 1 teaspoon oil in 12-inch nonstick skillet over medium heat until shimmering, 3 to 5 minutes. Using paper towels, wipe out oil, leaving thin film in skillet. Using ¼-cup measure, portion batter into skillet, spreading each into 4-inch round using back of spoon. Sprinkle each pancake with 1 rounded tablespoon blueberries. Cook until edges are set, first side is golden, and bubbles on surface are just beginning to break, 2 to 3 minutes.

4 Flip pancakes and cook until second side is golden, 1 to 3 minutes. Transfer to prepared rack and keep warm in oven. Repeat with remaining batter, whisking additional buttermilk into batter as needed to loosen, and adding remaining oil to pan as necessary. Serve.

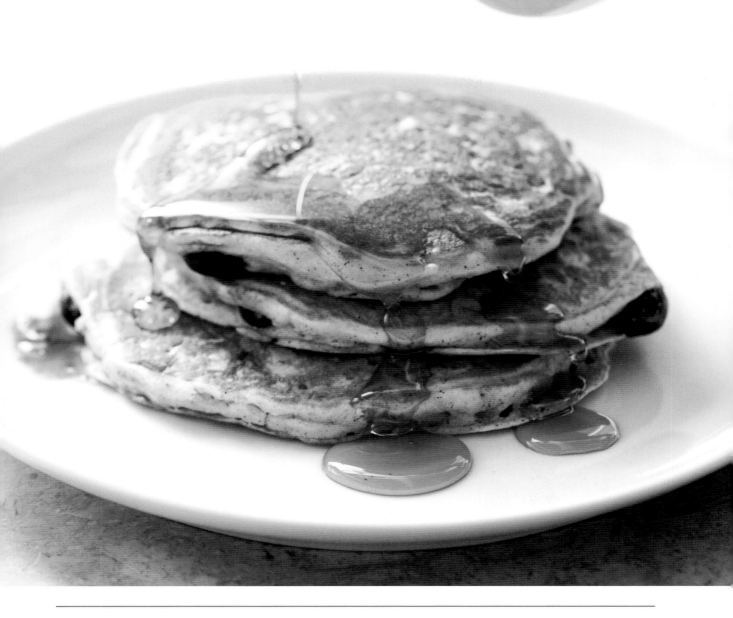

PER 3-PANCAKE SERVING

Dietary Fiber 6g **Cal** 350;
Total Fat 13g, **Sat Fat** 2g;
Chol 65mg; **Sodium** 390mg;
Total Carb 49g, **Total Sugars** 14g,
Added Sugars 6g; **Protein** 13g

LF **MAKE IT LOW FODMAP** Substitute dairy-free or lactose-free milk (see page 19) for buttermilk and add 2 tablespoons lemon juice to milk mixture. Substitute gluten-free flour blend (see page 31) for whole-wheat flour.

DF **MAKE IT DAIRY FREE** Substitute dairy-free milk (see page 19) for buttermilk and add 2 tablespoons lemon juice to milk mixture.

GF **MAKE IT GLUTEN FREE** Substitute gluten-free flour blend (see page 31) for whole-wheat flour.

PUMPKIN SPICE WAFFLES

MAKES FOUR 7-INCH WAFFLES

WHY THIS RECIPE WORKS While we love a plain waffle with its crisp exterior and custardy interior, we didn't hesitate to try a pumpkin-spice version. If the nutrients and fiber that canned pumpkin brings weren't enough incentive, the waffle's sunset-orange color, sweet earthy flavor, and autumnal aroma were. However, pumpkin also brings moisture, which initially softened our crispy edges. Blotting the puree with paper towels eliminated excess moisture, producing a batter that wasn't overly wet and crisped up while retaining the waffle's custardy center. To get extra fiber with flour, we traded out all-purpose flour for mild oat flour and a little whole-wheat flour. We prefer using store-bought oat flour, but you can grind your own in a pinch: Grind 2½ cups (7½ ounces) old-fashioned rolled oats in a food processor to a fine meal, about 2 minutes; waffles will be denser if using DIY ground oats. Do not use toasted oat flour in this recipe. Serve with maple syrup and fruit, if desired.

2½ cups (7½ ounces) oat flour (see page 18)

½ cup (2¾ ounces) whole-wheat flour

1 teaspoon ground cinnamon

1 teaspoon baking powder

½ teaspoon baking soda

½ teaspoon table salt

¼ teaspoon ground nutmeg

¼ teaspoon ground cardamom

1 (15-ounce) can unsweetened pumpkin puree

1¼ cups plain yogurt

2 large eggs

¼ cup canola oil, plus extra for brushing

¼ cup (1¾ ounces) sugar

1 teaspoon grated fresh ginger

1 Adjust oven rack to middle position and heat oven to 200 degrees. Whisk oat flour, whole-wheat flour, cinnamon, baking powder, baking soda, salt, nutmeg, and cardamom together in large bowl.

2 Line rimmed baking sheet with triple layer of paper towels. Spread pumpkin on paper towels in even layer. Cover pumpkin with second triple layer of paper towels and press firmly until paper towels are saturated. Peel back top layer of towels and discard. Grasp bottom towels and fold pumpkin in half; peel back towels. Transfer pumpkin to separate bowl and discard towels. Whisk in yogurt, eggs, oil, sugar, and ginger until combined. Whisk pumpkin mixture into flour mixture until well combined and smooth. Set wire rack in now-empty baking sheet and place in oven.

3 Heat waffle iron according to manufacturer's instructions and brush well with oil. Add mounded 1 cup batter to waffle iron and cook according to manufacturer's instructions until waffle is deep golden and has crisp, firm exterior. Serve immediately or transfer to wire rack in oven. Repeat with remaining batter, brushing waffle iron with additional oil.

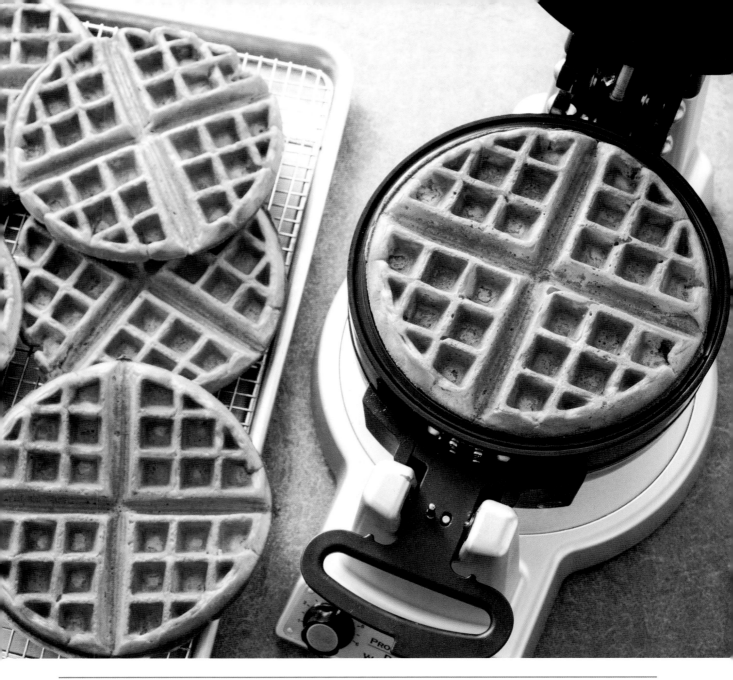

PER WAFFLE

Dietary Fiber 10g **Cal** 580;
Total Fat 24g, **Sat Fat** 4g;
Chol 105mg; **Sodium** 630mg;
Total Carb 74g, **Total Sugars** 21g,
Added Sugars 12g; **Protein** 19g

LF **MAKE IT LOW FODMAP** Substitute gluten-free flour blend (see page 31) for whole-wheat flour. Substitute dairy-free or lactose-free yogurt (see page 19) for plain yogurt.

DF **MAKE IT DAIRY FREE** Substitute dairy-free yogurt (see page 19) for plain yogurt.

GF **MAKE IT GLUTEN FREE** Substitute gluten-free flour blend (see page 31) for whole-wheat flour.

POWER SMOOTHIES

SERVES 2

WHY THIS RECIPE WORKS Rich and subtly sweet, avocado is a great choice for blending into creamy dairy-free smoothies and helps this green smoothie earn its "power" title. Kale, avocado, pineapple, and banana taste great together while also making you feel virtuous by giving you fiber by the sip. In addition to having impressive amounts of fiber and nutrients, we also wanted this smoothie to have enough protein to hold you over until lunch. We turned to a surprising source: hemp seed hearts. They pack a nutritional punch and their neutral flavor doesn't overwhelm the produce in the drink. The hulled center of the hemp seed, a soft, waxy nugget, blends beautifully, leaving just a trace of pleasantly grassy, sweet flavor. We like the neutral flavor and color of hemp seed hearts, but you can use 2 tablespoons almond butter or ¼ cup wheat germ in their place; with the latter, the smoothie will no longer be gluten-free. Do not use frozen chopped kale for this recipe.

1 cup baby kale

1 cup frozen pineapple chunks

1 cup water

1 ripe banana, peeled and halved lengthwise

½ cup pineapple juice

½ ripe avocado, cut into quarters

2 tablespoons hemp seed hearts

⅛ teaspoon table salt

Process all ingredients in blender on low speed until mixture is combined but still coarse in texture, about 10 seconds. Increase speed to high and process until completely smooth, about 1 minute. Serve.

PER SERVING

Dietary Fiber 7g **Cal** 270;
Total Fat 12g, **Sat Fat** 1.5g;
Chol 0mg; **Sodium** 160mg;
Total Carb 40g, **Total Sugars** 16g,
Added Sugars 0g; **Protein** 6g

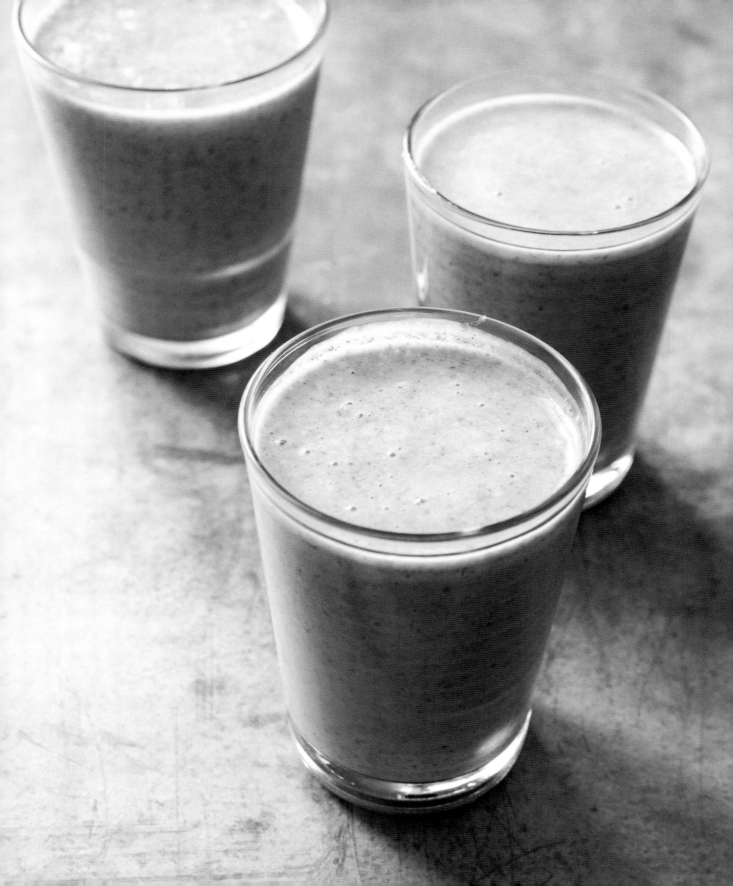

BERRY SMOOTHIES

SERVES 2

WHY THIS RECIPE WORKS Fruit is sweet and easy to blend, so making a great-tasting fruit smoothie is simple. But we didn't want our berry smoothie to just taste great—it also had to be filling enough to call it breakfast. Yogurt was an easy addition; it provided some protein and created a smooth, creamy texture. For an additional protein boost (without adding distracting flavors or textures) we took a cue from our Power Smoothie (page 66) and incorporated hemp seed hearts, the hulled center of the hemp seed. Blended into this smoothie they're hardly perceptible, and 2 tablespoons is enough to contribute an additional 6 grams of filling protein. For a flavor combination that everyone could get behind, we chose a mix of blueberries, raspberries, and strawberries, plus a whole banana. We like the neutral flavor and color of hemp seed hearts, but you can use 2 tablespoons almond butter or ¼ cup wheat germ in their place; with the latter, the smoothie will no longer be gluten-free.

10 ounces (2 cups) frozen blueberries, raspberries, and/or strawberries

 1 cup plain yogurt

 1 cup water

 1 ripe banana, peeled and halved lengthwise

 2 tablespoons hemp seed hearts

⅛ teaspoon table salt

Process all ingredients in blender on low speed until mixture is combined but still coarse in texture, about 10 seconds. Increase speed to high and process until completely smooth, about 1 minute. Serve.

PER SERVING

Dietary Fiber 8g **Cal** 250;
Total Fat 9g, **Sat Fat** 3g;
Chol 15mg; **Sodium** 210mg;
Total Carb 38g, **Total Sugars** 21g,
Added Sugars 0g; **Protein** 9g

 MAKE IT LOW FODMAP Serve 4 half-size portions of smoothies as between-meal snacks.

 MAKE IT DAIRY-FREE Substitute dairy-free yogurt (see page 19) for plain yogurt.

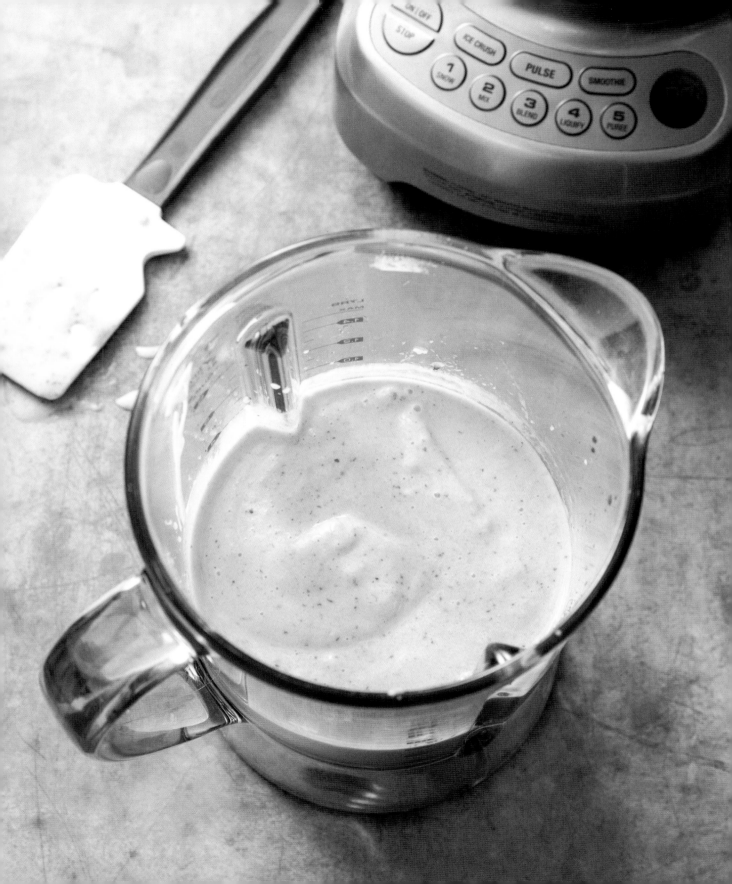

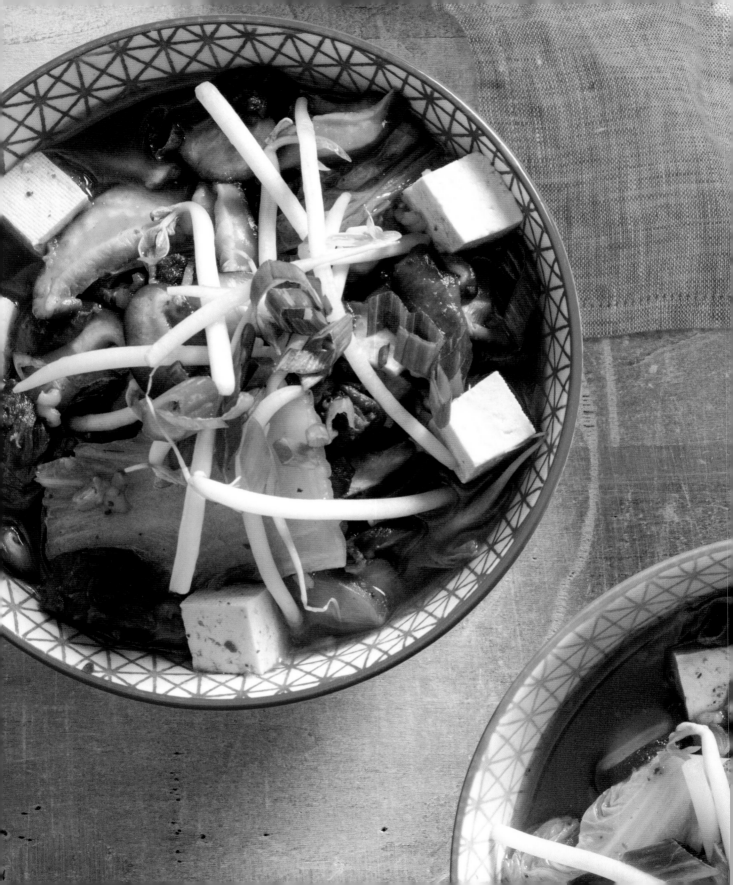

2 Soups & Stews

CHICKEN AND VEGETABLE SOUP

SERVES 6

WHY THIS RECIPE WORKS Onion, celery, and carrot: This trinity of aromatic vegetables is the start of most soups (and sauces and braises), supposedly providing a sweet, complexly flavored backbone to reinforce savory broths. It's an elementary lesson in cooking, but do we really need the high-FODMAP celery and onion to make a good soup? We tried making our chicken and vegetable soup without them and it turned out that with so many flavorful vegetables included—sweet ones like parsnips and cherry tomatoes, plus earthy kale—and our perfected homemade chicken broth, it was as good as our favorite chicken soup. In addition to flavoring the soup, all of those vegetables bring far more fiber than your standard chicken soup for a warmer whose healing elements are more than just anecdotal. We've developed low-FODMAP broth recipes for use here and throughout the chapter; note that supermarket broths will work but many include FODMAPs.

2 (12-ounce) bone-in split chicken breasts, trimmed

1 tablespoon canola oil

12 ounces parsnips, peeled, halved lengthwise, and sliced ¼ inch thick

4 carrots, peeled and sliced ¼ inch thick

1 tablespoon minced fresh thyme or 1 teaspoon dried

8 cups chicken broth (see page 18)

2 bay leaves

¼ teaspoon pepper

8 ounces baby kale, chopped

8 ounces cherry tomatoes, halved

¼ cup chopped fresh parsley

1 Pat chicken dry with paper towels. Heat oil in Dutch oven over medium-high heat until just smoking. Brown chicken, 3 to 5 minutes per side; transfer to plate.

2 Add parsnips and carrots to fat left in pot and cook over medium heat until softened and lightly browned, 5 to 7 minutes. Stir in thyme and cook until fragrant, about 30 seconds. Stir in broth, bay leaves, and pepper, scraping up any browned bits, and bring to boil.

3 Nestle chicken into pot and add any accumulated juices. Cover, reduce heat to low, and simmer gently until chicken registers 160 degrees, 15 to 20 minutes.

4 Discard bay leaves. Transfer chicken to cutting board, let cool slightly, then shred into bite-size pieces using 2 forks; discard skin and bones.

5 Stir shredded chicken, kale, and tomatoes into soup and cook over medium heat until heated through, 2 to 3 minutes. Stir in parsley and season with salt and pepper to taste. Serve.

PER 2-CUP SERVING

Dietary Fiber 6g **Cal** 220;
Total **Fat** 6g, **Sat Fat** 1g;
Chol 65mg; **Sodium** 860mg;
Total **Carb** 18g, **Total Sugars** 7g,
Added Sugars 0g; **Protein** 25g

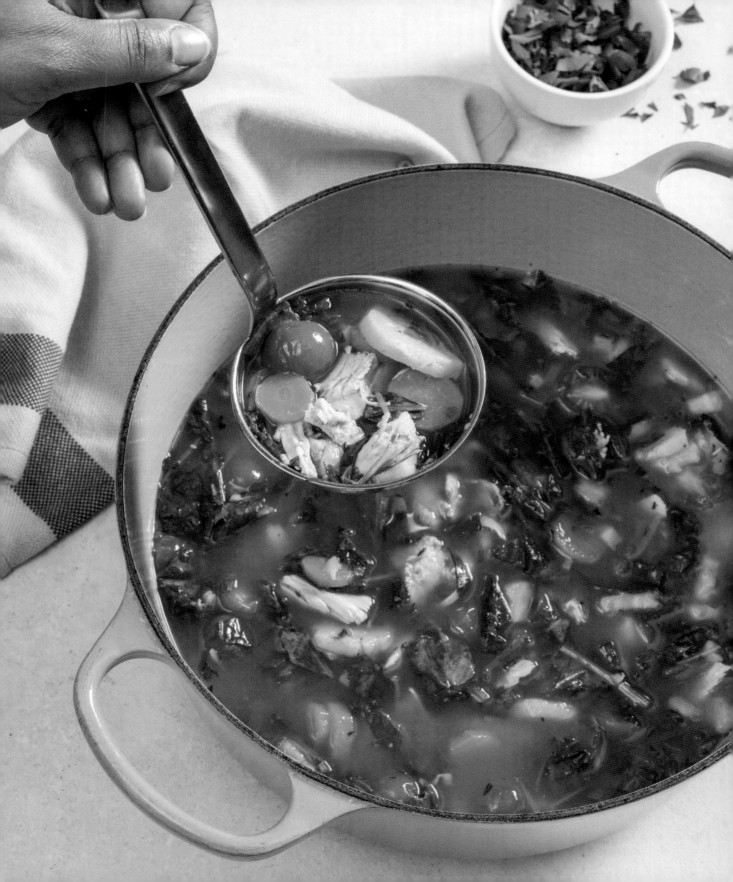

SMOKY CHICKEN AND LENTIL SOUP WITH SWISS CHARD

SERVES 6

WHY THIS RECIPE WORKS A simmered chicken-in-chicken-broth soup is a flavorful jumping off point, as many hearty and healthful additions can make soup a stellar meal. Here we add lentils, along with green bell pepper and Swiss chard, for fiber and substance and then offset their earthiness with brightness and smoke in the form of lemon zest, fire-roasted tomatoes, and smoked paprika. The process takes barely any more effort than making a chicken and vegetable soup (see page 72): We simply start simmering the lentils, add browned chicken partway through, remove the chicken when it's done, and add it back to the pot once it's shredded into bite-size pieces. The Swiss chard stems go in at the beginning of the process to adequately soften them; the leaves just need 2 minutes to wilt at the end so they're hearty and verdant. A generous amount of minced parsley—¼ cup—gets stirred in at the end to freshen everything up.

2 (12-ounce) bone-in split chicken breasts, trimmed

5 tablespoons garlic oil (see page 20), divided

12 ounces Swiss chard, stemmed, ½ cup stems chopped fine, leaves cut into 2-inch pieces

2 green bell peppers, stemmed, seeded, and chopped fine

4 teaspoons smoked paprika

4 cups chicken broth (see page 18)

1 (14.5-ounce) can fire-roasted diced tomatoes

1 cup green or brown lentils, picked over and rinsed

2 (2-inch) strips lemon zest, plus lemon wedges for serving

2 bay leaves

¼ teaspoon table salt

¼ teaspoon pepper

¼ cup minced fresh parsley

1 Pat chicken dry with paper towels. Heat 1 tablespoon oil in Dutch oven over medium-high heat until just smoking. Brown chicken, 3 to 5 minutes per side; transfer to plate.

2 Add chard stems and bell peppers to fat left in pot and cook over medium heat until softened and lightly browned, 5 to 7 minutes. Stir in paprika and cook until fragrant, about 30 seconds. Stir in broth, diced tomatoes and their juice, lentils, lemon zest, bay leaves, salt, and pepper, scraping up any browned bits, and bring to boil.

3 Nestle chicken into pot and add any accumulated juices. Cover, reduce heat to low, and simmer gently until chicken registers 160 degrees, 15 to 20 minutes.

4 Transfer chicken to cutting board, let cool slightly, then shred into bite-size pieces using 2 forks; discard skin and bones. Meanwhile, continue to simmer lentils, covered, until tender, 15 to 30 minutes.

5 Discard lemon zest and bay leaves. Stir in chicken and chard leaves and cook until chicken is heated through and chard is wilted, about 2 minutes. Off heat, stir in parsley and season with salt and pepper to taste. Drizzle each individual portion with 2 teaspoons oil and serve with lemon wedges.

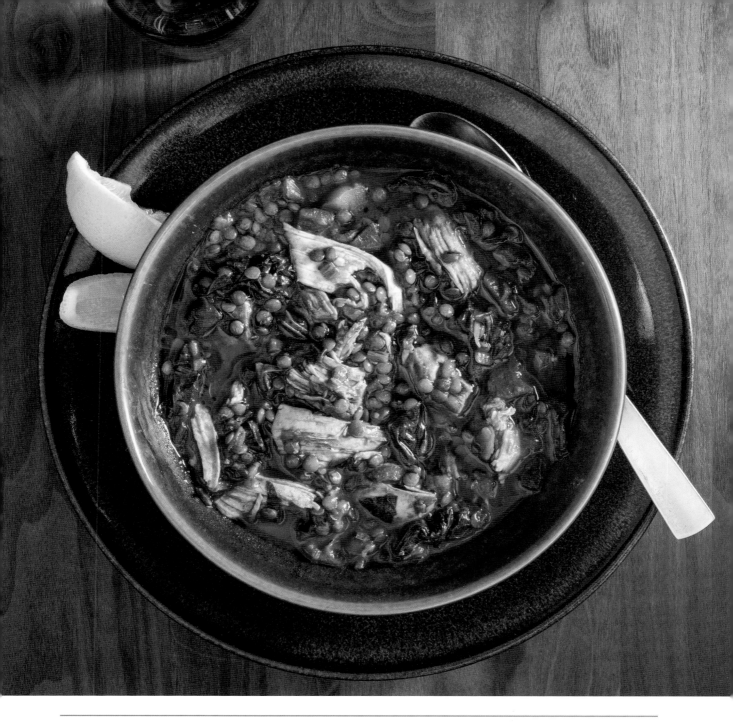

PER 1½-CUP SERVING

Dietary Fiber 8g **Cal** 360;
Total Fat 15g, **Sat Fat** 2g;
Chol 65mg; **Sodium** 770mg;
Total Carb 27g, **Total Sugars** 5g,
Added Sugars 0g; **Protein** 32g

 MAKE IT LOW FODMAP Substitute 1½ cups drained canned lentils for dried lentils; stir canned lentils into soup with chicken in step 5.

BEEF AND OAT BERRY SOUP

SERVES 4

WHY THIS RECIPE WORKS Comforting, earthy, deeply flavored beef and barley soup is a classic for a reason, but barley, a type of wheat, isn't the only hearty grain that's a match for robust beef. Low-FODMAP and gluten-free oat berries have substance, chew, a whole lot of fiber, and a cooking time that works for a simmered soup to boot. This soup typically takes some time to make while the beef braises to tenderness, as it traditionally calls for a connective tissue–heavy cut. To speed things up, we turned to sirloin steak tips, a cut that's already tender and full of flavor. By cutting the meat into ½-inch pieces, we were able to brown it in a skillet while the soup base simmered and then stir it in at the end to cook through quickly. Enhancing the broth with sautéed aromatics, porcini, tomato paste, and soy sauce took our soup to the next level. Sirloin steak tips, also known as flap meat, can be sold as whole steaks, cubes, and strips; we prefer to purchase whole steaks and cut them ourselves.

3 tablespoons garlic oil (see page 20), divided

4 carrots, peeled and cut into ¼-inch pieces

¼ ounce dried porcini mushrooms, rinsed and minced

1 tablespoon minced fresh thyme or 1 teaspoon dried

2 teaspoons tomato paste

4 cups beef broth (see page 18)

2 cups water

1 cup oat berries (groats), rinsed

¼ teaspoon table salt

1 pound sirloin steak tips, trimmed and cut into ½-inch pieces

¼ teaspoon pepper

2 tablespoons minced fresh parsley

1 Heat 1 tablespoon oil in Dutch oven over medium-high heat until shimmering. Add carrots and cook until softened and lightly browned, about 8 minutes. Stir in porcini, thyme, and tomato paste and cook until fragrant, about 30 seconds. Stir in broth, water, oat berries, and salt, scraping up any browned bits. Simmer until oat berries are tender, about 30 minutes.

2 Meanwhile, heat 1 tablespoon oil in 12-inch skillet over medium-high heat until just smoking. Pat beef dry with paper towels and sprinkle with pepper. Brown half of beef on all sides, about 8 minutes; transfer to bowl. Repeat with remaining 1 tablespoon oil and remaining beef; transfer to bowl.

3 Add browned beef and any accumulated juices to soup and let heat through, about 1 minute. Stir in parsley and season with salt and pepper to taste. Serve.

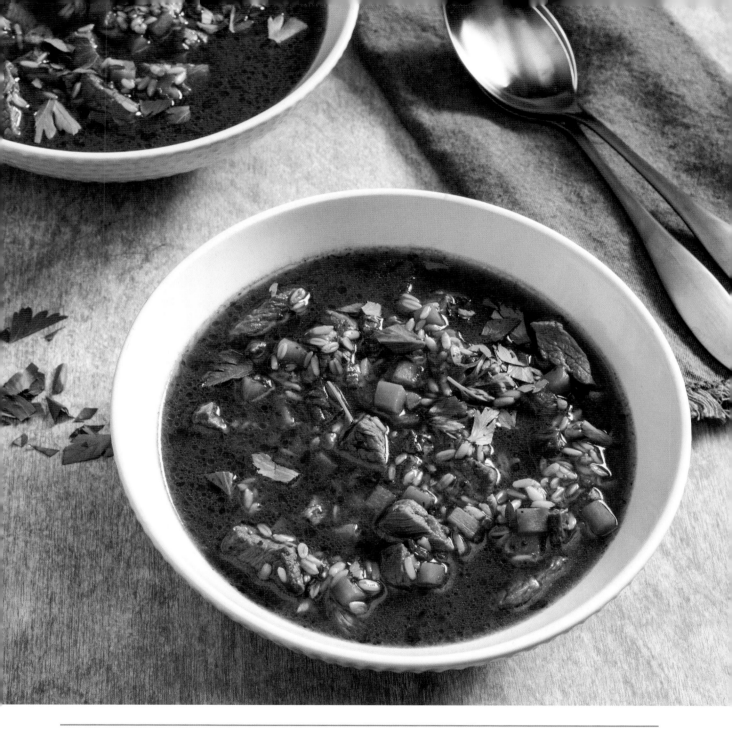

PER 1½-CUP SERVING

Dietary Fiber 7g Cal 520;
Total Fat 25g, Sat Fat 5g;
Chol 75mg; Sodium 750mg;
Total Carb 37g, Total Sugars 4g,
Added Sugars 0g; Protein 35g

BEEF, CABBAGE, AND TOFU SOUP WITH GOCHUGARU

SERVES 4

WHY THIS RECIPE WORKS This warming soup with Korean flavors will fill you up with protein from both beef and tofu, a remarkable amount of cabbage and mushrooms, plus supporting brown rice and a sprout-scallion topping. They simmer in a perky brew with a nuanced spice flavor from gochugaru pepper flakes. If gochugaru is unavailable, a combination of 1 tablespoon ancho chile powder and pinch cayenne pepper for every 1 tablespoon gochugaru is a good substitute. For a milder soup, use the lesser amount of gochugaru. Sirloin steak tips, also known as flap meat, can be sold as whole steaks, cubes, and strips; we prefer to purchase whole steaks and cut them ourselves.

14 ounces firm tofu, cut into ½-inch pieces

8 ounces sirloin steak tips, trimmed and cut into ½-inch pieces

2 tablespoons garlic oil (see page 20), divided

1 tablespoon grated fresh ginger

1–3 tablespoons gochugaru

4 cups beef broth (see page 18)

3 cups water

¼ cup long-grain brown rice, rinsed

1 tablespoon fish sauce, plus extra as needed

½ small head (12 ounces) napa cabbage, cored and cut into 2-inch pieces

1 pound shiitake mushrooms, stemmed and sliced thin

2 ounces (1 cup) bean sprouts

4 scallions, green parts only, sliced thin on bias

1 tablespoon toasted sesame oil, divided

¼ cup unseasoned rice vinegar

1 Spread tofu on paper towel–lined baking sheet and let drain for 20 minutes. Pat beef dry with paper towels. Heat 1 tablespoon oil in Dutch oven over medium-high heat until just smoking. Brown beef well on all sides, 5 to 7 minutes; transfer to bowl.

2 Add remaining 1 tablespoon oil, ginger, and gochugaru to now-empty pot and cook over medium heat until fragrant, about 30 seconds. Stir in broth and water, scraping up any browned bits. Stir in beef and any accumulated juices, rice, and fish sauce and bring to simmer. Cover, reduce heat to medium-low, and cook until beef and rice are tender, 45 to 50 minutes.

3 Stir in cabbage and mushrooms, return to simmer, and cook, uncovered, until vegetables are tender, about 5 minutes.

4 Meanwhile, toss bean sprouts, scallions, and 1 teaspoon sesame oil together in bowl; set aside. Off heat, stir tofu, vinegar, and remaining 2 teaspoons sesame oil into soup. Season with extra fish sauce to taste. Top individual portions evenly with bean sprout mixture. Serve.

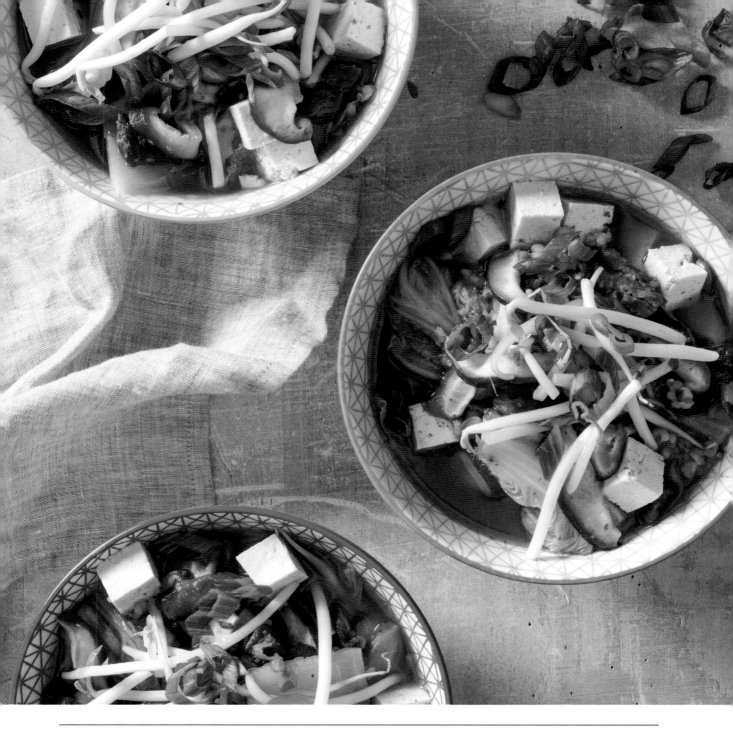

PER 2-CUP SERVING

Dietary Fiber 6g **Cal** 400;
Total Fat 22g, **Sat Fat** 3.5g;
Chol 40mg; **Sodium** 710mg;
Total Carb 24g, **Total Sugars** 5g,
Added Sugars 0g; **Protein** 29g

 MAKE IT LOW FODMAP Substitute oyster mushrooms for shiitake mushrooms.

MISO-GINGER SOUP WITH HALIBUT AND ZUCCHINI NOODLES

SERVES 4

WHY THIS RECIPE WORKS Packed with more ingredients than miso-based soups you may have encountered, this delicate ginger-soy broth (which comes together in minutes) is filled with tender, meaty chunks of halibut, crisp-tender carrots and edamame, refreshing daikon radish matchsticks, and noodles of spiralized zucchini for gut-friendly slurping. Yes, the soup is chock-full of goodness, but nothing overwhelms the broth or makes the dish feel heavy. We prefer to spiralize our own zucchini, but you can substitute store-bought spiralized raw zucchini. Mahi-mahi, red snapper, striped bass, or swordfish are good substitutes for the halibut. Yellow, red, or brown miso can be used instead of white, if desired. If you can't find daikon radish, you can substitute 8 medium radishes.

1 pound zucchini, trimmed

2 tablespoons garlic oil (see page 20)

2 tablespoons grated fresh ginger

4 cups water

4 carrots, peeled, halved lengthwise, and sliced ¼ inch thick

1 cup frozen edamame

1 tablespoon soy sauce (see page 18), plus extra for seasoning

1 pound skinless halibut fillets, 1 inch thick, cut into 2-inch pieces

3 tablespoons white miso

8 ounces daikon radish, peeled and cut into 2-inch-long matchsticks

4 scallions, green parts only, sliced thin

2 teaspoons sesame seeds, toasted

2 teaspoons toasted sesame oil (optional)

1 Using spiralizer, cut zucchini into ⅛-inch-thick noodles, then cut noodles into 6-inch lengths; set aside.

2 Heat oil in Dutch oven over medium heat until shimmering. Add ginger and cook until fragrant, about 30 seconds. Stir in water, carrots, edamame, and soy sauce and bring to simmer. Stir in zucchini noodles, then submerge halibut in soup and return to simmer. Reduce heat to medium-low, cover, and cook until halibut flakes apart when gently prodded with paring knife, 5 to 8 minutes.

3 Transfer 1 cup hot broth to liquid measuring cup and whisk in miso. Gently stir miso mixture into soup, return to simmer, then immediately remove from heat. Stir in radish and season with extra soy sauce to taste. Sprinkle individual portions evenly with scallion greens and sesame seeds and drizzle with sesame oil, if using. Serve.

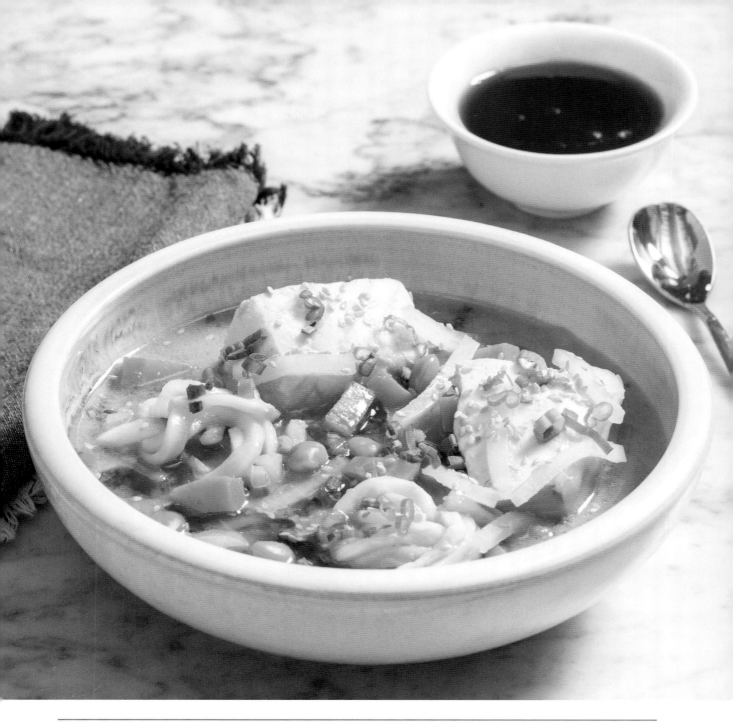

PER 2-CUP SERVING

Dietary Fiber 6g **Cal** 320;
Total Fat 14g, **Sat Fat** 1.5g;
Chol 55mg; **Sodium** 750mg;
Total Carb 21g, **Total Sugars** 10g;
Added Sugars 0g; **Protein** 29g

LF **MAKE IT LOW FODMAP** Decrease zucchini to 12 ounces and increase edamame to 1¼ cups.

GF **MAKE IT GLUTEN FREE** Substitute gluten-free soy sauce or tamari (see page 18) for soy sauce.

NEW ENGLAND–STYLE FISH AND VEGETABLE CHOWDER

SERVES 4

WHY THIS RECIPE WORKS Chowder might mean a dairy-laden once-in-a-while summer treat to you, but you can enjoy chowder with frequency, no matter your relationship with lactose or dairy, with this honestly creamy, secretly dairy-free fish chowder. Why? The creamy broth is created with super-smooth pureed cauliflower rather than milk or cream; the cauliflower's low-insoluble (high-soluble) fiber content helps it break down and blend beautifully (and chunk-free), unlike other vegetables. All the other requisite chowder players have a role: smoky bacon, chunky potatoes, tender cod. Some extra characters—chopped spinach, sweet corn, plus some florets reserved from the bulk cauliflower—add fiber without seeming out of place in a chowder. Haddock and striped bass are good substitutes for the cod.

4 slices bacon, chopped

1 teaspoon minced fresh thyme or ¼ teaspoon dried

1 pound cauliflower florets, cut into ½-inch pieces, divided

3 (8-ounce) bottles clam juice, divided

¼ teaspoon pepper

1 bay leaf

1 cup water

1½ pounds red potatoes, unpeeled, cut into ¾-inch pieces

1 pound skinless cod fillets, 1 inch thick, cut into 2-inch pieces

4 ounces (4 cups) baby spinach, chopped

1 cup frozen corn

1 teaspoon lemon juice

1 tablespoon minced fresh parsley

1 Cook bacon in Dutch oven over medium heat until crispy, 5 to 7 minutes. Using slotted spoon, transfer bacon to paper towel–lined plate; set aside for serving.

2 Add thyme to fat left in pot and cook until fragrant, about 30 seconds. Stir in half of cauliflower, 2 bottles clam juice, pepper, and bay leaf and bring to simmer. Reduce heat to medium-low, cover, and cook until cauliflower falls apart easily when poked with fork, about 12 minutes.

3 Off heat, discard bay leaf and let cauliflower mixture cool slightly, about 10 minutes. Working in batches, process cauliflower mixture in blender until smooth, about 1 minute, scraping down sides of blender jar as needed; return to now-empty pot. Stir in remaining 1 bottle clam juice, water, and potatoes and bring to simmer over medium-high heat. Cover, reduce heat to medium-low, and cook until potatoes are just tender, 15 to 20 minutes.

4 Stir in remaining cauliflower florets, then submerge cod in soup. Bring to simmer, cover, and reduce heat to medium-low. Simmer until cod flakes apart when gently prodded with paring knife, 5 to 8 minutes.

5 Gently stir in spinach and corn and simmer until spinach is wilted and corn is heated through, about 2 minutes. Off heat, break up any remaining large pieces of cod, stir in lemon juice, and season with salt and pepper to taste. Sprinkle individual portions evenly with parsley and bacon. Serve.

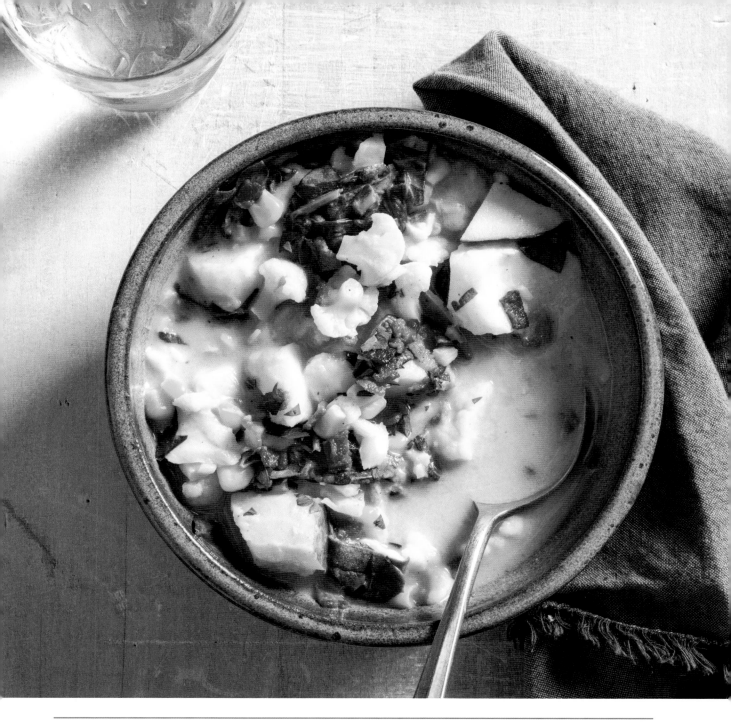

PER 2-CUP SERVING

Dietary Fiber 7g **Cal** 400;
Total Fat 13g, **Sat Fat** 4g;
Chol 75mg; **Sodium** 720mg;
Total Carb 42g, **Total Sugars** 6g,
Added Sugars 0g; **Protein** 32g

MUSHROOM AND WHEAT BERRY SOUP

SERVES 6

WHY THIS RECIPE WORKS Mushroom soups are so often cream based, which seems unnecessary to us: Mushrooms are among the most flavorful vegetables, boasting a deep umami flavor that bolsters any broth. This combination of mushrooms and wheat berries (a nice change from often-used rice) is rich and substantial but not heavy, and full of satisfying, savory flavors. To bring out the nutty flavor of fiber- and nutrient-rich wheat berries, we toast them in a dry Dutch oven. Next, we slowly cook our cremini mushrooms in a covered pot to concentrate their flavors and extract their juices. To amplify the earthiness of the wheat berries and cremini, we build a flavorful base from ground dried shiitake mushrooms (grinding ensures their flavor permeates the broth) and tomato paste in a dry sherry and chicken broth. After simmering our wheat berries, we finish the soup with arugula, whose peppery flavor complements the mushrooms; lemon zest provides welcome brightness to cut through the deep savor of all of these ingredients. White mushrooms can be substituted for the cremini. We used a spice grinder to grind the dried shiitake mushrooms, but a blender also works.

1½ **cups wheat berries, rinsed**

3 **tablespoons garlic oil (see page 20), divided**

2 **pounds cremini mushrooms, trimmed and sliced thin**

¼ **teaspoon table salt, divided**

1 **tablespoon tomato paste**

1 **cup dry sherry**

6 **cups chicken broth (see page 18)**

2 **cups water**

1 **sprig fresh thyme**

1 **bay leaf**

½ **ounce dried shiitake mushrooms, finely ground using spice grinder**

8 **ounces (8 cups) baby arugula**

¼ **teaspoon grated lemon zest**

1 Toast wheat berries in Dutch oven over medium heat, stirring often, until fragrant and beginning to darken, about 5 minutes; transfer to bowl.

2 Heat 2 tablespoons oil in now-empty pot over medium heat until shimmering. Add cremini mushrooms and salt, cover, and cook until mushrooms have released their liquid, about 5 minutes. Uncover, increase heat to medium-high, and cook until mushrooms begin to brown, 8 to 10 minutes; transfer to plate.

3 Heat remaining 1 tablespoon oil in now-empty pot over medium heat until shimmering. Stir in tomato paste and cook until slightly darkened, about 2 minutes. Stir in sherry, scraping up any browned bits, and cook until nearly evaporated, about 2 minutes.

4 Stir in wheat berries, broth, water, thyme, bay leaf, and ground shiitakes and bring to simmer. Cover, reduce heat to low, and cook until wheat berries are tender but still chewy, 45 minutes to 1 hour. Discard bay leaf and thyme sprig.

5 Off heat, stir in cremini and any accumulated juices, arugula, and lemon zest. Cover and let sit until greens are wilted, about 5 minutes. Season with salt and pepper to taste. Serve.

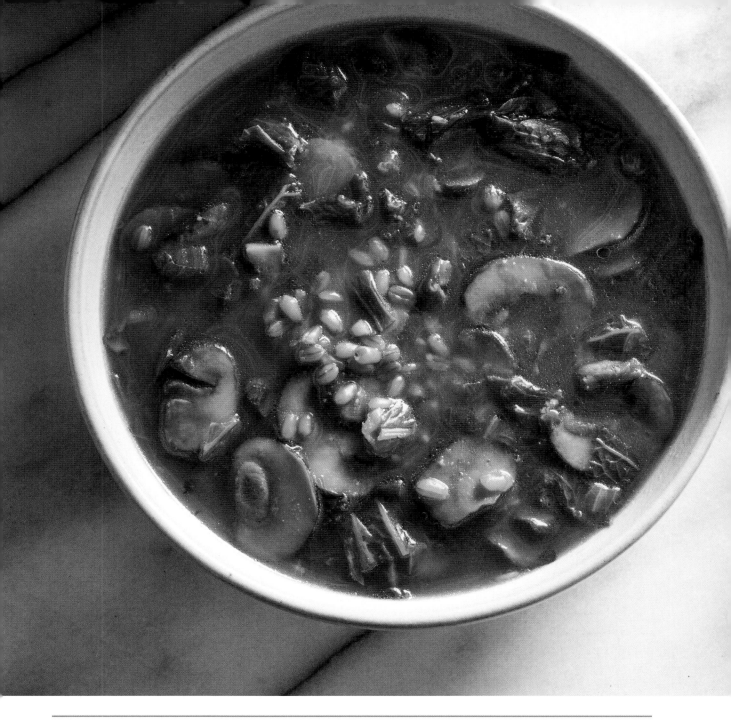

PER 1½-CUP SERVING

Dietary Fiber 8g **Cal** 320;
Total Fat 8g, **Sat Fat** 0g;
Chol 0mg; **Sodium** 710mg;
Total Carb 45g, **Total Sugars** 5g,
Added Sugars 0g; **Protein** 11g

LF **MAKE IT LOW FODMAP** Substitute oat berries (groats) for wheat berries and 1 pound oyster mushrooms, trimmed and cut into 1-inch pieces, for cremini mushrooms. Cook oat berries for 30 to 45 minutes in step 4.

GF **MAKE IT GLUTEN FREE** Substitute oat berries (groats) for wheat berries and cook for 30 to 45 minutes in step 4.

CHICKPEA AND ESCAROLE SOUP WITH FENNEL AND ORANGE

SERVES 6 TO 8

WHY THIS RECIPE WORKS We frequently turn to chickpeas to add heft and fiber to dishes, and while we often choose canned for ease, dried chickpeas are particularly well suited to soup; they hold their shape beautifully, remain firm while also becoming creamy, and take on all the flavor of the broth. Here we were inspired by the flavors of Sicily, and we combined the bean with slightly bitter escarole. Fennel, cooked in some garlic oil with oregano and red pepper flakes, served as our aromatic; its mild anise bite complemented the nutty chickpeas. A single strip of orange zest—a nod to the island's abundant citrus fruit crop—added a subtle citrusy note, and a Parmesan rind bolstered the nutty richness and complexity of the broth. The Parmesan rind can be replaced with a 2-inch chunk of Parmesan cheese.

3 tablespoons table salt for brining

1 pound (2¾ cups) dried chickpeas, picked over and rinsed

2 tablespoons garlic oil (see page 20), plus extra for drizzling

2 fennel bulbs, stalks discarded, bulbs halved, cored, and chopped fine

2 teaspoons minced fresh oregano or ½ teaspoon dried

¼ teaspoon red pepper flakes (optional)

4 cups vegetable or chicken broth (see page 20)

1 Parmesan cheese rind, plus grated Parmesan for serving

2 bay leaves

1 (3-inch) strip orange zest

1 large head escarole (1½ pounds), trimmed and cut into 1-inch pieces

2 tomatoes, cored and chopped

1 Dissolve salt in 4 quarts cold water in large container. Add chickpeas and soak at room temperature for at least 8 hours or up to 24 hours. Drain and rinse well.

2 Heat oil in Dutch oven over medium heat until shimmering. Add fennel and cook until softened, 8 to 10 minutes. Stir in oregano and pepper flakes, if using, and cook until fragrant, about 30 seconds.

3 Stir in soaked chickpeas, 8 cups water, broth, Parmesan rind, bay leaves, and orange zest and bring to boil. Reduce to simmer and cook until chickpeas are tender, 1¼ to 1¾ hours.

4 Stir in escarole and tomatoes and cook until escarole is wilted, 5 to 10 minutes. Off heat, discard bay leaves, orange zest, and Parmesan rind (scraping off any cheese that has melted and adding it back to pot). Season with salt and pepper to taste. Drizzle individual portions with extra oil and sprinkle with grated Parmesan. Serve.

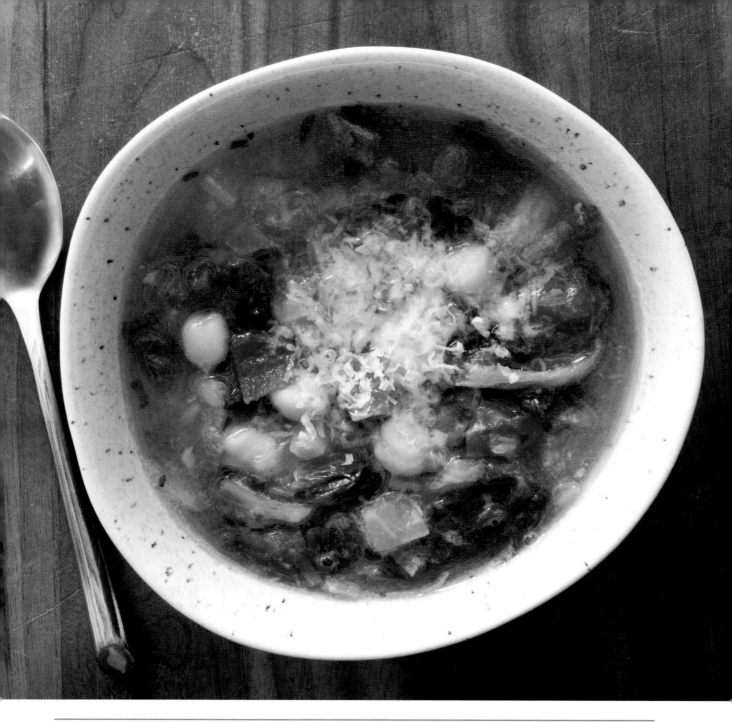

PER 2-CUP SERVING

Dietary Fiber 15g **Cal** 280;
Total Fat 7g, **Sat Fat** 0g;
Chol 0mg; **Sodium** 520g;
Total Carb 45g, **Total Sugars** 10g,
Added Sugars 0g; **Protein** 14g

 MAKE IT DAIRY FREE Omit Parmesan cheese.

CHICKEN STEW WITH COLLARD GREENS AND BLACK-EYED PEAS

SERVES 6

WHY THIS RECIPE WORKS Chicken stew often conjures thoughts of stodgy chicken soup, dull on flavor, with a thick flour-based broth—not this one. This take, with collard greens, black-eyed peas, and tomato is a far more flavorful and fresh approach. Hearty greens and smoky pork products are a classic combination, so these give the soup a backbone of fiber and richness. Cooking the aromatics in rendered bacon fat infuses the soup with that flavor. Simmering the collard greens for 15 to 20 minutes allows them to absorb the flavors of the stew and retain their texture without becoming mushy. Canned black-eyed peas, which work well with collards, were obvious fiber-boosters as well; what's more, there were benefits to also including the liquid in the can, as it helped thicken our soup just enough and give the broth a velvety texture without flour. Stirring fresh tomatoes in at the end added a bright acidity, and the reserved bacon bits boasted a meaty crunch. Kale can be substituted for collard greens. Use a Dutch oven that holds 6 quarts or more for this recipe.

1½ pounds boneless, skinless chicken thighs, trimmed and cut into 1-inch pieces

1 tablespoon garlic oil (see page 20)

4 ounces bacon, chopped

2 red bell peppers, stemmed, seeded, and chopped fine

1 tablespoon tomato paste

¼ teaspoon cayenne pepper (optional)

3 cups water

1 cup chicken broth (see page 18)

1 bay leaf

¼ teaspoon table salt

¼ teaspoon pepper

2 pounds collard greens, stemmed and cut into 1-inch pieces

1 (15-ounce) can black-eyed peas

2 tomatoes, cored, seeded, and chopped

1 Pat chicken dry with paper towels. Heat oil in Dutch oven over medium-high heat until just smoking. Brown half of chicken on all sides, 8 to 10 minutes; transfer to bowl. Repeat with remaining chicken; transfer to bowl.

2 Add bacon to fat left in pot and cook over medium heat until crispy, 5 to 7 minutes. Using slotted spoon, transfer bacon to paper towel–lined plate.

3 Add bell pepper to fat left in pot and cook over medium heat until softened, about 5 minutes. Stir in tomato paste and cayenne, if using, and cook until fragrant, about 1 minute. Stir in water, broth, bay leaf, salt, and pepper, scraping up any browned bits, and bring to simmer.

4 Add collard greens, one handful at a time, and cook, stirring occasionally, until wilted, about 2 minutes. Stir in black-eyed peas with their liquid and chicken, along with any accumulated juices. Return to simmer and cook, uncovered, until chicken is tender, 15 to 20 minutes.

5 Off heat, discard bay leaf. Stir in tomatoes and bacon; let sit until heated through, about 5 minutes. Season with salt and pepper to taste. Serve.

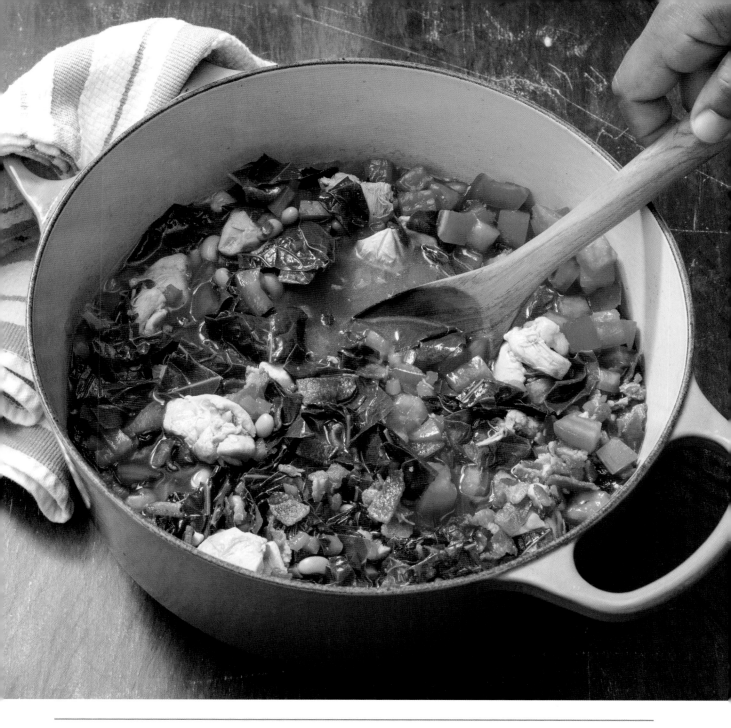

PER 1½-CUP SERVING

Dietary Fiber 7g **Cal** 340;
Total Fat 16g, **Sat Fat** 4g;
Chol 120mg; **Sodium** 680mg;
Total Carb 19g, **Total Sugars** 4g,
Added Sugars 0g; **Protein** 32g

LF **MAKE IT LOW FODMAP** Increase broth to 1½ cups and substitute 1 (15-ounce) can lentils, rinsed, for peas.

VEGETABLE AND BEEF STEW

SERVES 6

LOW FODMAP

DAIRY FREE

GLUTEN FREE

WHY THIS RECIPE WORKS Beef stew doesn't have to be a heavy carnivore's delight. We like a stew with a mix of root vegetables that share equal billing, like the potatoes, parsnips, and carrots here. The veggies contribute mildly sweet, earthy flavors to complement the robust umami notes of beef braised in red wine and broth. The size we cut the vegetables proved key—too small, and they disappeared into the stew; too large, and they didn't cook through. Kale, peas, and parsley offered welcome freshness, vibrant color, and textural contrast to the root vegetables and beef. To add body and balance the flavors in the finished stew, in lieu of a roux made with flour, we mashed a portion of the cooked vegetables and stirred them back in for a beef stew anyone can take comfort in.

2 pounds boneless beef chuck-eye roast, trimmed and cut into 1½-inch pieces

½ teaspoon table salt

¼ teaspoon pepper

1 tablespoon garlic oil (see page 20), divided

1 tablespoon tomato paste

1 tablespoon minced fresh thyme or 1 teaspoon dried

1½ cups dry red wine

4 cups beef broth (see page 18)

2 bay leaves

12 ounces red potatoes, unpeeled, cut into 1-inch pieces

4 carrots, peeled, halved lengthwise, and sliced 1 inch thick

4 parsnips, peeled, halved lengthwise, and sliced 1 inch thick

1 pound kale, stemmed and chopped

¼ cup frozen peas

¼ cup minced fresh parsley

1 Adjust oven rack to lower-middle position and heat oven to 300 degrees. Pat beef dry with paper towels and sprinkle with salt and pepper. Heat 1½ teaspoons oil in Dutch oven over medium-high heat until just smoking. Brown half of meat on all sides, 5 to 10 minutes; transfer to bowl. Repeat with remaining 1½ teaspoons oil and remaining beef; transfer to bowl.

2 Stir tomato paste and thyme into fat left in pot and cook until fragrant, about 30 seconds. Slowly whisk in wine, scraping up any browned bits. Stir in beef, broth, and bay leaves and bring to simmer. Cover, transfer pot to oven, and cook for 1½ hours.

3 Remove pot from oven and stir in potatoes, carrots, and parsnips. Return pot to oven and cook, covered, until meat and vegetables are tender, about 1 hour.

4 Remove pot from oven and discard bay leaves. Transfer 1½ cups cooked potatoes, carrots, and parsnips to bowl and mash with potato masher until mostly smooth. Stir mashed vegetables and kale into stew and simmer over medium heat, stirring occasionally, until kale is tender, about 10 minutes.

5 Off heat, stir in peas and let sit until peas are heated through, about 5 minutes. Stir in parsley and season with salt and pepper to taste. Serve.

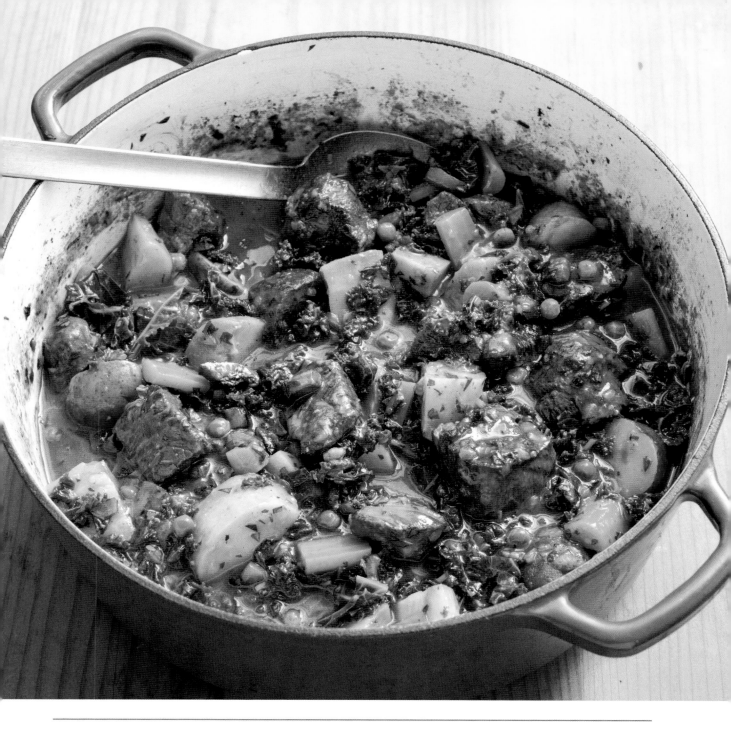

PER 1½-CUP SERVING

Dietary Fiber 8g **Cal** 430;
Total Fat 10g, **Sat Fat** 2.5g;
Chol 100mg; **Sodium** 790mg;
Total Carb 34g, **Total Sugars** 9g,
Added Sugars 0g; **Protein** 41g

FISH TAGINE

SERVES 4

WHY THIS RECIPE WORKS This warm-spiced stew of chickpeas and halibut, cooked in a Dutch oven in the style of North African tagines, is a little sweet (from red bell peppers, carrots, and tomato paste), a little piquant (from pops of oil-cured olives and sherry vinegar), and altogether good for you (namely from the chickpeas, fish, and abundant vegetables). To give the stew a clear seafood backnote, we employ a bottle of clam juice, with smoky fire-roasted tomatoes making up the remainder of the braising liquid. Ras el hanout, orange zest, and mint give the stew an incredibly alluring quality. Meaty halibut is a great choice for the fish here; it has a pleasantly firm texture so it holds its shape while simmering in the pot and readily soaks up the stew's multidimensional flavors. Mahi-mahi, red snapper, striped bass, or swordfish are good substitutes for the halibut.

2 tablespoons garlic oil (see page 20)

3 carrots, peeled, halved lengthwise, and sliced ¼ inch thick

2 red bell peppers, stemmed, seeded, and chopped

1 tablespoon tomato paste

1 tablespoon ras el hanout

1 (14.5-ounce) can fire-roasted diced tomatoes

1 (15-ounce) can chickpeas, rinsed

1 (8-ounce) bottle clam juice

2 (2-inch) strips orange zest

1 pound skinless halibut fillets, 1 inch thick

¼ cup pitted oil-cured black olives, chopped

2 tablespoons chopped fresh mint, divided

1 teaspoon sherry vinegar

1 Heat oil in Dutch oven over medium heat until shimmering. Add carrots and bell peppers and cook until softened and lightly browned, 10 to 12 minutes.

2 Stir in tomato paste and ras el hanout and cook until fragrant, about 30 seconds. Stir in tomatoes and their juice, chickpeas, clam juice, and orange zest, scraping up any browned bits, and bring to simmer. Reduce heat to medium-low, cover, and cook until flavors meld, about 5 minutes.

3 Cut halibut into 4 even pieces. Nestle halibut into stew and spoon some of broth over top. Return to simmer, cover, and cook over medium-low heat until halibut flakes apart when gently prodded with paring knife, 6 to 8 minutes.

4 Off heat, discard orange zest. Transfer halibut to individual serving bowls. Stir olives, 1 tablespoon mint, and vinegar into stew and season with salt and pepper to taste. Ladle stew evenly over halibut and sprinkle with remaining 1 tablespoon mint. Serve.

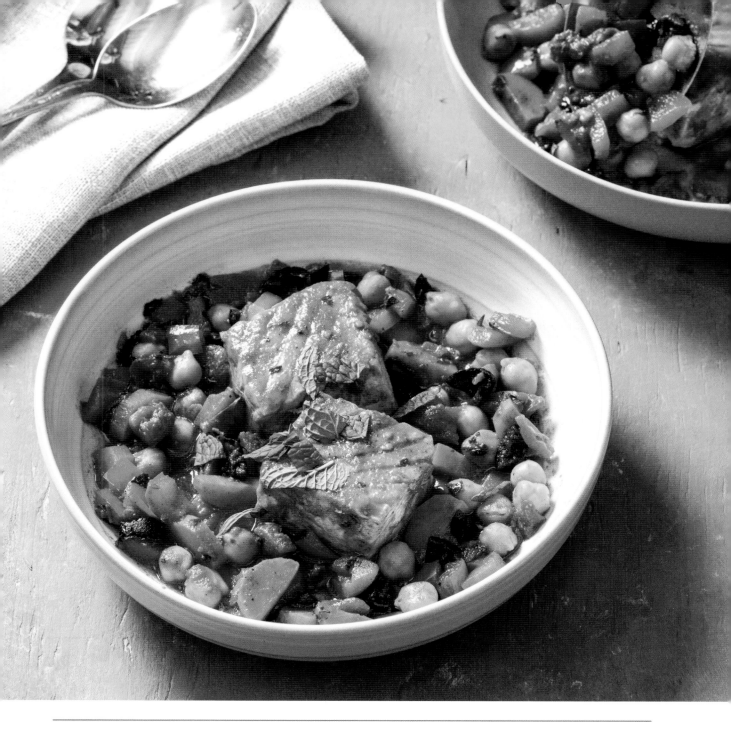

PER 2-CUP SERVING

Dietary Fiber 7g **Cal** 310;
Total Fat 11g, **Sat Fat** 1g;
Chol 55mg; **Sodium** 800mg;
Total Carb 26g, **Total Sugars** 8g,
Added Sugars 0g; **Protein** 27g

 MAKE IT LOW FODMAP Reduce chickpeas to 1 cup and increase carrots to 4.

OKRA PEPPER POT

SERVES 6

WHY THIS RECIPE WORKS This pepper pot is inspired by those of the Caribbean made with beef, mutton, or pork and aggressively flavored with hot peppers. But it forgoes the meat and stands as a shining example of how flavorful low-FODMAP cooking can be. Okra and cassava are traditional pepper pot vegetables, so we used a liberal amount of fiber-packing okra assisted by sweet potatoes and also hearty collard greens, which made this a colorful one-pot meal. One Scotch bonnet chile was all it took to give the stew its heat, while allspice and thyme produced an incredibly complex aroma. The okra helped thicken the dish, and a little coconut milk provided nice richness. We prefer the flavor and texture of fresh okra in this recipe, but you can substitute thawed, frozen, cut okra; thoroughly pat it dry and skip step 1. Kale can be substituted for collard greens, and a habanero chile can be substituted for the Scotch bonnet. We recommend wearing rubber gloves to protect your hands while prepping the chile.

12 ounces okra, trimmed

¼ teaspoon table salt, plus salt for salting okra

2 tablespoons garlic oil (see page 20)

2 red bell peppers, stemmed, seeded, and chopped fine

2 tablespoons tomato paste

2 teaspoons minced fresh thyme or ½ teaspoon dried

½ teaspoon ground allspice

4 cups vegetable broth (see page 18)

1 Scotch bonnet chile, stemmed, seeded, and minced (optional)

1 pound sweet potatoes, peeled and cut into 2-inch pieces

2 pounds collard greens, stemmed and chopped into 1-inch pieces

½ cup canned coconut milk

¼ cup minced fresh cilantro

Lime wedges

1 Toss okra with 1 teaspoon salt in colander and let sit for 1 hour, tossing again halfway through. Rinse well, cut into ½-inch pieces, and set aside.

2 Heat oil in Dutch oven over medium heat until shimmering. Add bell peppers and ¼ teaspoon salt and cook until softened, about 5 minutes. Stir in tomato paste, thyme, and allspice and cook until fragrant, about 30 seconds. Stir in broth, Scotch bonnet, if using, and sweet potatoes, scraping up any browned bits, and bring to simmer. Cover, reduce heat to medium-low, and cook until sweet potatoes are just tender, 15 to 20 minutes.

3 Add collard greens, one handful at a time, and cook, stirring occasionally, until wilted, about 2 minutes. Stir in okra, return to simmer, and cook until potatoes and okra are fully tender, 5 to 10 minutes. Off heat, stir in coconut milk and cilantro and season with salt and pepper to taste. Serve with lime wedges.

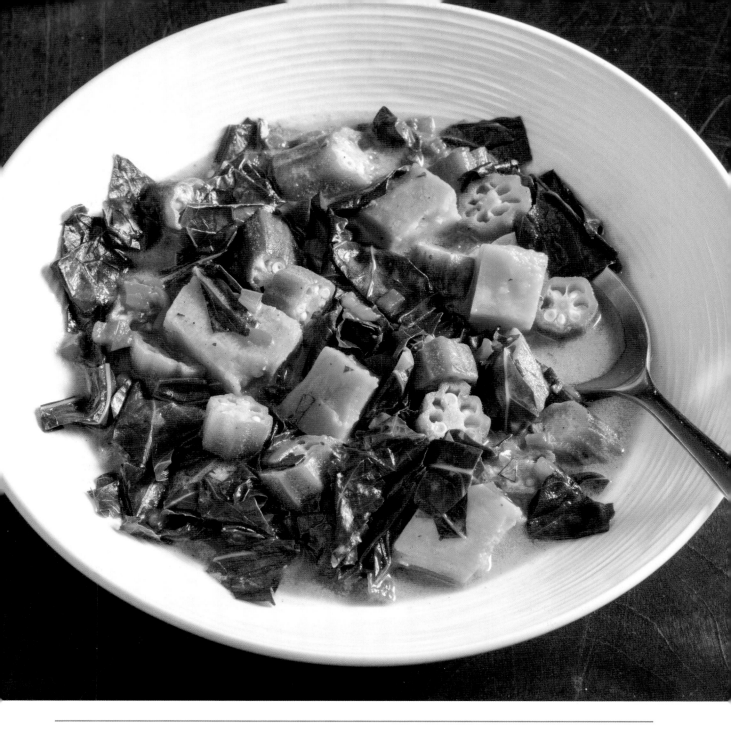

PER 1½-CUP SERVING

Dietary Fiber 9g **Cal** 200;
Total Fat 9g, **Sat Fat** 4g;
Chol 0mg; **Sodium** 750mg;
Total Carb 27g, **Total Sugars** 7g;
Added Sugars 0g; **Protein** 6g

TUSCAN BEAN STEW

SERVES 8

WHY THIS RECIPE WORKS This bean stew, made in the style of bean stews from Tuscany, provides 22 grams of fiber per serving; moreover, it's a delicious way to get that fiber, with its aromatic base, the creamiest of white beans, and complementary hearty greens. Bean perfection is paramount here, so we started from dried. Soaking the beans overnight was important to soften them so that their interiors cooked up creamy. And salting the soaking water—essentially brining—softened the skins until barely perceptible for ultratender beans. After experimenting with cooking times and temperatures, we found that a vigorous simmer caused some beans to explode, so we gently cooked them in a 250-degree oven for even results. A beautiful broth is guaranteed with aromatic vegetables, pancetta, a Parmesan cheese rind, bay leaves, and rosemary in the pot. Adding the tomatoes toward the end of cooking ensured their acidity wouldn't toughen the beans. If pancetta is unavailable, substitute four slices of bacon. The Parmesan rind can be replaced with a 2-inch chunk of Parmesan cheese.

3 tablespoons table salt, for soaking

1 pound (2½ cups) dried cannellini beans, picked over and rinsed

1 tablespoon garlic oil (see page 20), plus extra for serving

3 ounces pancetta, cut into ¼-inch pieces

2 carrots, peeled and cut into ½-inch pieces

2 celery ribs, cut into ½-inch pieces

4 cups chicken broth (see page 18)

3 cups water

1 Parmesan cheese rind, plus grated Parmesan for serving

2 bay leaves

1 pound kale or collard greens, stemmed and chopped

1 (14.5-ounce) can diced tomatoes, drained

1 sprig fresh rosemary

1 Dissolve salt in 4 quarts cold water in large container. Add beans and soak at room temperature for at least 8 hours or up to 24 hours. Drain and rinse well.

2 Adjust oven rack to lower-middle position and heat oven to 250 degrees. Cook oil and pancetta in Dutch oven over medium heat, stirring occasionally, until pancetta is lightly browned and fat has rendered, 6 to 10 minutes. Add carrots and celery and cook, stirring occasionally, until softened and lightly browned, 10 to 16 minutes. Stir in beans, broth, water, Parmesan rind, and bay leaves and bring to boil. Cover, transfer pot to oven, and cook until beans are almost tender (very center of beans will still be firm), 45 minutes to 1 hour.

3 Remove pot from oven and stir in kale and tomatoes. Cover, return pot to oven, and cook until beans and greens are fully tender, 30 to 40 minutes.

4 Remove pot from oven and submerge rosemary sprig in stew. Cover and let sit for 15 minutes. Discard Parmesan rind, bay leaves, and rosemary sprig and season stew with salt and pepper to taste. If desired, use back of spoon to press some beans against side of pot to thicken stew. Serve, passing extra oil and grated Parmesan separately.

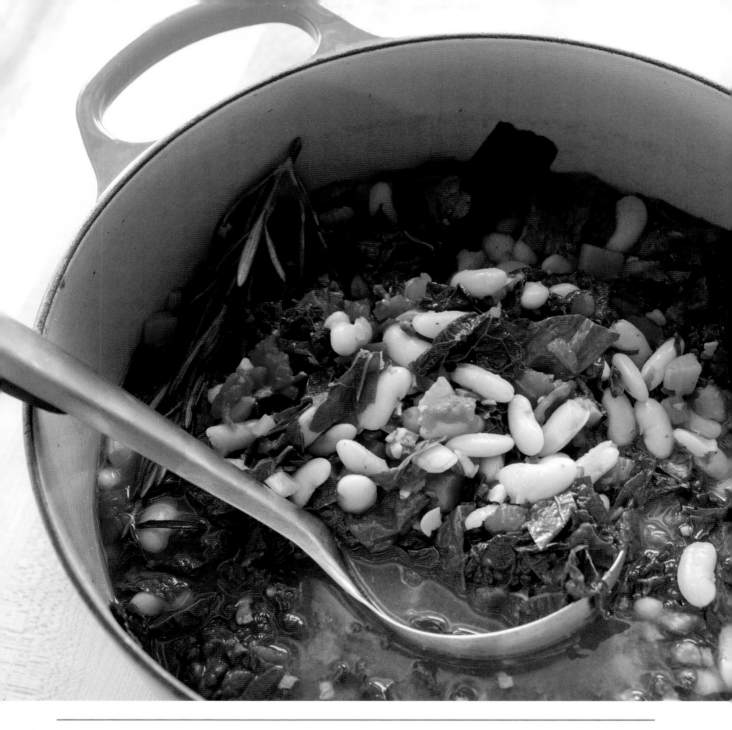

PER 1½-CUP SERVING

Dietary Fiber 22g **Cal** 290;
Total Fat 6g, **Sat Fat** 1.5g;
Chol 10mg; **Sodium** 700mg;
Total Carb 43g, **Total Sugars** 4g,
Added Sugars 0g; **Protein** 17g

DF **MAKE IT DAIRY FREE** Omit Parmesan rind and
grated Parmesan.

PUMPKIN TURKEY CHILI

SERVES 6

WHY THIS RECIPE WORKS If you want a lighter turkey chili to alternate with more common beef chilis, you might find that existing recipes lack depth and richness. We wanted to add a satisfying turkey chili to our repertoire that wouldn't leave us missing beef. And of course we wanted it to meet our fiber goals. To safeguard against rubbery turkey, we treated the meat with salt and baking soda, which helped it hold on to moisture. Then, to give our dish a smoky, aromatic backbone, we made our own chili powder with spices that complemented the more mild turkey. We ground toasted ancho chiles, cumin, coriander, paprika, and oregano together, then loaded the chili with red bell peppers and black beans for extra fiber and protein. Still, our chili was missing something. We found the answer in a unique ingredient—canned pumpkin puree. Folding this into the chili gave it a rich, silky texture and subtle squash-y flavor—and even more fiber gains. Be sure to use ground turkey, not ground turkey breast (also labeled 99 percent fat-free) in this recipe.

1 pound ground turkey

2 cups plus 1 tablespoon water, divided

¾ teaspoon table salt, divided

¼ teaspoon baking soda

4 dried ancho chiles, stemmed, seeded, and torn into 1-inch pieces (1 cup)

1½ tablespoons ground cumin

1½ teaspoons ground coriander

1½ teaspoons dried oregano

1½ teaspoons paprika

1 teaspoon pepper

1 (28-ounce) can whole peeled tomatoes

2 tablespoons garlic oil (see page 20)

2 red bell peppers, stemmed, seeded, and cut into ½-inch pieces

1 cup canned unsweetened pumpkin puree

2 (15-ounce) cans black beans, rinsed

¼ cup chopped fresh cilantro

Lime wedges

1 Toss turkey, 1 tablespoon water, ¼ teaspoon salt, and baking soda in bowl until thoroughly combined; set aside for 20 minutes.

2 Toast anchos in Dutch oven over medium-high heat, stirring frequently, until fragrant, 4 to 6 minutes; transfer to food processor and let cool slightly. Add cumin, coriander, oregano, paprika, and pepper and process until finely ground, about 2 minutes; transfer to bowl. Process tomatoes and their juice in now-empty food processor until smooth, about 30 seconds.

3 Heat oil in now-empty pot over medium heat until shimmering. Add bell peppers and remaining ½ teaspoon salt and cook until softened, 8 to 10 minutes. Increase heat to medium-high, add turkey mixture, and cook, breaking up meat with wooden spoon, until no longer pink, 4 to 6 minutes. Stir in ancho mixture and cook until fragrant, about 30 seconds. Stir in pureed tomatoes, pumpkin, and remaining 2 cups water and bring to simmer. Reduce heat to low, cover, and simmer gently, stirring occasionally, for 1 hour.

4 Stir in beans, cover, and cook until chili is slightly thickened, about 45 minutes. (If chili begins to stick to bottom of pot or looks too thick, stir in extra water as needed.) Season with salt and pepper to taste. Sprinkle individual portions with cilantro and serve with lime wedges.

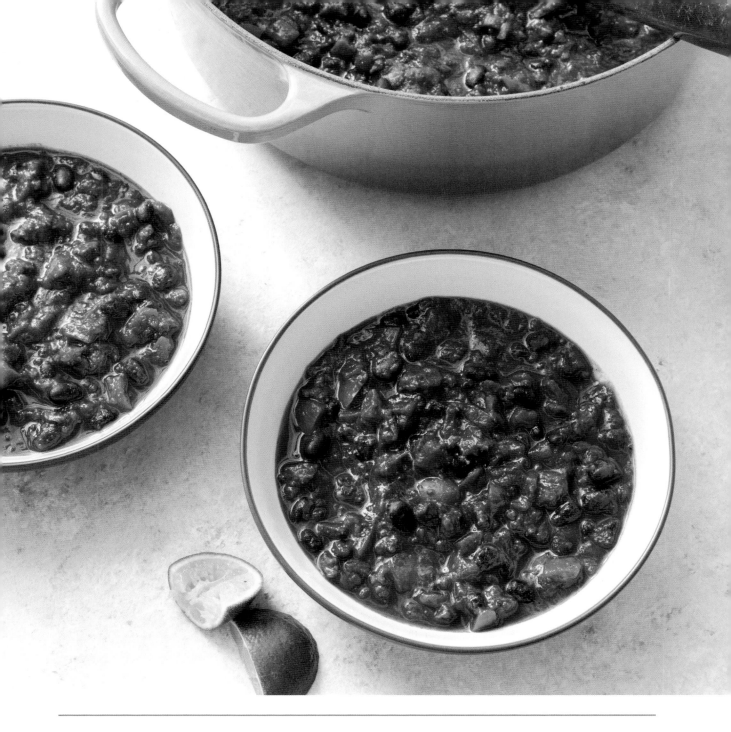

PER 1½-CUP SERVING

Dietary Fiber 10g **Cal** 290;
Total Fat 8g, **Sat Fat** 2g;
Chol 30mg; **Sodium** 700mg;
Total Carb 30g, **Total Sugars** 6g,
Added Sugars 0g; **Protein** 27g

WHITE CHICKEN CHILI

SERVES 6

WHY THIS RECIPE WORKS White chicken chili is a fresher cousin of thick red chili, with vibrant, pleasantly grassy notes from green chiles. However, many white chicken chili recipes lack bold chile flavor. To remedy this, we used a trio of fresh chiles: poblano, Anaheim, and jalapeño. We pureed some of our sautéed chile mixture with beans and chicken broth to thicken the base. To avoid rubbery chicken, we browned, poached, and shredded bone-in, skin-on chicken breasts, which gave the chicken a hearty texture and full flavor. To finish, we garnished with avocado which brought richness and fiber to the bright, vegetal chili. If you can't find Anaheim chiles, add an additional poblano and jalapeño.

3 poblano chiles, stemmed, seeded, and chopped

3 Anaheim chiles, stemmed, seeded, and chopped

3 jalapeño chiles, stemmed, seeded, and minced, divided

2 pounds bone-in split chicken breasts, trimmed

2 tablespoons canola oil

1 tablespoon ground cumin

1½ teaspoons ground coriander

¼ teaspoon table salt

¼ teaspoon pepper

2 (15-ounce) cans cannellini beans, rinsed, divided

4 cups chicken broth (see page 18), divided

2 cups frozen corn

2 tablespoons lime juice, plus lime wedges for serving

¼ cup minced fresh cilantro

4 scallions, green part only, sliced thin

1 tablespoon minced fresh oregano

2 ripe avocados, halved, pitted, and cut into 1-inch pieces (2 cups)

1 Toss poblanos, Anaheims, and two-thirds of jalapeños together in bowl. Working in two batches, pulse chiles in food processor until coarsely chopped, about 5 pulses; set aside.

2 Pat chicken dry with paper towels. Heat oil in Dutch oven over medium-high heat until just smoking. Brown chicken, 3 to 5 minutes per side; transfer to plate and discard skin.

3 Add processed chile mixture, cumin, coriander, salt, and pepper to fat left in pot and cook over medium heat, stirring often, until chiles are softened, about 10 minutes. Remove pot from heat.

4 Process ½ cup cooked chile mixture, 1 cup beans, and 1 cup broth in food processor until smooth, about 20 seconds, scraping down sides of bowl as needed. Return pureed mixture to pot and stir in remaining 3 cups broth, scraping up any browned bits. Nestle chicken into pot, add any accumulated juices, and bring to simmer. Reduce heat to medium-low, cover, and cook until chicken registers 160 degrees, 10 to 15 minutes.

5 Transfer chicken to cutting board, let cool slightly, then shred into bite-size pieces using 2 forks; discard bones.

6 Stir corn and remaining beans into chili, bring to simmer over medium heat, and cook, uncovered, until chili has thickened slightly, about 10 minutes. Off heat, stir in chicken and let sit until heated through, about 5 minutes. Stir in lime juice, cilantro, scallions, oregano, and remaining jalapeños and season with salt and pepper to taste. Top individual portions with ⅓ cup avocado and serve with lime wedges.

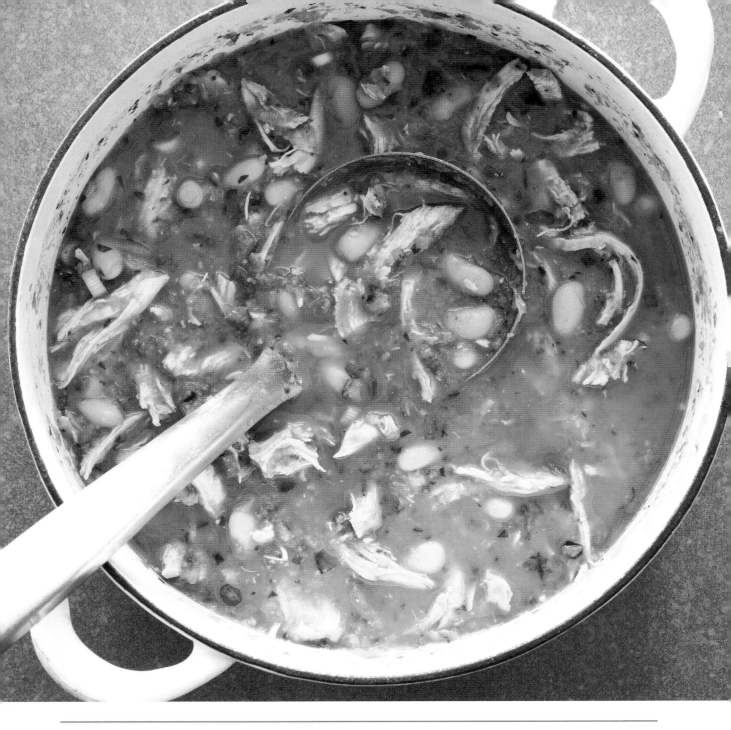

PER 1½-CUP SERVING

Dietary Fiber 12g Cal 450;
Total Fat 19g, **Sat Fat** 2.5g;
Chol 90mg; **Sodium** 790mg;
Total Carb 36g, **Total Sugars** 6g,
Added Sugars 0g; **Protein** 38g

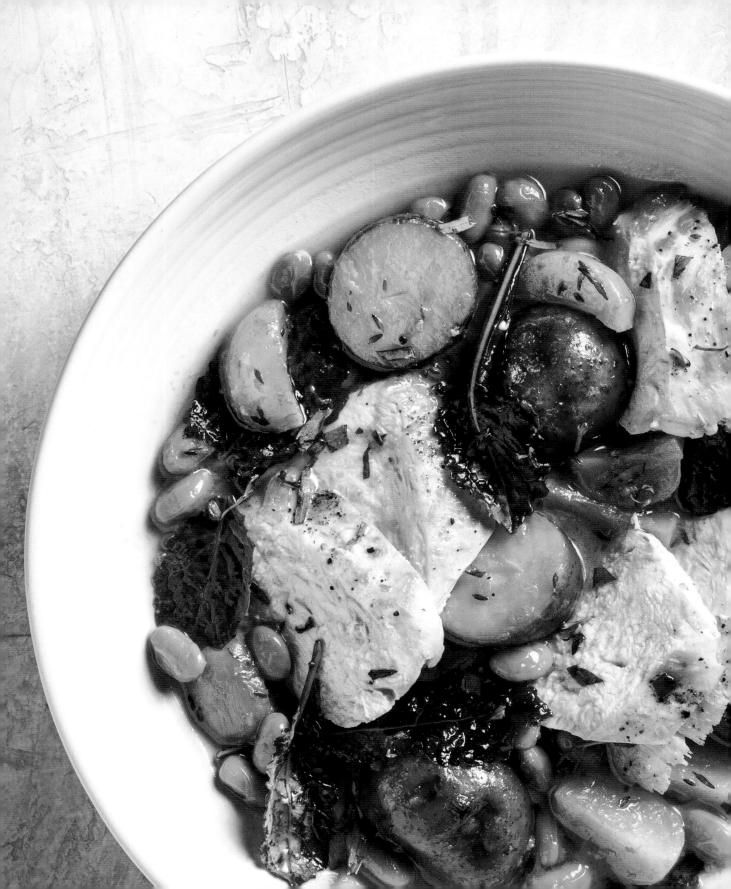

3 Poultry

Chicken

Turkey

POACHED CHICKEN BREASTS WITH WARM TOMATO-GINGER VINAIGRETTE

SERVES 4

WHY THIS RECIPE WORKS When you're looking for a protein to fill you up without slowing or disrupting digestion, poached lean chicken breasts are a great choice. While high-heat methods like sautéing or broiling can make the meat dry or stringy, poaching, by contrast, is reliable, forgiving, and dead simple—and it doesn't create bland spa food. Poached chicken can be incredibly flavorful when you use a highly seasoned poaching liquid. Salt, soy sauce, and a little sugar amp up ours, which also serves as a brine. Allowing the chicken to gently poach, elevated in a steamer basket, ensures even cooking and moist, savory breasts, ready to be paired with a bold sauce like our aromatic but allium-free ginger-infused vinaigrette with softened cherry tomatoes. Pair it with a fresh side like Sautéed Green Beans with Fresh Herbs (page 266), or add to salads or sandwiches. You can omit the tomato-ginger vinaigrette and instead serve the chicken with one of the sauces on pages 21–25.

CHICKEN

- 4 (6-ounce) boneless, skinless chicken breasts, trimmed
- ½ cup soy sauce (see page 18) for poaching
- ¼ cup table salt for poaching
- 2 tablespoons granulated sugar for poaching

VINAIGRETTE

- 2 tablespoons extra-virgin olive oil, divided
- 1 teaspoon grated fresh ginger
- Pinch ground cumin
- Pinch ground fennel
- 6 ounces cherry tomatoes, halved
- ⅛ teaspoon table salt
- 1½ teaspoons red wine vinegar
- ½ teaspoon light brown sugar
- 1 tablespoon chopped fresh cilantro or parsley

1 For the chicken: Cover chicken breasts with plastic wrap and pound thick ends gently with meat pounder until ¾ inch thick. Whisk 4 quarts water, soy sauce, salt, and granulated sugar together in Dutch oven until salt and sugar are dissolved. Arrange breasts skinned side up in steamer basket, making sure not to overlap them. Submerge steamer basket in brine and let sit at room temperature for 30 minutes.

2 Heat pot over medium heat, stirring liquid occasionally to even out hot spots, until water registers 175 degrees, 15 to 20 minutes. Turn off heat, cover pot, remove from burner, and let sit until chicken registers 160 degrees, 17 to 22 minutes. Transfer breasts to cutting board, tent with aluminum foil, and let rest while preparing vinaigrette.

3 For the vinaigrette: Cook 1 tablespoon oil, ginger, cumin, and fennel in 10-inch nonstick skillet over medium heat until fragrant, about 1 minute. Stir in tomatoes and salt and cook, stirring frequently, until tomatoes have softened, 3 to 5 minutes. Off heat, stir in vinegar and brown sugar and season with salt and pepper to taste.

4 Slice chicken on bias into ¼-inch-thick slices and transfer to serving platter or individual plates. Stir cilantro and remaining 1 tablespoon oil into vinaigrette and serve with chicken.

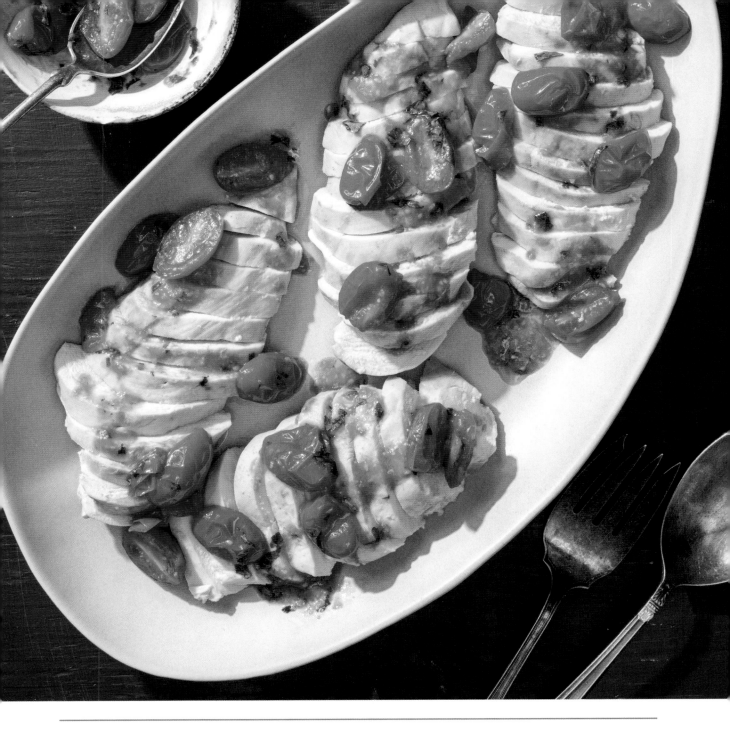

PER SERVING

Dietary Fiber 1g **Cal** 280;
Total Fat 12g, **Sat Fat** 2g;
Chol 125mg; **Sodium** 310mg;
Total Carb 2g, **Total Sugars** 1g,
Added Sugars 0g; **Protein** 39g

 MAKE IT GLUTEN FREE Substitute gluten-free soy sauce or tamari (see page 18) for soy sauce.

PARMESAN CHICKEN WITH BITTER GREENS AND FENNEL

SERVES 4

WHY THIS RECIPE WORKS Crispy, tender, juicy breaded chicken cutlets are a multipurpose standby to enjoy as a main dish, in salads, or on sandwiches. Oftentimes, however, they come out dripping with oil; sometimes they're draped with a distracting amount of cheese. For a version we feel good about eating often, we pair whole-wheat panko with a mindful amount of Parmesan, a low-lactose cheese that adds both flavor and crispness to our coating. Cooking the cutlets in a non-stick skillet means that we can use a moderate amount of oil. We serve the chicken alongside a salad with a bright vinaigrette that contrasts with the salty richness of the breading. Softened fennel and tomatoes slightly wilt our multidimensional salad of radicchio, frisée, and arugula.

½ cup all-purpose flour

2 large eggs

½ cup 100 percent whole-wheat panko bread crumbs

1 ounce Parmesan cheese, grated (½ cup)

½ teaspoon dried oregano

4 (6-ounce) boneless, skinless chicken breasts, trimmed

5 tablespoons garlic oil (see page 20), divided

1 tablespoon white wine vinegar

½ teaspoon Dijon mustard

¼ teaspoon table salt

Pinch pepper

2 fennel bulbs, stalks discarded, bulbs halved, cored, and sliced thin

1 pound cherry tomatoes, halved

½ head radicchio (5 ounces), cored and sliced thin

1 head frisée (6 ounces), trimmed and cut into bite-size pieces

3 ounces (3 cups) baby arugula

1 Adjust oven rack to middle position and heat oven to 200 degrees. Set wire rack in rimmed baking sheet. Spread flour in shallow dish. Beat eggs in second shallow dish. Combine panko, Parmesan, and oregano in third shallow dish. Cover chicken breasts with plastic wrap and pound to uniform thickness as needed, then pat dry with paper towels. Working with 1 breast at a time, dredge in flour, dip in egg, then coat with panko mixture, pressing gently to adhere.

2 Heat 3 tablespoons oil in 12-inch nonstick skillet over medium heat until shimmering. Add 2 breasts and cook until chicken is tender, golden brown, and crisp, 3 to 4 minutes per side. Transfer to prepared rack and transfer sheet to oven to keep warm. Repeat with remaining 2 breasts; transfer to prepared rack in oven.

3 Whisk 1 tablespoon oil, vinegar, mustard, salt, and pepper together in large bowl. Wipe skillet clean with paper towels. Heat remaining 1 tablespoon oil in now-empty skillet over medium heat until shimmering. Add fennel and cook until softened and lightly browned, 5 to 7 minutes. Add tomatoes and cook until beginning to soften, about 2 minutes. Transfer to bowl with vinaigrette along with radicchio, frisée, and arugula and gently toss to combine. Season with pepper to taste. Serve with chicken.

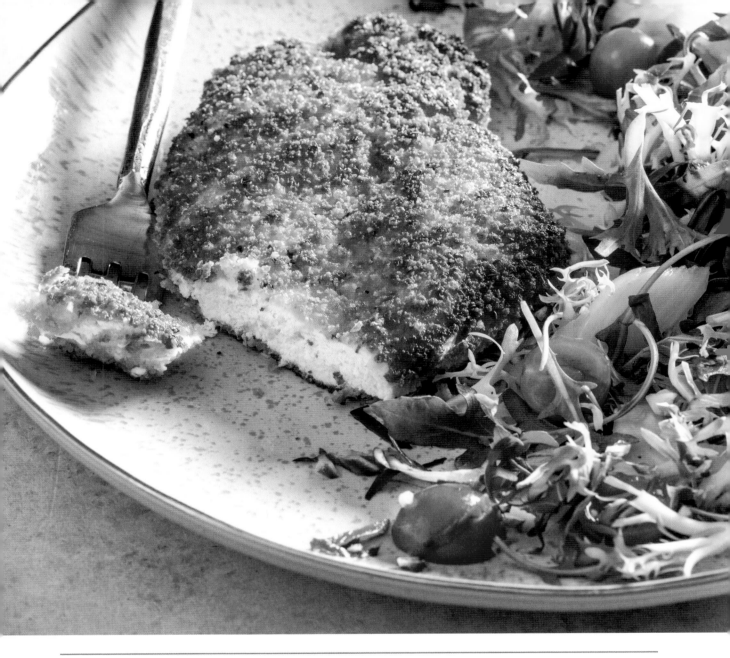

PER SERVING

Dietary Fiber 7g **Cal** 570;
Total Fat 27g, **Sat Fat** 5g;
Chol 220mg; **Sodium** 490mg;
Total Carb 29g, **Total Sugars** 9g,
Added Sugars 0g; **Protein** 51g

LF **MAKE IT LOW FODMAP** Substitute gluten-free flour blend (see page 31) for all-purpose flour and gluten-free panko bread crumbs for whole-wheat panko. Reduce fennel to 1 small bulb and increase frisée to 2 heads.

DF **MAKE IT DAIRY FREE** Omit Parmesan and increase panko to 1 cup.

GF **MAKE IT GLUTEN FREE** Substitute gluten-free flour blend for all-purpose flour and gluten-free panko bread crumbs for whole-wheat panko.

PAN-SEARED CHICKEN BREASTS WITH ARTICHOKE, TOMATO, AND BULGUR PILAF

SERVES 4

WHY THIS RECIPE WORKS Don't sleep on bulgur: If you eat wheat, it's a great whole grain to choose, as it is high in fiber and one of the easiest grains to cook. A robustly flavored artichoke (also a fiber heavy hitter), tomato, olive, and feta-filled bulgur pilaf makes a dish of perfectly cooked pan-seared chicken breasts far from boring. A cumin rub on the chicken helps it fit in with the bold pilaf. Since the bulgur takes only 5 minutes to cook, we were able to use just one skillet. After cooking the chicken in the skillet, we sauté baby artichokes until they're nicely browned. We then steam the bulgur directly in the skillet to take advantage of the flavorful fond that we built from sautéing the chicken. While we prefer the flavor and texture of jarred whole baby artichoke hearts in this recipe, you can substitute 9 ounces frozen artichoke hearts, thawed and patted dry, for the jarred. Do not confuse bulgur with cracked wheat, which has a much longer cooking time and will not work in this recipe. Serve with lemon wedges, if desired.

½ teaspoon ground cumin

¼ teaspoon plus ⅛ teaspoon table salt, divided

⅛ teaspoon pepper

4 (6-ounce) boneless, skinless chicken breasts, trimmed

¼ cup extra-virgin olive oil, divided

1½ cups jarred whole baby artichokes packed in water, rinsed, patted dry, and quartered

2¼ cups water

1½ cups medium-grind bulgur

10 ounces cherry tomatoes, halved

3 ounces feta cheese, crumbled (¾ cup)

¾ cup minced fresh parsley

⅓ cup pitted kalamata olives, chopped

1 tablespoon lemon juice

1 Combine cumin, ¼ teaspoon salt, and pepper in bowl. Cover chicken breasts with plastic wrap and pound to uniform thickness as needed. Pat dry with paper towels and sprinkle with cumin mixture.

2 Heat 1 tablespoon oil in 12-inch skillet over medium-high heat until just smoking. Cook breasts, turning as needed, until golden brown and register 160 degrees, about 10 minutes. Transfer breasts to plate, tent with aluminum foil, and let rest while preparing pilaf.

3 Heat 1 tablespoon oil in now-empty skillet over medium-high heat until shimmering. Add artichoke hearts and cook, without stirring, until spotty brown, about 2 minutes. Stir in water, scraping up any browned bits, and bring to boil. Stir in bulgur and remaining ⅛ teaspoon salt. Off heat, cover and let sit until grains are softened and liquid is fully absorbed, about 5 minutes.

4 Add tomatoes, feta, parsley, olives, lemon juice, and remaining 2 tablespoons oil to pilaf and gently fluff with fork to combine. Season with pepper to taste. Serve chicken with pilaf.

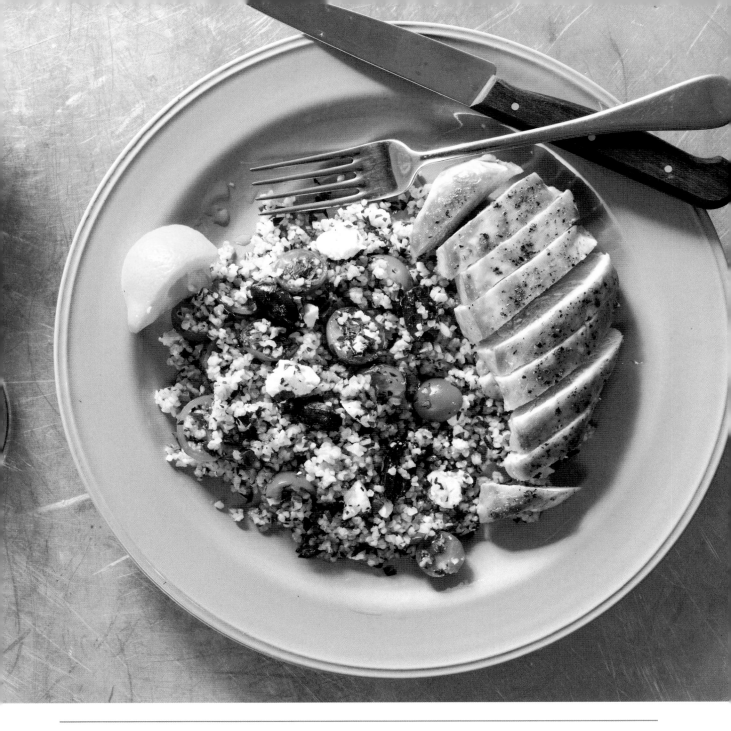

PER SERVING

Dietary Fiber 8g **Cal** 610;
Total Fat 25g, **Sat Fat** 6g;
Chol 145mg; **Sodium** 700mg;
Total Carb 48g, **Total Sugars** 4g,
Added Sugars 0g; **Protein** 80g

 MAKE IT DAIRY FREE Omit feta.

ONE-POT CHICKEN WITH BRAISED SPRING VEGETABLES

SERVES 4

WHY THIS RECIPE WORKS There's no need to reserve braising for tough, collagen-rich cuts of meat in rich sauces. It's a snap to create a delicate dish featuring chicken breasts in an aromatic broth surrounded by the most vibrant of vegetables. The moist heat technique cooks our lean boneless, skinless chicken breasts and spring vegetables gently and evenly. We start by browning just one side of the chicken breasts in a Dutch oven before removing them from the pot. We then cook fresh thyme and red pepper flakes in garlic oil to create a fragrant cooking medium for the vegetables. Radishes enter the pot with chunks of red potatoes and water, as these heartier vegetables need a head start. Next, we place the chicken on top of these vegetables, cover the pot, and let the contents simmer. After removing the chicken, we add verdant asparagus, some frozen peas, and lemon and orange zests and cook the mixture until tender. Look for asparagus that is approximately ½ inch thick at base.

4 (6-ounce) boneless, skinless chicken breasts, trimmed

1 teaspoon table salt, divided

⅛ teaspoon pepper

3 tablespoons garlic oil (see page 20)

3 sprigs fresh thyme

Pinch red pepper flakes (optional)

12 ounces red potatoes, unpeeled, cut into 1-inch pieces

8 radishes, trimmed and halved if small or quartered lengthwise if large

1¼ cups water

1½ pounds asparagus, trimmed and cut into 2-inch lengths

2 cups frozen peas

2 teaspoons grated lemon zest

2 teaspoons grated orange zest

1 tablespoon chopped fresh tarragon

1 Cover chicken breasts with plastic wrap and pound to uniform thickness as needed. Pat chicken dry with paper towels and sprinkle with ¼ teaspoon salt and pepper. Heat 1 tablespoon oil in Dutch oven over medium-high heat until shimmering. Add chicken skinned side down and cook until browned on 1 side, about 5 minutes. Transfer chicken to plate browned side up.

2 Add thyme sprigs, pepper flakes, if using, and 1 tablespoon oil to now-empty pot and cook over medium heat until fragrant, about 30 seconds. Stir in potatoes, radishes, water, and ¼ teaspoon salt and bring to boil. Place chicken browned side up on top of potato mixture. Reduce heat to medium-low, cover, and simmer until chicken registers 160 degrees, about 10 minutes.

3 Transfer chicken to plate, tent with aluminum foil, and let rest while finishing vegetables. Stir asparagus, peas, lemon zest, orange zest, and remaining ½ teaspoon salt into potato mixture. Cook, covered, until vegetables are tender, 7 to 10 minutes, stirring halfway through cooking. Remove from heat.

4 Discard thyme sprigs. Slice chicken on bias ½ inch thick. Place chicken browned side up on top of vegetables in pot, adding any accumulated chicken juices. Sprinkle with tarragon and drizzle with remaining 1 tablespoon oil. Serve.

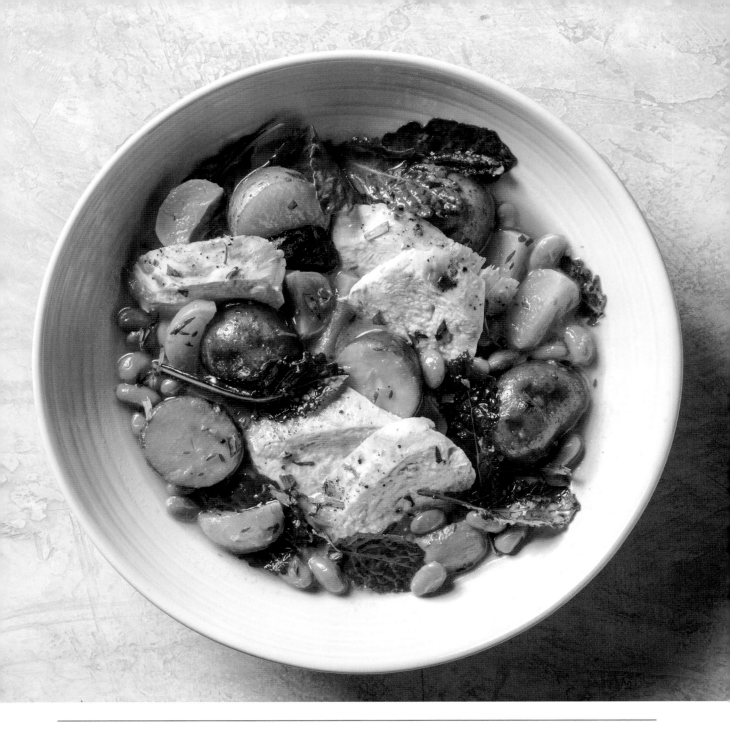

PER SERVING

Dietary Fiber 7g **Cal** 430;
Total Fat 15g, **Sat Fat** 2.5g;
Chol 125mg; **Sodium** 680mg;
Total Carb 27g, **Total Sugars** 6g,
Added Sugars 0g; **Protein** 46g

 MAKE IT LOW FODMAP Omit asparagus. Substitute frozen edamame for peas. After discarding thyme sprigs, stir 2 cups baby kale or spinach into braising liquid and let sit until slightly wilted, about 2 minutes.

PAN-ROASTED CHICKEN BREASTS WITH VERMOUTH PAN SAUCE

SERVES 4

WHY THIS RECIPE WORKS Boneless, skinless chicken breasts are lean, quick-cooking, and convenient; bone-in chicken breasts are richly flavored and offer skin that we can crisp appealingly. Both have a place in a healthy gut diet, and here we tackled perfect bone-in chicken breasts with a deeply flavored pan sauce—one that doesn't require foundational ingredients of minced garlic or shallot. Pan-roasting—browning in a skillet on the stovetop and then sliding the skillet into a hot oven to finish—achieved tender chicken with crispy skin. Along with this method, brining the chicken beforehand ensured the meat stayed moist and flavorful. For a shining sauce, we made a vermouth-based pan sauce with sage using the savor-boosting browned bits left behind by the chicken. With a swirl of emulsifying butter, this sauce was so flavorful we didn't miss the allium. It's great for adorning the chicken and perhaps an accompanying side dish like comforting Mashed Potatoes and Root Vegetables (page 278) for a winner chicken dinner. If using kosher chicken, do not brine. You can omit the sage-vermouth sauce and instead serve with one of the sauces on pages 21–25.

CHICKEN

- ½ cup table salt for brining
- 2 (12-ounce) bone-in split chicken breasts, trimmed and halved crosswise
- ⅛ teaspoon pepper
- 1 tablespoon canola oil

SAUCE

- 4 fresh sage leaves, each leaf torn in half
- ¾ cup chicken broth (see page 18)
- ½ cup dry vermouth
- 3 tablespoons unsalted butter, cut into 3 pieces

1 **For the chicken:** Dissolve salt in 2 quarts cold water in large container. Submerge chicken pieces in brine, cover, and refrigerate for at least 30 minutes or up to 1 hour.

2 Adjust oven rack to middle position and heat oven to 450 degrees. Remove chicken from brine and pat dry with paper towels. Sprinkle chicken with pepper. Heat oil in 12-inch ovensafe skillet over medium-high heat until just smoking. Cook chicken skin side down until well browned, 6 to 8 minutes, reducing heat if skillet begins to scorch. Flip chicken and brown lightly on second side, about 3 minutes. Flip chicken skin side down, transfer skillet to oven, and roast until chicken registers 160 degrees, about 10 minutes.

3 Using potholder, remove skillet from oven. Transfer chicken to serving platter and let rest while making sauce.

4 **For the sauce:** Being careful of hot skillet handle, pour off all but 1 teaspoon fat left in skillet. Add sage and cook over medium-high heat until fragrant, about 30 seconds. Stir in broth and vermouth, scraping up any browned bits, and simmer until thickened and measures ⅔ cup, about 6 minutes. Stir in any accumulated chicken juices. Reduce heat to low and whisk in butter, one piece at a time. Off heat, season with salt and pepper to taste. Spoon sauce over chicken and serve.

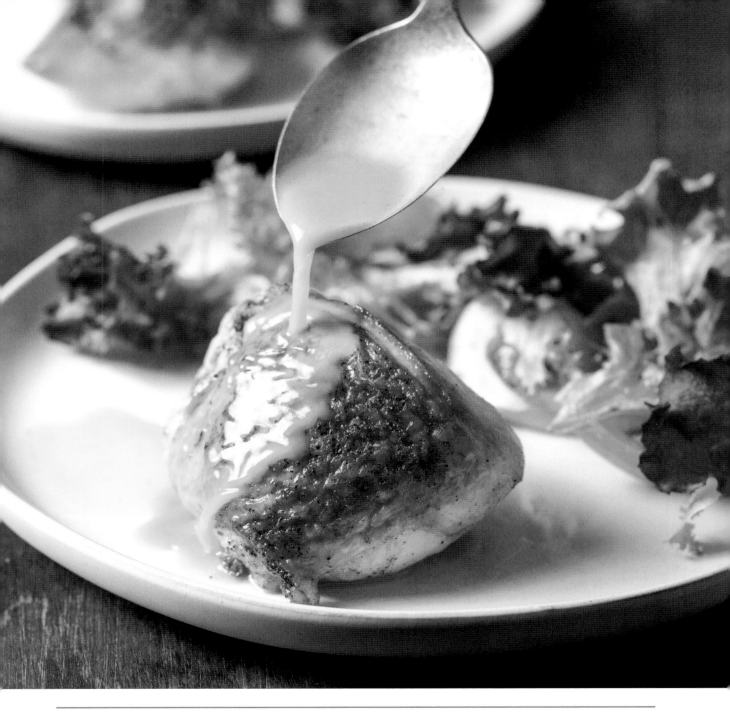

PER SERVING

Dietary Fiber 6g **Cal** 380;
Total Fat 24g, **Sat Fat** 9g;
Chol 110mg; **Sodium** 530mg;
Total Carb 2g, **Total Sugars** 2g,
Added Sugars 0g; **Protein** 20g

ROASTED CHICKEN BREASTS WITH KABOCHA SQUASH AND KALE

SERVES 4

WHY THIS RECIPE WORKS Two roasted vegetables (both hearty and fiber-packed) and bone-in chicken breasts make a satisfying meal—but we wanted to make them in one sheet pan. Roasted squash turns out tender, golden, and sweet—we chose kabocha. The squash that looks like a squat pumpkin is just as sweet as others but, unlike butternut or similarly honeylike sweet potatoes, is completely free of FODMAPs. Another bonus: You can forget about all that peeling and eat the tender skin for additional fiber and ease of prep and serving. For a decidedly contrasting texture, we paired the squash pieces with earthy-tasting kale. A simple mixture of garlic oil, sage, and paprika seasoned the chicken, and halving the bone-in split breasts assisted in even cooking—as did starting the chicken and squash before the kale. In just 25 minutes, we had crisp-skinned chicken; tender, not mushy, squash; and pleasantly tender-crispy kale. We topped our chicken with a drizzle of a light, creamy yogurt sauce accented with orange zest to bring the dish's components into harmony. Both curly and Lacinato kale will work in this recipe.

5 tablespoons garlic oil (see page 20)

2 tablespoons minced fresh sage

¾ teaspoon table salt

½ teaspoon pepper

¾ cup plain yogurt

1 tablespoon water

1 teaspoon grated orange zest

1 kabocha squash (2 pounds), halved lengthwise and seeded

2 teaspoons paprika

2 (12-ounce) bone-in split chicken breasts, trimmed and halved crosswise

1 pound kale, stemmed and cut into 2-inch pieces

1 Adjust oven rack to upper-middle position and heat oven to 475 degrees. Combine oil, sage, salt, and pepper in bowl. Combine 1 tablespoon of the sage oil with yogurt, water, and orange zest in separate bowl. Season with salt and pepper to taste and refrigerate yogurt sauce until ready to serve.

2 Cut each squash half into 2½- to 3-inch pieces. Combine squash and 3 tablespoons sage oil in large bowl; set aside. Stir paprika into remaining sage oil. Pat chicken dry with paper towels. Using your fingers, gently loosen skin covering each breast piece, then rub paprika-sage oil evenly under skin.

3 Spread squash in single layer over three-quarters of rimmed baking sheet. Place chicken pieces skin side up on empty portion of sheet and roast for 15 minutes.

4 Meanwhile, vigorously squeeze and massage kale with hands in now-empty bowl until leaves are uniformly darkened and slightly wilted, about 1 minute. Rotate sheet, stir kale into squash, and roast until vegetables are browned and tender and chicken registers 160 degrees, 10 to 20 minutes, stirring vegetables halfway through roasting. Toss vegetables with any accumulated chicken juices. Serve, passing yogurt sauce separately.

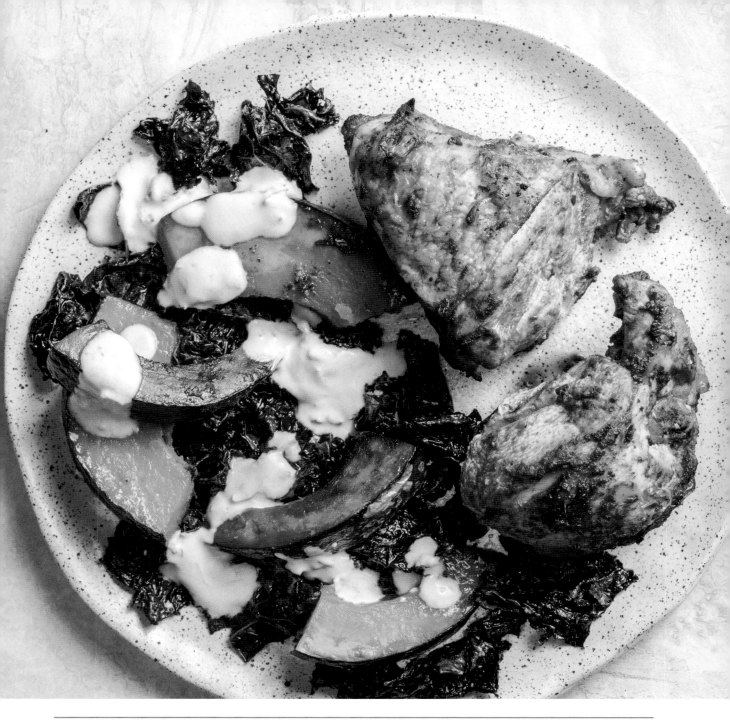

PER SERVING

Dietary Fiber 6g **Cal** 510;
Total Fat 28g, **Sat Fat** 6g;
Chol 90mg; **Sodium** 560mg;
Total Carb 29g, **Total Sugars** 12g,
Added Sugars 0g; **Protein** 38g

 MAKE IT LOW FODMAP Substitute dairy-free or lactose-free yogurt (see page 19) for plain yogurt.

 MAKE IT DAIRY FREE Substitute dairy-free yogurt (see page 19) for plain yogurt.

BRAISED CHICKEN BREASTS WITH CHICKPEAS, FENNEL, AND CHERMOULA

SERVES 4

WHY THIS RECIPE WORKS As with our One-Pot Chicken with Braised Spring Vegetables (page 110), this braise not only conveniently cooks a complete meal at one time in one vessel but also results in a remarkable exchange of flavors, here among flavorful bone-in chicken breasts, licorice-y fennel, and hearty, nutty chickpeas. Aromatic fennel helps to quickly develop flavor during the braise's relatively fast cooking time. And the chickpeas add a starchy component that increases the fiber and soaks up all the flavorful jus of the braise. The sturdy beans soften slightly but hold their shape. We finish the dish by drizzling homemade chermoula on top; the Moroccan green sauce adds bright, potent freshness. If you can't find fennel bulbs with their fronds intact, omit the fronds or use minced parsley instead.

1½ cups fresh cilantro leaves

6 tablespoons garlic oil (see page 20), divided

3 tablespoons lemon juice, plus lemon wedges for serving

1 teaspoon ground cumin

1 teaspoon paprika

¼ teaspoon cayenne pepper

½ teaspoon table salt, divided

2 (12-ounce) bone-in split chicken breasts, trimmed and halved crosswise

¼ teaspoon pepper

2 fennel bulbs, 2 tablespoons fronds minced, stalks discarded, bulbs halved, cored, and sliced thin

¾ cup chicken broth (see page 18)

2 (15-ounce) cans chickpeas, rinsed

1 Process cilantro, ¼ cup oil, lemon juice, cumin, paprika, cayenne, and ¼ teaspoon salt in food processor until finely ground, about 1 minute, scraping down sides of bowl as needed. Transfer chermoula to bowl and set aside for serving.

2 Pat chicken dry with paper towels and sprinkle with remaining ¼ teaspoon salt and pepper.

3 Heat 1 tablespoon oil in Dutch oven over medium-high heat until just smoking. Cook chicken pieces skin side down in pot until well browned, 6 to 8 minutes, reducing heat if pot begins to scorch; transfer to plate.

4 Heat remaining 1 tablespoon oil in now-empty pot over medium heat until shimmering. Add fennel and cook until softened, about 5 minutes. Stir in broth, scraping up any browned bits. Stir in chickpeas and bring to simmer. Nestle chicken into pot and add any accumulated juices. Reduce heat to medium-low, cover, and cook until chicken registers 160 degrees, 15 to 20 minutes.

5 Transfer chicken to plate and discard skin, if desired. Stir minced fennel fronds and 1 tablespoon chermoula into chickpea mixture. Top individual portions of chicken and chickpea mixture evenly with remaining chermoula. Serve with lemon wedges.

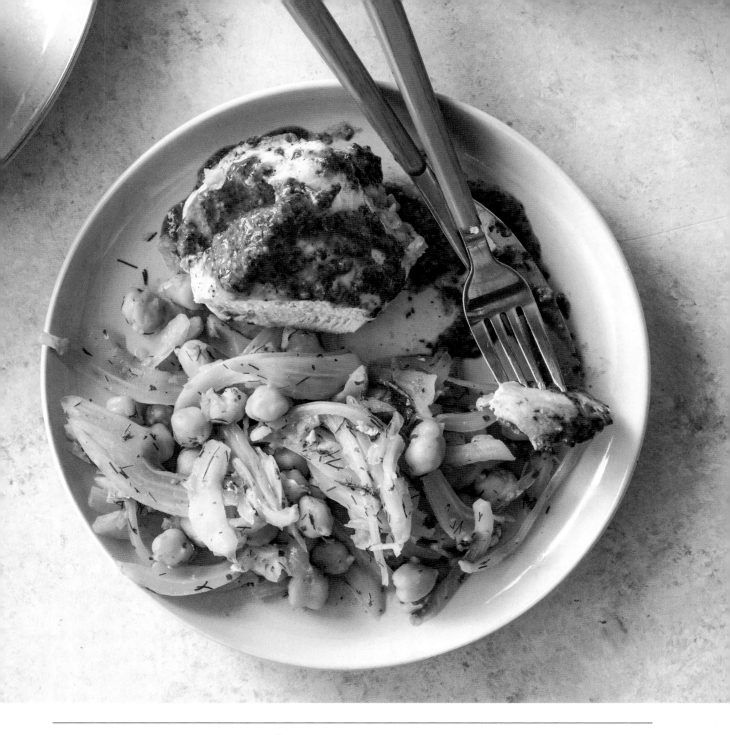

PER SERVING

Dietary Fiber 10g **Cal** 540;
Total Fat 26g, **Sat Fat** 4g;
Chol 100mg; **Sodium** 480mg;
Total Carb 34g, **Total Sugars** 6g,
Added Sugars 0g; **Protein** 41g

 MAKE IT LOW FODMAP Substitute 1½ pounds of carrots, quartered lengthwise and cut into 2-inch lengths, for fennel. Reduce chickpeas to 1 cup.

GRILLED YOGURT CHICKEN AND WARM OAT BERRY SALAD

SERVES 4

WHY THIS RECIPE WORK Grilling chicken breasts and vegetables simultaneously, on the hotter and cooler sides of a grill, is a quick way to a fresh complete summer meal. But here we don't just cook vegetables to serve plain; we chop grilled zucchini and bell pepper to add further complexity to a lively oat berry salad. The healthful components are married with a bright lemon-yogurt dressing.

4 (6-ounce) boneless, skinless chicken breasts, trimmed

½ cup plain yogurt, divided

5 tablespoons garlic oil (see page 20), divided

1 teaspoon table salt, divided, plus salt for cooking oat berries

½ teaspoon ground cumin

¼ teaspoon ground cinnamon

¼ teaspoon pepper, divided

¾ cup oat berries (groats) (see page 18), rinsed

3 zucchini, trimmed and quartered lengthwise

2 red bell peppers, quartered, stemmed, and seeded

½ teaspoon lemon zest plus 1 tablespoon juice

½ cup chopped fresh parsley

1 Cover chicken breasts with plastic wrap and pound to uniform thickness as needed. Combine ¼ cup yogurt, 2 tablespoons oil, ½ teaspoon salt, cumin, cinnamon, and ⅛ teaspoon pepper in large bowl. Add chicken and toss to coat; refrigerate until ready to cook.

2 Bring 2 quarts water to boil in large saucepan. Add oat berries and 1½ teaspoons salt and cook until grains are tender with slight chew, 45 to 50 minutes. Drain oat berries, spread over large plate, and let cool completely, about 15 minutes.

3A For a charcoal grill: Open bottom vent completely. Light large chimney starter filled with charcoal briquettes (6 quarts). When top coals are partially covered with ash, pour two-thirds evenly over half of grill, then pour remaining coals over other half of grill. Set cooking grate in place, cover, and open lid vent completely. Heat grill until hot, about 5 minutes.

3B For a gas grill: Turn all burners to high, cover, and heat grill until hot, about 15 minutes. Leave primary burner on high and turn other burner(s) to medium. (Adjust burners as needed to maintain hot fire and medium fire on separate sides of grill.)

4 Brush zucchini and bell peppers with 1 tablespoon oil and sprinkle with ¼ teaspoon salt. Clean and oil cooking grate. Remove chicken from marinade, allowing excess to drip off, and place on hotter side of grill. Place zucchini and bell peppers on cooler side of grill. Cook (covered if using gas), turning chicken and vegetables as needed, until chicken is browned and registers 160 degrees and vegetables are tender and charred in spots, 8 to 12 minutes. Transfer chicken and vegetables to cutting board as they finish cooking. Tent chicken with aluminum foil and coarsely chop vegetables.

5 Whisk lemon zest and juice, remaining ¼ cup yogurt, remaining 2 tablespoons oil, remaining ¼ teaspoon salt, and remaining ⅛ teaspoon pepper together in small bowl. Transfer ¼ cup yogurt mixture to large bowl, add oat berries, chopped vegetables, and parsley and toss to combine. Season with salt and pepper to taste. Serve chicken with salad, passing remaining yogurt mixture separately.

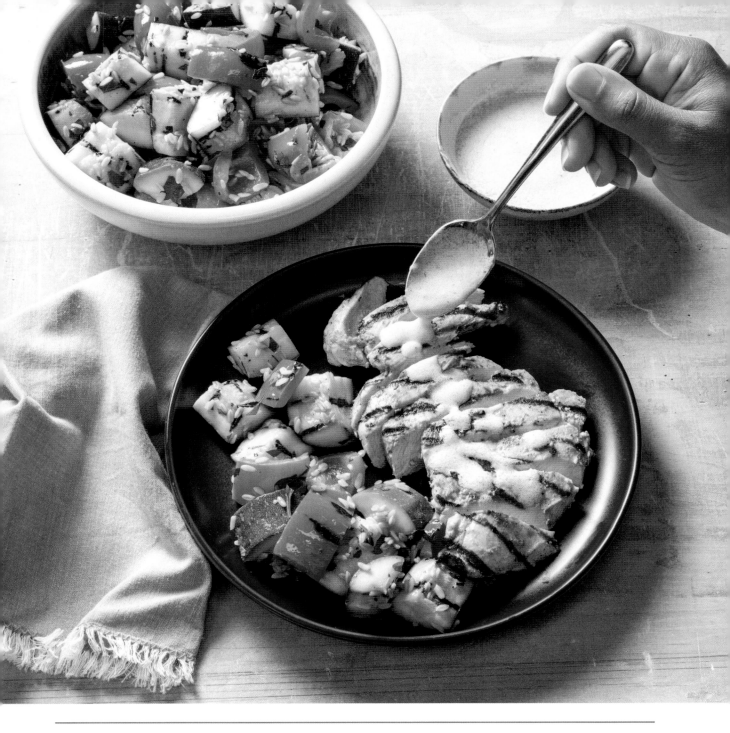

PER SERVING

Dietary Fiber 7g **Cal** 570;
Total Fat 26g, **Sat Fat** 3.5g;
Chol 130mg; **Sodium** 770mg;
Total Carb 35g, **Total Sugar**s 9g,
Added Sugar 0g; **Protein** 48g

LF **MAKE IT LOW FODMAP** Substitute dairy-free or lactose-free yogurt (see page 19) for plain yogurt.

DF **MAKE IT DAIRY FREE** Substitute dairy-free yogurt (see page 19) for plain yogurt.

ROASTED CHICKEN THIGHS WITH ROOT VEGETABLES

SERVES 4

WHY THIS RECIPE WORKS Sometimes we like to indulge in the richer, darker meat of chicken thighs, which hold up nicely in a one-pan roast with a one-two fiber punch of flavorful root vegetables and Brussels sprouts. To ensure even cooking, we're careful not to smother the vegetables underneath the chicken; we place the thighs on top of the vegetables along the perimeter of the sheet, where the heat is more intense for the long-cooking thighs. A similar placement strategy for the vegetables—leafy Brussels sprouts in the middle, hardier potatoes and carrots on the outside—is also effective. A sprinkle of sugar over the vegetables ensures deep, flavorful browning, and an herb-enhanced garlic oil flavors all of the components for a lovely, cool-weather chicken dinner. Use Brussels sprouts no bigger than golf balls, as larger ones are often tough and woody.

12 ounces red potatoes, unpeeled, cut into 1-inch pieces

12 ounces Brussels sprouts, trimmed and halved

4 carrots, peeled, cut into 2-inch pieces, thick ends halved lengthwise

¼ cup garlic oil (see page 20), divided

4 teaspoons minced fresh thyme or 1½ teaspoons dried, divided

2 teaspoons minced fresh rosemary or ½ teaspoon dried, divided

4 (5- to 7-ounce) bone-in chicken thighs, trimmed

¾ teaspoon table salt, divided

⅛ teaspoon plus ¼ teaspoon pepper, divided

1 teaspoon sugar

1 Adjust oven rack to upper-middle position and heat oven to 475 degrees. Toss potatoes, Brussels sprouts, and carrots with 2 tablespoons oil, half the thyme, and half the rosemary in bowl. Toss chicken with remaining 2 tablespoons oil, remaining thyme, remaining rosemary, ¼ teaspoon salt, and ⅛ teaspoon pepper in second bowl.

2 Spread vegetables in single layer on rimmed baking sheet, discarding any excess liquid and arranging Brussels sprouts cut sides down in center. Sprinkle vegetables with sugar, remaining ½ teaspoon salt, and remaining ¼ teaspoon pepper.

3 Place chicken thighs skin side up on top of vegetables around perimeter of sheet. Roast until chicken registers 175 degrees, 35 to 40 minutes, rotating sheet halfway through roasting.

4 Transfer chicken to serving platter, tent with aluminum foil, and let rest while finishing vegetables. Return vegetables to oven and continue to roast until lightly browned, 5 to 10 minutes. Toss vegetables with any accumulated chicken juices and transfer to platter with chicken. Serve.

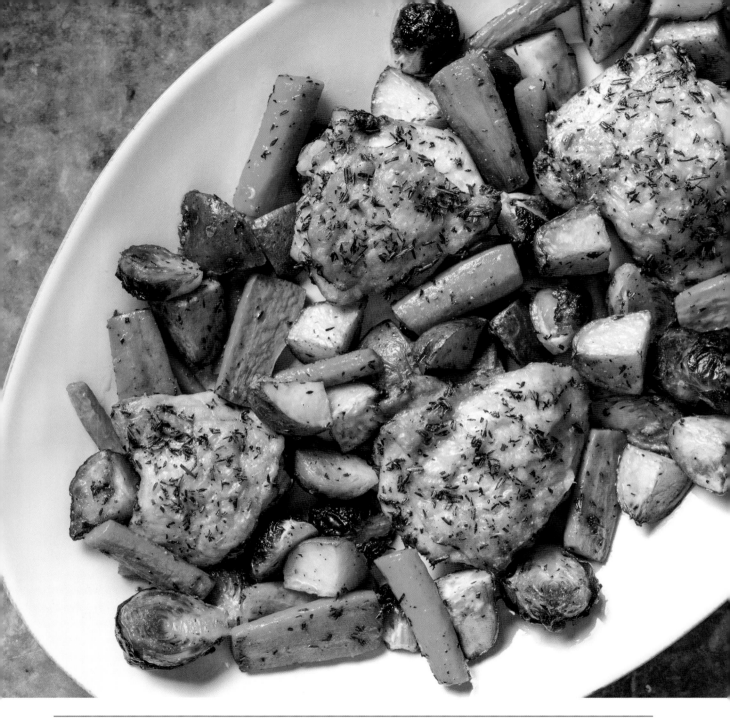

PER SERVING

Dietary Fiber 7g **Cal** 520;
Total Fat 35g; **Sat Fat** 8g;
Chol 120mg; **Sodium** 620mg;
Total Carb 29g, **Total Sugars** 7g,
Added Sugars 1g; **Protein** 25g

 MAKE IT LOW FODMAP Omit Brussels sprouts and increase carrots to 6; spread vegetable mixture evenly on baking sheet.

CHICKEN MOLE WITH CILANTRO-LIME RICE AND BEANS

SERVES 4

WHY THIS RECIPE WORKS Sauces might scare those cooking for their gut health—they can be overly rich, or allium- or dairy-heavy—but a deeply flavored Mexican mole is not only a treat but very practical when eating for your gut. There's plenty of flavor without any offending ingredients. Moles take many, many forms depending on the region they come from, but they typically gain complexity from dried chiles and long, slow cooking. The sauce here is decidedly quick—but it gives you the fruity, nutty, spicy flavors that moles carry with chili powder, cocoa powder, tomato, and raisins, plus peanut butter for thickening. The flavors of this lush sauce imbue chicken thighs as they simmer to tenderness. We turn this chicken dish into a full, fiberful meal by serving it with brown rice and black beans that bake in the oven while the chicken simmers on the stove. We fluff in some cilantro and lime zest to make it a lively side. For an accurate measurement of boiling water, bring a full kettle of water to a boil and then measure out the desired amount.

2⅓ cups plus ¾ cup boiling water, divided

1½ cups long-grain brown rice, rinsed

4 teaspoons vegetable oil, divided

½ teaspoon table salt, divided

3 tablespoons raisins

1 tablespoon chili powder

1 tablespoon unsweetened cocoa powder

1 tomato, cored and chopped

1 tablespoon creamy peanut butter

1 pound boneless, skinless chicken thighs, trimmed

1 (15-ounce) can black beans, rinsed

½ cup chopped fresh cilantro, divided

1 teaspoon lime zest and 1 tablespoon juice, plus lime wedges for serving

1 Adjust oven rack to middle position and heat oven to 375 degrees. Combine 2⅓ cups boiling water, rice, 2 teaspoons oil, and ¼ teaspoon salt in 8-inch square baking dish. Cover dish tightly with aluminum foil and bake until rice is tender and no water remains, about 1 hour.

2 Meanwhile, combine raisins, chili powder, cocoa, and remaining 2 teaspoons oil in small bowl. Microwave, stirring occasionally, until fragrant, 30 to 45 seconds. Process raisin mixture, tomato, peanut butter, remaining ¾ cup water, and remaining ¼ teaspoon salt in blender until smooth, about 1 minute, scraping down sides of blender jar as needed. Transfer puree to 12-inch skillet.

3 Nestle chicken into sauce. Bring to simmer over medium heat, then reduce heat to medium-low, cover, and cook until chicken registers at least 175 degrees, 20 to 25 minutes, flipping chicken halfway through cooking.

4 Remove rice from oven and fluff with fork, scraping up any rice that has stuck to bottom of dish. Add beans in even layer over rice, cover, and let sit until beans are heated through, about 10 minutes.

5 Transfer chicken to cutting board, tent with foil, and let rest while finishing sauce and rice. Return sauce to simmer over medium heat and cook until thickened slightly, about 5 minutes. Whisk sauce to recombine and season with salt and pepper to taste. Add ¼ cup cilantro and lime zest and juice to rice and beans, fluff with fork to combine, and season with salt and pepper to taste. Slice chicken ½ inch thick and serve with rice and beans, sauce, lime wedges, and remaining ¼ cup cilantro.

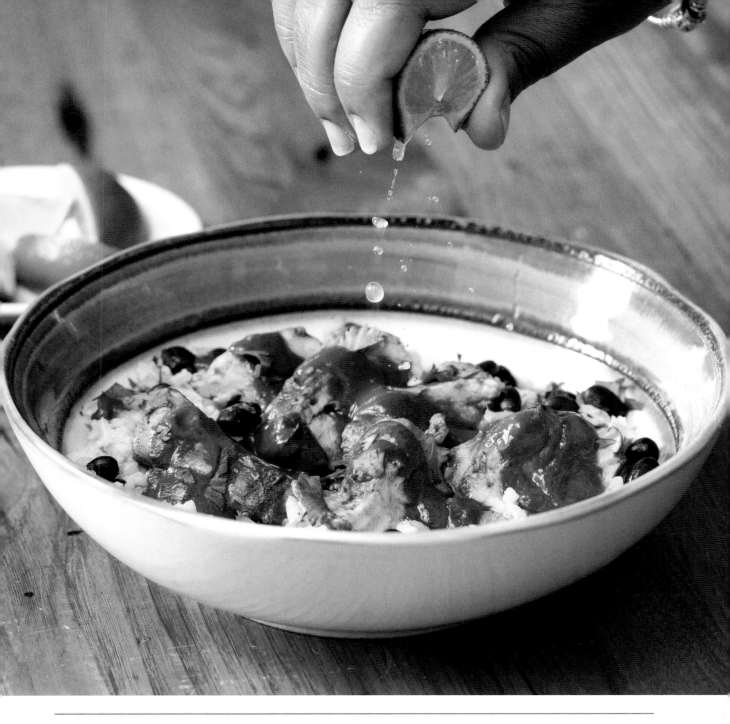

PER SERVING

Dietary Fiber 9g **Cal** 520;
Total Fat 15g, **Sat Fat** 2g;
Chol 105mg; **Sodium** 700mg;
Total Carb 72g, **Total Sugars** 7g,
Added Sugars 0g; **Protein** 32g

 MAKE IT LOW FODMAP Substitute canned lentils for black beans.

STIR-FRIED GINGER-ORANGE CHICKEN AND LONG BEANS

SERVES 4

WHY THIS RECIPE WORKS A stir-fry can be one of the ultimate complete, good-for-you meals: Through the power of high heat, you quickly bring together lean protein and a ton of vegetables for a harmony of flavors and textures. Here, hearty charred long beans, with their meaty, slightly chewy texture, get the spotlight, their trademark earthy flavor brightened with ginger and orange. In addition to the plentiful ginger and orange, toasted sesame oil brings nutty flavor supported also by a sesame seed finish. To make the chicken easier to slice, freeze it for 15 minutes. Long beans are available at most Asian markets. If you can't find them, substitute haricots verts or thin green beans; trim but do not halve. You will need a 12-inch nonstick skillet or 14-inch flat-bottomed wok for this recipe.

½ teaspoon water

⅛ teaspoon baking soda

1 pound boneless, skinless chicken breasts, trimmed, halved lengthwise, and sliced thin crosswise

3 tablespoons soy sauce (see page 18), divided

1 tablespoon Shaoxing wine or dry sherry

½ teaspoon cornstarch

1 tablespoon toasted sesame oil

1 teaspoon grated fresh ginger

½ teaspoon grated orange zest

2 pounds long beans, trimmed and halved

3 tablespoons canola oil, divided

2 teaspoons sesame seeds, toasted

1 Combine water and baking soda in bowl. Add chicken and toss to coat; let sit for 5 minutes. Add 1 tablespoon soy sauce, Shaoxing wine, and cornstarch and toss until well combined; let sit for 15 minutes. Combine sesame oil, ginger, and orange zest in small bowl; set aside.

2 Rinse long beans, but do not dry. Place in large bowl, cover, and microwave until tender, 6 to 12 minutes, tossing every 3 minutes. Transfer long beans to paper towel–lined plate and let drain.

3 Heat 1 tablespoon canola oil in 12-inch nonstick skillet or 14-inch flat-bottomed wok over medium-high heat until just smoking. Add chicken mixture and increase heat to high. Cook, tossing chicken slowly but constantly, until no longer pink, 2 to 6 minutes; transfer to large bowl.

4 Heat 1 tablespoon canola oil in now-empty pan over medium-high heat until just smoking. Add half of long beans and increase heat to high. Cook, tossing slowly but constantly, until green beans are softened and charred, 5 to 10 minutes. Transfer to bowl with chicken and tent with aluminum foil. Repeat with remaining 1 tablespoon canola oil and remaining long beans; transfer to bowl.

5 Add ginger-zest mixture to again-empty pan and cook over medium-high heat, mashing mixture into skillet, until fragrant, about 15 seconds. Add chicken–long bean mixture and remaining 2 tablespoons soy sauce and cook, tossing constantly, until chicken and green beans are well combined and heated through, about 1 minute. Transfer to serving platter and sprinkle with sesame seeds. Serve.

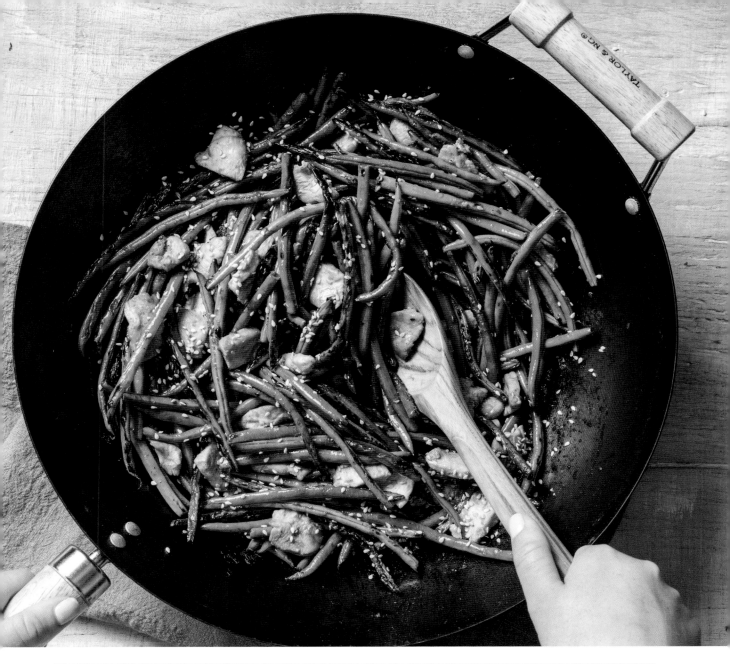

PER SERVING

Dietary Fiber 6g **Cal** 340;
Total Fat 18g, **Sat Fat** 2g;
Chol 85mg; **Sodium** 790mg;
Total Carb 15g, **Total Sugars** 7g,
Added Sugars 0g; **Protein** 31g

LF **MAKE IT LOW FODMAP** Substitute 12 ounces green beans for long beans and cook in 1 batch. Then cook 1 red bell pepper, stemmed, seeded, and sliced thin, with remaining 1 tablespoon oil in empty pan over medium-high heat until tender, about 5 minutes. Transfer to bowl with chicken and beans and proceed with step 5.

GF **MAKE IT GLUTEN FREE** Substitute gluten-free soy sauce or tamari (see page 18) for soy sauce.

GRILLED CHICKEN FAJITAS

SERVES 4

DAIRY FREE

WHY THIS RECIPE WORKS Sweet, crisp, low-FODMAP bell peppers rarely get star status in dishes, usually added with aromatics or as a contrasting stir-in—except in fajitas, where the smoky grilled vegetable is paired with strips of meat (here, chicken) and wrapped in a warm tortilla. Fajitas are either highly flavorful or not at all, and we wanted to achieve the former so we incorporated a lime-and-jalapeño marinade. Do not marinate the chicken for longer than an hour. You can use any color bell peppers in this recipe. Serve the fajitas with your favorite toppings, if desired.

6 tablespoons garlic oil (see page 20), divided

⅓ cup lime juice (3 limes)

1 jalapeño chile, stemmed, seeded, and minced

¼ cup minced fresh cilantro

1 tablespoon soy sauce

1½ teaspoons packed brown sugar

1½ teaspoons table salt, divided

¾ teaspoon pepper

1½ pounds boneless, skinless chicken breasts, trimmed

4 large bell peppers, quartered, stemmed, and seeded

12 (6-inch) 100 percent whole-wheat flour tortillas

4 scallions, green parts only, sliced thin

1 Whisk ¼ cup oil, lime juice, jalapeño, cilantro, soy sauce, sugar, ½ teaspoon salt, and pepper together in bowl. Measure out and reserve ¼ cup marinade separately for serving. Whisk remaining 1 teaspoon salt into remaining marinade and transfer to 1-gallon zipper-lock bag. Cover chicken breasts with plastic wrap and pound to uniform thickness as needed. Add chicken to bag and toss to coat; press out as much air as possible and seal bag. Refrigerate for at least 30 minutes or up to 1 hour, flipping bag every 15 minutes.

2A For a charcoal grill: Open bottom vent completely. Light large chimney starter filled with charcoal briquettes (6 quarts). When top coals are partially covered with ash, pour coals over two-thirds of grill, leaving remaining one-third empty. Set cooking grate in place, cover, and open lid vent completely. Heat grill until hot, about 5 minutes.

2B For a gas grill: Turn all burners to high, cover, and heat grill until hot, about 15 minutes. Leave primary burner on high and turn other burner(s) to medium. (Adjust burners as needed to maintain hot fire and medium fire on separate sides of grill.)

3 Brush bell peppers with remaining 2 tablespoons oil. Clean and oil cooking grate. Remove chicken from marinade and place on hotter side of grill. Place bell peppers on cooler side of grill. Cook (covered if using gas), turning chicken and bell peppers as needed, until chicken is browned and registers 160 degrees and bell peppers are tender and charred in spots, 8 to 12 minutes. Transfer chicken and bell pepper to cutting board as they finish cooking and tent with aluminum foil.

4 Working in batches, grill tortillas, turning as needed, until warm and lightly browned, about 40 seconds; transfer to plate and cover with foil.

5 Slice bell peppers into ¼-inch strips and toss with 2 tablespoons reserved marinade and scallions in bowl. Slice chicken on bias into ¼-inch-thick slices and toss with remaining 2 tablespoons marinade in second bowl. Transfer chicken and vegetables to platter and serve with warmed tortillas.

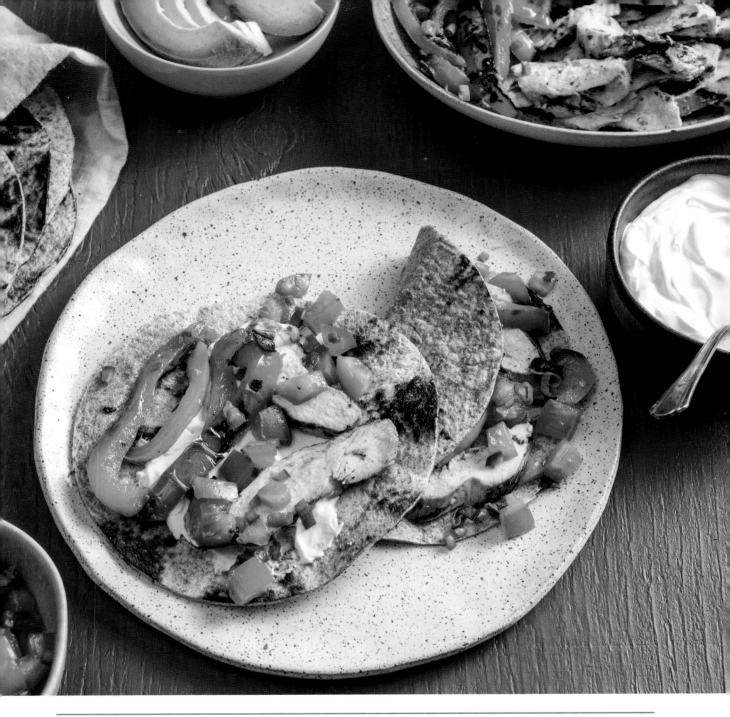

PER SERVING

Dietary Fiber 11g **Cal** 690;
Total Fat 24g, **Sat Fat** 5g;
Chol 125mg; **Sodium** 810mg;
Total Carb 66g, **Total Sugars** 12g,
Added Sugars 1g; **Protein** 49g

 MAKE IT LOW FODMAP Substitute gluten-free or corn tortillas for whole-wheat flour tortillas or serve without tortillas.

 MAKE IT GLUTEN FREE Substitute gluten-free soy sauce or tamari (see page 18) for soy sauce. Substitute gluten-free tortillas for whole-wheat flour tortillas or serve without tortillas.

WEEKNIGHT SKILLET ROAST CHICKEN

SERVES 4 TO 6

WHY THIS RECIPE WORKS For some, roast chicken is one of the most comforting dishes; the chicken's rich flavor and juicy meat need little adornment and pair with most any vegetable, grain, or bean side you can think of (see pages 226–259). But the process of cooking just chicken isn't as simple as we'd like, and recipes often call for brining or salting the bird to ensure juiciness, complicated trussing techniques, and rotating the bird multiple times during cooking. After systematically testing the various components and steps of a typical recipe, we found we could just tie the legs together and tuck the wings underneath. We also discovered we could skip the V-rack by using a preheated skillet and placing the chicken breast side up; this method gave the thighs a jump-start on cooking. Starting the chicken in a 450-degree oven and then turning the oven off while the chicken finished cooking slowed the evaporation of juices, ensuring moist, tender meat to serve with sides like Pan-Steamed Kale (page 262) or a richness-cutting Escarole and Orange Salad with Green Olive Vinaigrette (page 274). We prefer to use a 3½- to 4-pound chicken for this recipe. If roasting a larger bird, increase the time when the oven is on in step 2 to 35 to 40 minutes. Serve with one of the sauces on pages 21–25, if desired.

1 tablespoon kosher salt

½ teaspoon pepper

1 (3½- to 4-pound) whole chicken, giblets discarded, brined if desired

1 tablespoon canola oil

1 Adjust oven rack to middle position, place 12-inch ovensafe skillet on rack, and heat oven to 450 degrees. Combine salt and pepper in bowl. Pat chicken dry with paper towels. Rub entire surface with oil. Sprinkle with salt mixture and rub in mixture with hands to coat evenly. Tie legs together with twine and tuck wing tips behind back.

2 Transfer chicken breast side up to hot skillet in oven. Roast chicken until breast registers 120 degrees and thighs register 135 degrees, 25 to 35 minutes. Turn oven off and leave chicken in oven until breast registers 160 degrees and thighs register 175 degrees, 25 to 35 minutes. Transfer chicken to carving board and let rest for 20 minutes. Carve chicken and serve.

PER SERVING

Dietary Fiber 0g **Cal** 300;
Total Fat 17g, **Sat Fat** 5g;
Chol 110mg; **Sodium** 660mg;
Total Carb 0g, **Total Sugars** 0g,
Added Sugars 0g; **Protein** 34g

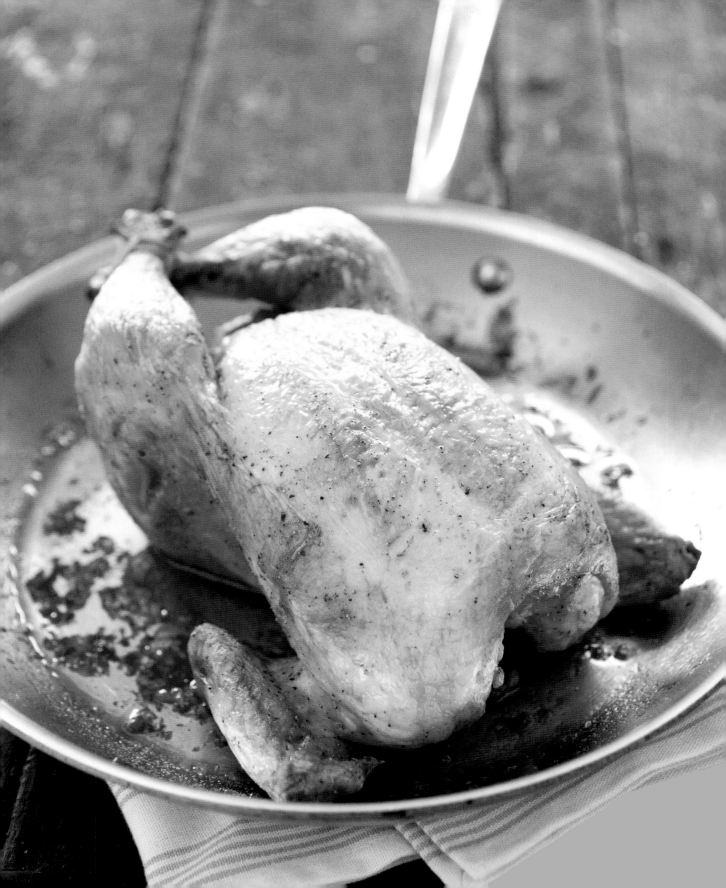

ROAST CHICKEN WITH RAS EL HANOUT AND CARROTS

SERVES 4 TO 6

LOW FODMAP

DAIRY FREE

GLUTEN FREE

WHY THIS RECIPE WORKS Weeknight Skillet Roast Chicken (page 128) gives you room to play with pairings, but we also love roasting chicken on a bed of vegetables. Choosing carrots means you can eat plenty and get fiber even if you follow a low-FODMAP diet. By butterflying the chicken so that it lies flat, we're able to roast it relatively quickly. You might think of onion and garlic aromas when roasting chicken, but allium are unnecessary with the smart rub of ras el hanout and garlic oil that adds sweet, warm spice to the chicken and complements the carrot side. And the carrots truly become a complex accompaniment: Flavored throughout from the spice rub and chicken drippings, they then get a pre-serving toss with bright cilantro and lemon juice to balance their richness.

2 tablespoons ras el hanout

2 tablespoons garlic oil (see page 20), divided

2 teaspoons kosher salt, divided

1 (3½- to 4-pound) whole chicken, giblets discarded

3 pounds carrots, peeled, halved lengthwise, and cut into 2-inch lengths

1 tablespoon minced fresh cilantro

1 teaspoon lemon juice

1 Adjust oven rack to lower-middle position and heat oven to 450 degrees. Combine ras el hanout, 1 tablespoon oil, and 1½ teaspoons salt in bowl. With chicken breast side down on cutting board, use kitchen shears to cut through bones on either side of backbone. Discard backbone and trim away excess fat and skin around neck. Flip chicken, press firmly on breastbone to flatten, then pound breast to be same thickness as legs and thighs.

2 Pat chicken dry with paper towels. Gently loosen skin covering breast and thighs. Rub 2 teaspoons spice mixture underneath skin, then rub remaining spice mixture all over chicken. Tuck wingtips underneath.

3 Toss carrots with remaining 1 tablespoon oil and remaining ½ teaspoon salt in 12-inch ovensafe skillet. Place chicken skin side up on top of carrots. Transfer skillet to oven and roast chicken until breast registers 160 degrees and drumsticks/thighs register 175 degrees, 45 to 60 minutes. (If chicken begins to get too dark, cover loosely with aluminum foil.)

4 Using potholders, remove skillet from oven. Transfer chicken to carving board and let rest while finishing carrots. Being careful of hot skillet handle, return skillet to oven and roast carrots until softened, 12 to 16 minutes. Using slotted spoon, transfer carrots to serving bowl. Add cilantro and lemon juice and gently toss to coat. Season with salt and pepper to taste. Carve chicken and serve with carrots.

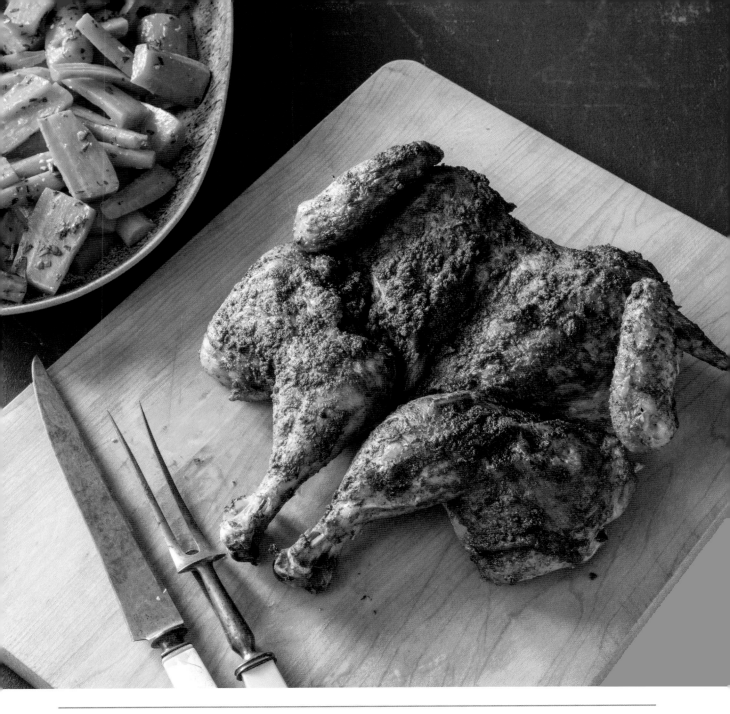

PER SERVING

Dietary Fiber 6g **Cal** 430;
Total Fat 22g, **Sat Fat** 6g;
Chol 110mg; **Sodium** 620mg;
Total Carb 20g, **Total Sugars** 10g,
Added Sugars 0g; **Protein** 36g

SUPER COBB SALAD

SERVES 4

WHY THIS RECIPE WORKS Stunning presentation aside, Cobb salad has all the markers of a powerhouse meal, including protein-rich eggs and lean chicken, high-fiber avocado, and nutritious tomato. Less great for digestion: all that bacon and cheese. We were sad to sacrifice bacon's smoky flavor until we tried sautéing shiitake mushrooms with smoked paprika and chili powder. This made mushroom marvels—mushrooms that were smoky and packed with umami meatiness, a not-at-all-sad substitute for bacon. Using kale (soaked in warm water to soften) in place of the romaine upped the fiber, and radicchio contributed beautiful color. For the dressing, just a bit of blue cheese whisked with yogurt, garlic oil, and lemon juice provided the tangy low-lactose blue cheese flavor we expected—a little of the pungent cheese goes a long way. We tossed some dressing with our greens and drizzled the rest over our complete mindfully updated Cobb salad.

12 ounces boneless, skinless chicken breasts, trimmed

¾ teaspoon table salt, divided

¼ teaspoon pepper, divided

4 teaspoons garlic oil (see page 20), divided

10 ounces shiitake mushrooms, stemmed and sliced thin

⅛ teaspoon smoked paprika

8 ounces kale, stemmed and cut into 1-inch pieces (8 cups)

¾ cup plain yogurt

¼ cup crumbled blue cheese

1 tablespoon lemon juice

½ small head radicchio (3 ounces), cored and cut into ½-inch pieces

3 hard-cooked large eggs, quartered

2 avocados, halved, pitted, and cut into ½-inch pieces

6 ounces cherry tomatoes, halved

1 Cover chicken breasts with plastic wrap and pound to uniform thickness as needed. Pat chicken dry with paper towels and sprinkle with ¼ teaspoon salt and ⅛ teaspoon pepper. Heat 1 teaspoon oil in 10-inch skillet over medium-high heat until just smoking. Brown chicken well on first side, about 6 minutes. Flip chicken, add ¼ cup water, and cover. Reduce heat to medium-low and continue to cook until chicken registers 160 degrees, 5 to 7 minutes.

2 Transfer chicken to cutting board, tent with aluminum foil, and let rest for 5 minutes. Cut chicken into ½-inch-thick slices; set aside.

3 Heat 2 teaspoons oil in now-empty skillet over medium heat until shimmering. Add mushrooms and ¼ teaspoon salt, cover, and cook until mushrooms have released their liquid, 4 to 6 minutes. Uncover and increase heat to medium-high. Stir in paprika and remaining ⅛ teaspoon pepper and cook until mushrooms are golden, 4 to 6 minutes. Transfer to plate and let cool.

4 Place kale in large bowl and cover with warm tap water (110 to 115 degrees). Swish kale around to remove grit. Let kale sit in warm water bath for 10 minutes. Remove kale from water and spin dry in salad spinner in multiple batches. Pat leaves dry with paper towels if still wet.

5 Whisk yogurt, blue cheese, lemon juice, remaining 2 teaspoons oil, and remaining ¼ teaspoon salt in bowl until well combined. Adjust consistency with water and season with salt and pepper to taste.

6 Toss kale and radicchio with ½ cup dressing to coat. Transfer to serving platter and mound in even layer. Arrange chicken, cooled mushrooms, eggs, avocado, and tomatoes in rows over greens. Drizzle remaining dressing over salad. Serve.

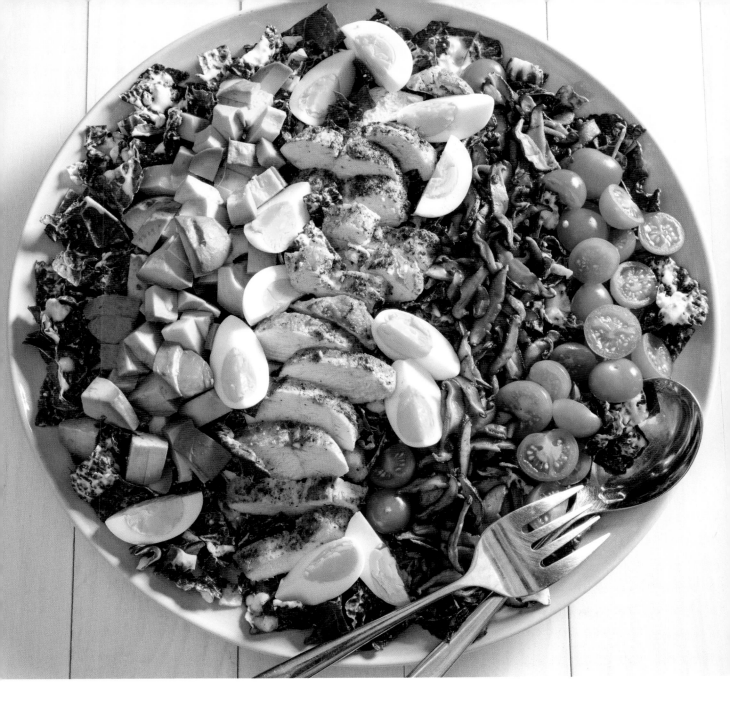

PER SERVING

Dietary Fiber 11g Cal 490;
Total Fat 29g, **Sat Fat** 6g;
Chol 210mg; **Sodium** 670mg;
Total Carb 25g, **Total Sugars** 8g,
Added Sugars 0g; **Protein** 34g

LF **MAKE IT LOW FODMAP** Substitute oyster mushrooms, trimmed and cut into 1-inch pieces, for shiitakes. Substitute dairy-free or lactose-free yogurt (see page 19) for plain yogurt. Omit avocado and increase tomatoes to 12 ounces.

DF **MAKE IT DAIRY FREE** Substitute dairy-free yogurt (see page 19) for plain yogurt and omit blue cheese.

CHOPPED SALAD WITH CHICKEN AND JÍCAMA

SERVES 4

WHY THIS RECIPE WORKS A great chopped salad is a lively mix of lettuce, vegetables, fruit, nuts, and cheese, offering a variety of tastes and textures, plus visual appeal. Unfortunately, the ingredients in most collections are often haphazardly selected or high in FODMAPs. We wanted to make careful selections of ingredients for a superlative salad that anyone could enjoy. Crisp, slightly sweet jícama, pleasantly bitter escarole, and juicy seared-then-poached chicken formed the bulk of our salad. For a fruity addition, grapes paired well, and some goat cheese—which despite being pleasantly creamy is perfectly low in lactose in normal servings—added richness and tang. Light and fresh were our aims, so we made an assertive dressing with a ratio that tipped toward the vinegar. Fresh tarragon perfumed the salad with its unique aroma.

12 ounces boneless, skinless chicken breasts, trimmed

¾ teaspoon table salt, divided

⅛ teaspoon pepper

4 teaspoons extra-virgin olive oil, divided

2 ounce goat cheese, crumbled (½ cup)

3 tablespoons cider vinegar

2 tablespoons minced fresh tarragon

1 pound jícama, peeled and cut into ½-inch pieces

1 head escarole (1 pound), trimmed and sliced ½ inch thick

8 ounces red or green grapes, halved

1 Cover chicken breasts with plastic wrap and pound to uniform thickness as needed. Pat chicken dry with paper towels and sprinkle with ¼ teaspoon salt and pepper. Heat 1 teaspoon oil in 10-inch skillet over medium-high heat until just smoking. Brown chicken well on first side, about 6 minutes. Flip chicken, add ¼ cup water, and cover. Reduce heat to medium-low and continue to cook until chicken registers 160 degrees, 5 to 7 minutes.

2 Transfer chicken to cutting board, let cool slightly, then cut into ½-inch pieces.

3 Whisk goat cheese, vinegar, tarragon, remaining 1 tablespoon oil, and remaining ½ teaspoon salt together in large bowl. Add chicken, jícama, escarole, and grapes and toss to combine. Season with salt and pepper to taste. Serve.

PER SERVING

Dietary Fiber 9g **Cal** 280;
Total Fat 10g, **Sat Fat** 3.5g;
Chol 70mg; **Sodium** 570mg;
Total Carb 23g, **Total Sugars** 11g,
Added Sugars 0g; **Protein** 24g

 MAKE IT DAIRY FREE Omit goat cheese.

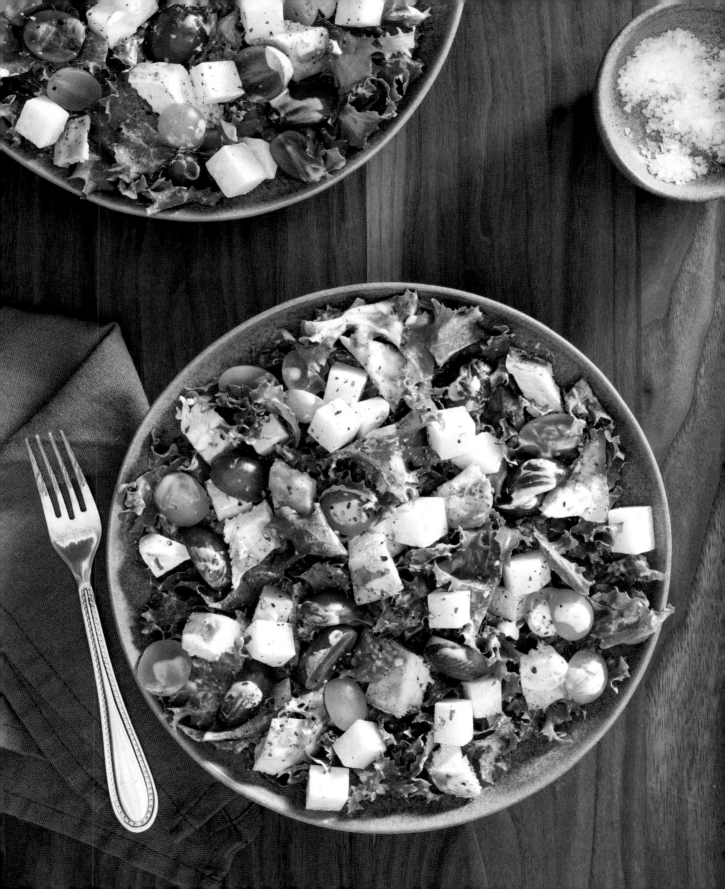

BLACK RICE AND CHICKEN SALAD WITH SNAP PEAS AND GINGER-SESAME VINAIGRETTE

SERVES 4

WHY THIS RECIPE WORKS Rice salad is good for reaching fiber and nutrition goals but still not our go-to grain salad—unless the rice is black. The ancient grain has a roasted, nutty taste and so it should be paired with lively ingredients like the fresh snap peas and gingery vinaigrette in this salad. The most foolproof method for making black rice is to cook it like pasta in lots of boiling water, giving it space to move around. Once it's done, we drain it, drizzle it with vinegar so it absorbs flavor, and let it cool completely on a baking sheet so the grains have the expected chew and no mushiness. Wild rice can be substituted for the black rice; increase cook time to 45 to 55 minutes. You can substitute snow peas for the sugar snap peas; incorporate them raw, with the bell pepper and radishes.

1½ cups black rice

¾ teaspoon table salt, divided, plus salt for cooking rice

¼ cup plus 1 teaspoon rice vinegar, divided

12 ounces boneless, skinless chicken breasts, trimmed

¼ teaspoon pepper, divided

3 tablespoons plus 1 teaspoon garlic oil (see page 20), divided

1 tablespoon toasted sesame oil

2 teaspoons grated fresh ginger

2 teaspoons honey

6 ounces sugar snap peas, strings removed, halved crosswise

1 red bell pepper, stemmed, seeded, and chopped fine

5 radishes, trimmed, halved, and sliced thin

¼ cup minced fresh cilantro

1 Bring 4 quarts water to boil in large pot over medium-high heat. Add rice and 1 tablespoon salt and cook until rice is tender, 20 to 25 minutes. Drain rice and spread onto rimmed baking sheet, drizzle with 1 teaspoon vinegar, and let cool for 15 minutes.

2 Meanwhile, cover chicken breasts with plastic wrap and pound to uniform thickness as needed. Pat chicken dry with paper towels and sprinkle with ¼ teaspoon salt and ⅛ teaspoon pepper. Heat 1 teaspoon oil in 10-inch skillet over medium-high heat until just smoking. Brown chicken well on first side, about 6 minutes. Flip chicken, add ¼ cup water, and cover. Reduce heat to medium-low and continue to cook until chicken registers 160 degrees, 5 to 7 minutes.

3 Transfer chicken to cutting board, let cool slightly, then shred into bite-size pieces using 2 forks; set aside.

4 Whisk sesame oil, ginger, honey, remaining ¼ cup vinegar, remaining 3 tablespoons garlic oil, remaining ½ teaspoon salt, and remaining ⅛ teaspoon pepper in large bowl. Add cooled rice, chicken, snap peas, bell pepper, radishes, and cilantro and toss to combine. Season with salt and pepper to taste. Serve.

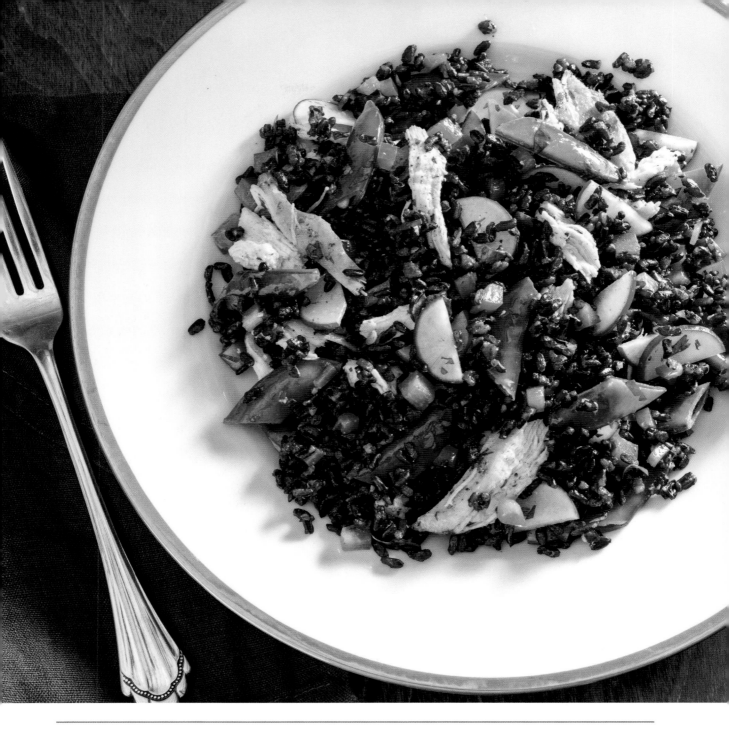

PER SERVING

Dietary Fiber 6g Cal 500;
Total Fat 20g, **Sat Fat** 2.5g;
Chol 60mg; **Sodium** 370mg;
Total Carb 58g, **Total Sugars** 6g,
Added Sugars 3g; **Protein** 27g

 MAKE IT LOW FODMAP Omit snap peas and use
2 bell peppers.

PASTA WITH KALE PESTO, TOMATOES, AND CHICKEN

SERVES 4

WHY THIS RECIPE WORKS Pasta dishes can certainly be gut-friendly for many especially when they're packed with fiber. For a luscious, creamy, bold-flavored pesto pasta with a fiber boost, we took a closer look at what goes into a classic pesto. To give our pesto more body, we deviated from using just traditional basil and added nutrient-rich kale and spinach to the mix. And though we love pine nuts in pesto, we opted for also-earthy roasted sunflower seeds for another slight twist on the classic. The new pesto's flavor stood up to the whole-wheat pasta it napped. But pasta alone isn't a complete meal: Sautéed chicken breasts and cherry tomatoes gave our dish more protein and bulk to ensure it was hearty enough to fill us up without us having to eat a mountain of pasta. You can use 12 ounces of any other 100 percent whole-wheat pasta shape instead of the farfalle, but the cup amount may vary.

1¼ ounces curly kale, stemmed and chopped (¾ cup)

½ cup fresh basil leaves

½ cup baby spinach

3 tablespoons roasted sunflower seeds

1½ tablespoons water

½ teaspoon table salt, divided, plus salt for cooking pasta

5 tablespoons garlic oil (see page 20), divided

¼ cup grated Parmesan cheese, plus extra for serving

1½ pounds boneless, skinless chicken breast, trimmed and cut into 1-inch pieces

¼ teaspoon pepper

12 ounces cherry tomatoes, halved

12 ounces (4½ cups) 100 percent whole-wheat farfalle

1 Process kale, basil, spinach, sunflower seeds, water, and ¼ teaspoon salt in food processor until smooth, about 30 seconds, scraping down sides of bowl as needed. With processor running, slowly add ¼ cup oil until incorporated. Transfer mixture to bowl, stir in Parmesan, and season with pepper to taste. (Pesto can be refrigerated with plastic wrap pressed flush to surface for up to 3 days.)

2 Pat chicken dry with paper towels and sprinkle with remaining ¼ teaspoon salt and pepper. Heat remaining 1 tablespoon oil in 12-inch nonstick skillet over medium-high heat until shimmering. Add chicken and cook, stirring occasionally, until lightly browned all over and cooked through, about 5 minutes. Add cherry tomatoes and cook until softened slightly, about 2 minutes.

3 Meanwhile, bring 4 quarts water to boil in large pot. Add pasta and 1 tablespoon salt and cook, stirring often, until al dente. Reserve ½ cup cooking water, then drain pasta and return it to pot. Add pesto and chicken-tomato mixture and toss to combine. Season with pepper to taste and adjust consistency with reserved cooking water as needed. Serve, passing extra Parmesan separately.

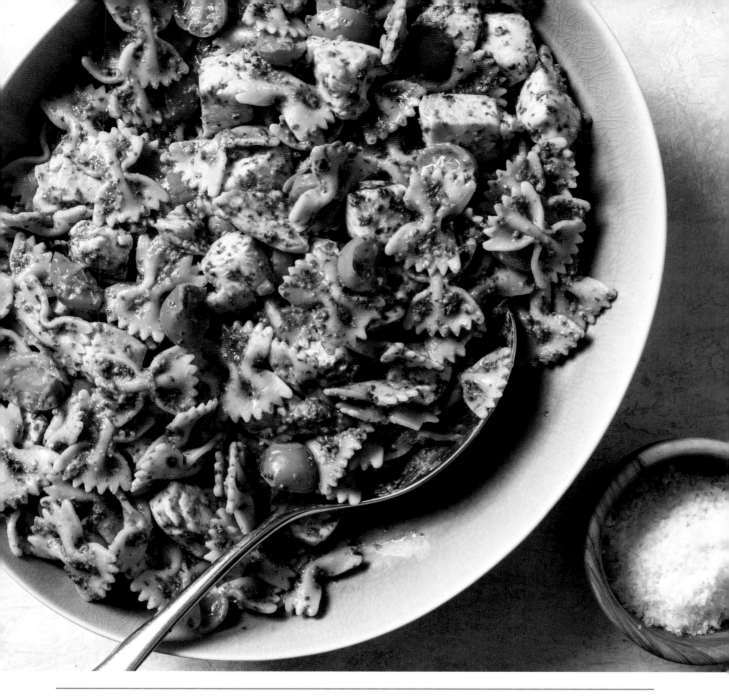

PER SERVING

Dietary Fiber 11g **Cal** 700;
Total Fat 28g, **Sat Fat** 4.5g;
Chol 125mg; **Sodium** 540mg;
Total Carb 58g, **Total Sugars** 4g,
Added Sugars 0g; **Protein** 53g

LF **MAKE IT LOW FODMAP** Substitute gluten-free pasta
(see page 19) for whole-wheat farfalle.

DF **MAKE IT DAIRY FREE** Omit Parmesan and increase sunflower
seeds to ¼ cup. Add 2 teaspoons nutritional yeast to food
processor with seeds.

GF **MAKE IT GLUTEN FREE** Substitute gluten-free pasta
(see page 19) for whole-wheat farfalle.

CHICKEN ENCHILADAS

SERVES 6

WHY THIS RECIPE WORKS You might not know that under the cheese and sauce of chicken enchiladas lives a gut-friendly, low-FODMAP, satisfying dish. It's even more friendly when chicken gets paired with plenty of hearty Swiss chard for a fresh fiber boost. A tomato-based sauce receives instant depth from chipotle chile powder, while boneless, skinless chicken thighs become tender and stay moist as they simmer in the sauce—perfect for shredding. Just a cup of Monterey Jack was plenty to add melty richness inside and on top of the corn tortilla roll-ups. For a milder dish, use the lesser amount of chipotle chile powder.

¼ cup garlic oil
(see page 20), divided

1 pound Swiss chard,
trimmed, stems chopped
fine, and leaves cut into
1-inch pieces

¼ teaspoon table salt

1–2 teaspoons chipotle
chile powder

1 teaspoon ground cumin

1 (15-ounce) can tomato
sauce (see page 18)

1 cup chicken broth
(see page 18)

1 pound boneless, skinless
chicken thighs, trimmed

4 ounces Monterey Jack
cheese, shredded (1 cup),
divided

½ cup plus 2 tablespoons
chopped fresh cilantro,
divided

12 (6-inch) corn tortillas
(see page 19)

Lime wedges

1 Adjust oven rack to middle position and heat oven to 350 degrees. Heat 1 tablespoon oil in Dutch oven over medium heat until shimmering. Add chard stems and salt and cook until softened, about 5 minutes. Stir in chard leaves and cook until tender, 4 to 6 minutes. Transfer to large bowl; set aside.

2 Heat 1 tablespoon oil in now-empty pot over medium heat until shimmering. Add chile powder and cumin and cook until fragrant, about 30 seconds. Stir in tomato sauce and broth, bring to simmer, and cook until slightly thickened, about 5 minutes. Nestle chicken into sauce. Bring to simmer over medium heat, then reduce heat to medium-low, cover, and cook until chicken registers at least 175 degrees, 20 to 25 minutes, flipping chicken halfway through cooking.

3 Transfer chicken to cutting board, let cool slightly, then shred into bite-size pieces using 2 forks. Add chicken, ½ cup sauce from the pot, ½ cup Monterey Jack, and ½ cup cilantro to bowl with chard and stir to combine. Season filling with salt and pepper to taste.

4 Spread ½ cup sauce over bottom of 13 by 9-inch baking dish. Brush both sides of tortillas with remaining 2 tablespoons oil. Stack tortillas, wrap in damp dish towel, and place on plate; microwave until warm and pliable, about 1 minute.

5 Working with 1 warm tortilla at a time, spread ¼ cup filling across center and roll tortilla tightly around filling. Place enchiladas seam side down in baking dish, arranging in 2 columns across width of dish. Pour remaining sauce over top to cover completely and sprinkle remaining ½ cup Monterey Jack down center of enchiladas.

6 Cover dish tightly with aluminum foil and bake until enchiladas are heated through and cheese is melted, about 20 minutes. Remove dish from oven and let cool for 10 minutes. Sprinkle with remaining 2 tablespoons cilantro and serve with lime wedges.

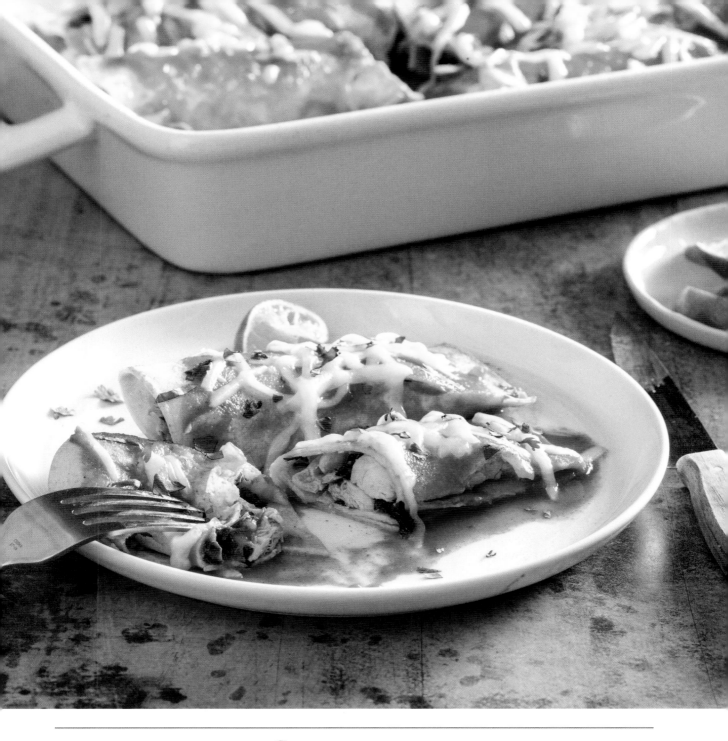

PER SERVING

Dietary Fiber 6g **Cal** 380;
Total Fat 21g, **Sat Fat** 5g;
Chol 90mg; **Sodium** 570mg;
Total Carb 29g, **Total Sugars** 4g,
Added Sugars 0g; **Protein** 24g

DF **MAKE IT DAIRY FREE** Omit Monterey Jack cheese.

TURKEY MEATBALLS WITH LEMONY WILD RICE AND ARTICHOKES

SERVES 4

DAIRY
FREE

WHY THIS RECIPE WORKS Think beyond pasta when serving meatballs for a simple, pleasing meal full of nutrition, like this skillet of turkey meatballs and wild rice. Both ground turkey and brown rice can be mild mannered, so we use lots of aromatic lemon (both zest and juice) and garlic oil in this one-skillet dish. Cooking the wild rice in a combination of chicken broth and water intensifies its richness and adds meaty backbone. Artichokes are an excellent vegetable addition, adding more bulk and fiber. Sweet cherry tomatoes contrast the brown rice and artichokes' earthiness; we scatter them atop the finished dish for a beautiful pop of red color and bright flavor. Be sure to use ground turkey, not ground turkey breast (also labeled 99 percent fat-free), in this recipe. Ground chicken can be substituted for the ground turkey.

½ cup 100 percent whole-wheat panko bread crumbs

1 large egg

¼ cup chopped fresh parsley

2 teaspoons grated lemon zest, divided, plus 2 tablespoons juice

½ teaspoon table salt, divided

½ teaspoon pepper

1 pound 93 percent lean ground turkey

2 tablespoons garlic oil (see page 20)

2 cups chicken broth (see page 18)

2 cups water

1 cup wild rice

8 ounces frozen artichoke hearts, thawed, patted dry, and quartered

6 ounces cherry tomatoes, halved

1 Combine panko, egg, 2 tablespoons parsley, 1½ teaspoons lemon zest, ¼ teaspoon salt, and pepper in large bowl. Add turkey and, using your hands, gently knead mixture until combined. Using wet hands, roll heaping tablespoons of mixture into meatballs and transfer to baking sheet. (You should have 20 meatballs.) Cover and refrigerate for 15 minutes.

2 Heat oil in 12-inch nonstick skillet over medium-high heat until shimmering. Brown meatballs on all sides, 5 to 7 minutes; transfer to paper towel–lined plate.

3 Add broth, water, remaining ½ teaspoon lemon zest and juice, and remaining ¼ teaspoon salt to now-empty skillet and bring to boil over medium-high heat. Stir in rice and return to boil. Reduce heat to medium-low, cover, and simmer for 40 minutes.

4 Stir in artichokes, then nestle meatballs into rice. Cover and cook until rice is tender and meatballs are cooked through, about 15 minutes. Scatter tomatoes over top, sprinkle with remaining 2 tablespoons parsley, and season with salt and pepper to taste. Serve.

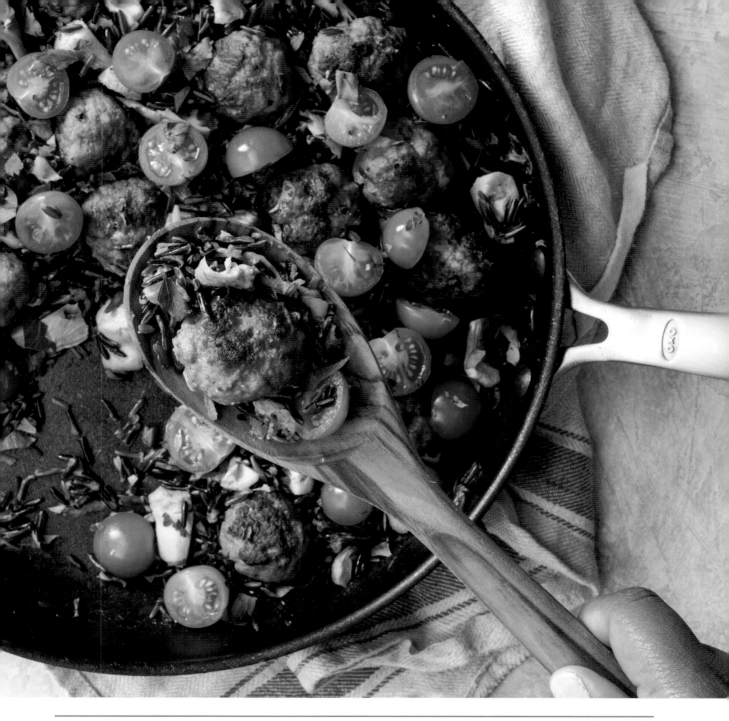

PER SERVING

Dietary Fiber 9g **Cal** 480;
Total Fat 12g, **Sat Fat** 3g;
Chol 90mg; **Sodium** 720mg;
Total Carb 56g, **Total Sugars** 4g,
Added Sugars 0g; **Protein** 41g

LF **MAKE IT LOW FODMAP** Omit artichoke hearts. Substitute gluten-free panko for whole-wheat panko. Before topping rice with tomatoes and parsley, fold in 4 cups baby arugula.

GF **MAKE IT GLUTEN FREE** Substitute gluten-free panko for whole-wheat panko.

TURKEY BURGERS

SERVES 4

WHY THIS RECIPE WORKS A lean, flavorful turkey burger is a classic, healthier alternative to a beef burger, but it has a bit of a second-best reputation. We wanted to create a satisfying patty that was as good as any beef burger. To start, we surveyed the ground turkey sold in supermarkets and found a few kinds: ground white meat, ground dark meat, and 93 percent lean ground turkey. We much preferred the cleaner flavor of 93 percent lean ground turkey so we made up for lost richness by incorporating some melted butter, which also ensured moist, juicy burgers. A little bit of Worcestershire and Dijon added plenty of flavor and a pleasant tang to the mild meat. We provide instructions for a grill or skillet so you can make these burgers anywhere, anytime, any season. Be sure to use ground turkey, not ground turkey breast (also labeled 99 percent fat-free), in this recipe.

1½ pounds 93 percent lean ground turkey

2 tablespoons unsalted butter, melted and cooled

2 teaspoons soy sauce

2 teaspoons Dijon mustard

¼ teaspoon table salt

¼ teaspoon pepper

2 teaspoons canola oil, if using skillet

4 thin slices deli sharp cheddar cheese

4 100 percent whole-wheat hamburger buns, lightly toasted

1 avocado, halved, pitted, and sliced ¼ inch thick

4 green leaf lettuce leaves

1 tomato, cored and sliced ¼ inch thick

1 Break ground turkey into small pieces in large bowl. Add melted butter, soy sauce, and mustard and gently knead with hands until well combined. Divide mixture into 4 equal portions, then gently shape each into ¾-inch-thick patty. Using your fingertips, press center of each patty down until about ½ inch thick, creating slight divot.

2A For a skillet: Sprinkle patties with salt and pepper. Heat oil in 12-inch skillet over medium heat until just smoking. Transfer patties to skillet divot side up and cook until well browned on first side, 4 to 6 minutes. Flip patties, top with cheese, and continue to cook until browned on second side and meat registers 160 degrees, 5 to 7 minutes. Transfer burgers to platter and let rest for 5 minutes.

2B For a charcoal grill: Open bottom vent completely. Light large chimney starter filled with charcoal briquettes (6 quarts). When top coals are partially covered with ash, pour evenly over grill. Set cooking grate in place, cover, and open lid vent completely. Heat grill until hot, about 5 minutes. Clean and oil cooking grate. Sprinkle patties with salt and pepper. Place patties on grill divot side up and cook until well browned on first side and meat easily releases from grill, 4 to 6 minutes. Flip patties, top with cheese, and continue to cook until browned on second side and meat registers 160 degrees, 5 to 7 minutes. Transfer burgers to platter and let rest for 5 minutes.

2C For a gas grill: Turn all burners to high, cover, and heat grill until hot, about 15 minutes. Turn all burners to medium. Clean and oil cooking grate. Sprinkle patties with salt and pepper. Place patties on grill divot side up and cook until well browned on first side and meat easily releases from grill, 4 to 6 minutes. Flip patties, top with cheese, and continue to cook until browned on second side and meat registers 160 degrees, 5 to 7 minutes. Transfer burgers to platter and let rest for 5 minutes.

3 Serve burgers on buns topped with avocado, lettuce, and tomato.

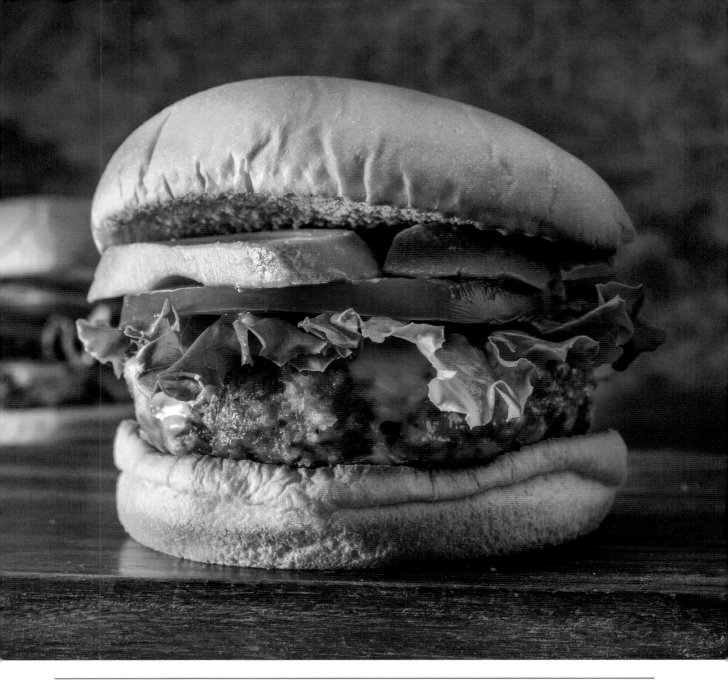

PER SERVING

Dietary Fiber 7g **Cal** 590;
Total Fat 28g, **Sat Fat** 14g;
Chol 115mg; **Sodium** 720mg;
Total Carb 30g, **Total Sugars** 4g,
Added Sugars 0g; **Protein** 51g

LF **MAKE IT LOW FODMAP** Omit bun or substitute low-FODMAP bread. Reduce avocado to ½ (4 ounces).

DF **MAKE IT DAIRY FREE** Omit cheddar. Substitute 1 tablespoon canola oil for melted butter.

GF **MAKE IT GLUTEN FREE** Substitute gluten-free soy sauce or tamari for soy sauce. Omit bun or substitute gluten-free bread.

EASY ROAST TURKEY BREAST

SERVES 10 TO 12

WHY THIS RECIPE WORKS Bone-in turkey breasts are an underutilized cut, and a perfectly roasted breast is, of course, a great option for a smaller gathering, especially if your guests prefer white meat, but it also makes great leftovers for healthful sandwiches and salads. Other benefits: A breast requires less cooking time than a whole bird, which can free up your oven for other dishes (maybe Roasted Kabocha Squash with Maple Vinaigrette, page 280, or Baked Wild Rice, page 282). And a breast is much easier to carve than a whole bird. To start, we removed the backbone so that the breast sat flat in the oven for even cooking and to make carving easier. The trick to moist, tender meat, we found, was to use two different oven temperatures. We elevated the breast in a V-rack and started it out in a blazing hot oven to kick-start the browning process. Dropping the temperature to 325 degrees after 30 minutes allowed the meat to gently finish cooking so that it stayed moist. Brining the turkey helped retain moisture too and efficiently seasoned the bird throughout. If using a self-basting turkey (such as a frozen Butterball) or a kosher turkey, do not brine. Serve with one of the sauces on pages 21–25.

1 (5-pound) bone-in turkey breast

¼ cup table salt for brining turkey

1 teaspoon pepper

1 To remove backbone, use kitchen shears to cut through ribs following vertical line of fat where breast meets back, from tapered end of breast to wing joint. Using your hands, bend back away from breast to pop shoulder joint out of socket. With paring knife, cut through joint between bones to separate back from breast; discard backbone. Trim excess fat from breast. Dissolve salt in 4 quarts cold water in large container. Submerge turkey breast in brine, cover, and refrigerate for at least 3 hours or up to 6 hours.

2 Adjust oven rack to middle position and heat oven to 425 degrees. Set V-rack inside roasting pan and spray with canola oil spray. Remove turkey from brine, pat dry with paper towels, and sprinkle with pepper. Place turkey skin side up on prepared V-rack and add 1 cup water to pan. Roast turkey for 30 minutes.

3 Reduce oven temperature to 325 degrees and continue to roast until turkey registers 160 degrees, about 1 hour. Transfer turkey to carving board and let rest for 20 minutes. Carve turkey and serve.

PER SERVING

Dietary Fiber 0g **Cal** 260;
Total Fat 10g, **Sat Fat** 3g;
Chol 100mg; **Sodium** 230mg;
Total Carb 0g, **Added Sugars** 0g,
Total Sugars 0g; **Protein** 39g

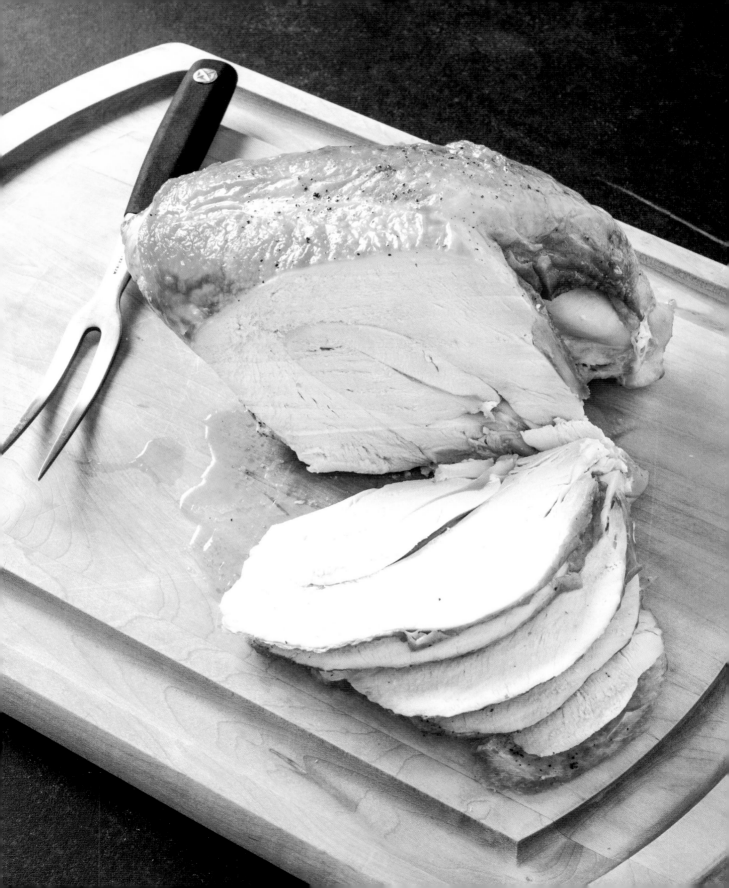

TURKEY SHEPHERD'S PIE

SERVES 6

WHY THIS RECIPE WORKS We wanted to refashion shepherd's pie, not known for its nutrients, into a high-fiber, good-for-your-gut dinner while keeping its hearty comforts. Substituting ground turkey for beef or lamb was a start. We seared mushrooms and tomato paste as the base for a rich gravy, and enriched the gravy with soy sauce (for umami flavor) and carrots (for a touch of natural sweetness)—no flour needed. For a more fiberful topping, we swapped out mashed potatoes for mild, fiber-rich cauliflower and parsnips. Be sure to use ground turkey, not ground turkey breast (also labeled 99 percent fat-free), in this recipe. You will need a 10-inch broiler-safe skillet.

- 3 tablespoons garlic oil (see page 20), divided
- 1 head cauliflower (2 pounds), cored and cut into ½-inch pieces
- 1 pound parsnips, peeled and cut into ½-inch pieces
- ½ cup plus 2 tablespoons water, divided
- ¾ teaspoon table salt, divided
- 1 large egg, lightly beaten
- 3 tablespoons minced fresh chives
- 1 pound 93 percent lean ground turkey
- ¼ teaspoon baking soda
- ¼ teaspoon pepper
- 8 ounces cremini mushrooms, trimmed and chopped
- 1 tablespoon tomato paste
- ¾ cup chicken broth (see page 18)
- 2 carrots, peeled and chopped
- 2 sprigs fresh thyme
- 1 tablespoon soy sauce (see page 18)
- 1 tablespoon cornstarch

1 Heat 2 tablespoons oil in Dutch oven over medium-low heat until shimmering. Add cauliflower and parsnips and cook, stirring occasionally, until softened and beginning to brown, 10 to 12 minutes. Stir in ½ cup water and ½ teaspoon salt, cover, and cook until cauliflower falls apart easily when poked with fork, about 10 minutes.

2 Transfer vegetables and any remaining liquid to food processor and let cool for 5 minutes. Process until smooth, about 45 seconds, scraping down sides of bowl as needed. Transfer to large bowl and stir in egg and chives; set aside.

3 Meanwhile, toss turkey, 1 tablespoon water, baking soda, remaining ¼ teaspoon salt, and pepper in bowl until thoroughly combined. Set aside for 20 minutes.

4 Heat remaining 1 tablespoon oil in 10-inch broiler-safe skillet over medium heat until shimmering. Add mushrooms and cook until liquid has evaporated and fond begins to form on bottom of skillet, 10 to 12 minutes. Stir in tomato paste and cook until bottom of skillet is dark brown, about 2 minutes. Stir in broth, scraping up any browned bits. Stir in carrots, thyme sprigs, and soy sauce, bring to simmer, and reduce heat to medium-low. Pinch off turkey in ½-inch pieces and add to skillet. Bring to gentle simmer, cover, and cook until turkey is cooked through, 8 to 10 minutes, stirring and breaking up meat into small pieces halfway through cooking.

5 Whisk cornstarch and remaining 1 tablespoon water together, then stir mixture into filling and continue to simmer until thickened, about 1 minute. Discard thyme sprigs and season with pepper to taste.

6 Adjust oven rack 5 inches from broiler element and heat broiler. Transfer vegetable mixture to 1-gallon zipper-lock bag. Using scissors, snip 1 inch off filled corner. Squeezing bag, pipe mixture in even layer over filling, making sure to cover entire surface. Smooth mixture with back of spoon, then use tines of fork to make ridges over surface. Place skillet on aluminum foil–lined rimmed baking sheet and broil until topping is golden brown and crusty and filling is bubbly, 10 to 15 minutes. Let cool for 10 minutes before serving.

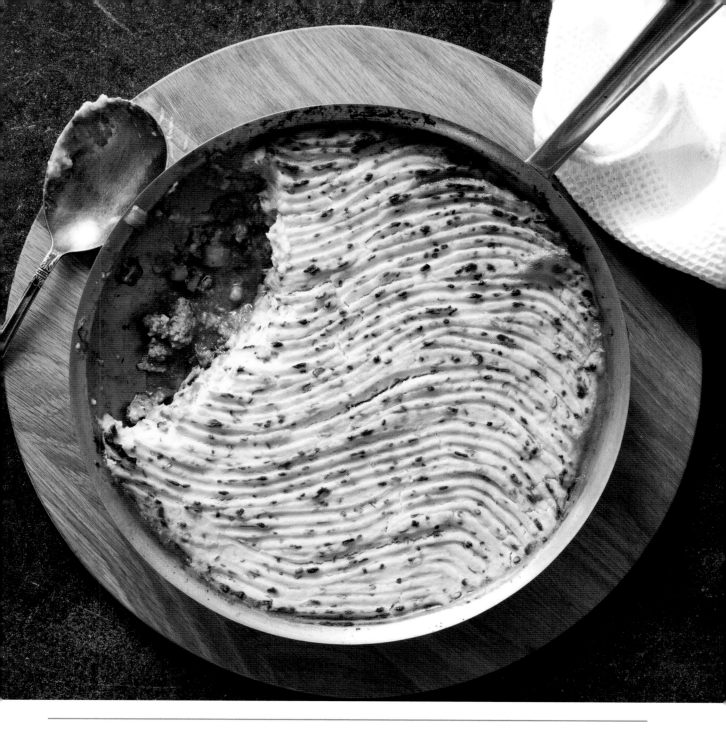

PER SERVING

Dietary Fiber 8g Cal 370;
Total Fat 14g, Sat Fat 4g;
Chol 90mg; Sodium 730mg;
Total Carb 29g, Total Sugars 11g,
Added Sugars 0g; Protein 35g

FARFALLE WITH BROCCOLI AND TURKEY SAUSAGE

SERVES 4

WHY THIS RECIPE WORKS Folded farfalle pasta is ideal for cradling chunky (read: hearty, good-for-you) ingredients, like the broccoli and turkey sausage in this preparation. We cook the pasta in the water used for cooking the broccoli, which makes the prep quite convenient. Turkey sausage often includes allium ingredients like garlic and onion or their respective powders, so we create our own flavored turkey sausage with just the spices. Including fresh fennel in addition to the ground fennel seed in the turkey mixture really drives home the sweet Italian sausage flavor and ups the fiber content. And paprika gives the sausage the smoky quality at home. Tossing the sausage, broccoli, and pasta with Parmesan and a bit of cooking water brings a touch of creamy consistency to the finished fiberful, deceptively healthful dish. Be sure to use ground turkey, not ground turkey breast (also labeled 99 percent fat-free), in this recipe. Ground chicken can be substituted for the ground turkey. You can use 12 ounces of any other 100 percent whole-wheat pasta shape instead of farfalle, but the cup amount may vary.

⅓ cup garlic oil (see page 20)

1 fennel bulb, 1 teaspoon fronds minced, stalks discarded, bulb halved, cored, and sliced thin

¾ teaspoon table salt, divided, plus salt for cooking broccoli and pasta

¼ teaspoon pepper

8 ounces 93 percent lean ground turkey

½ teaspoon ground fennel

¼ teaspoon dried thyme

¼ teaspoon smoked paprika

12 ounces broccoli florets, cut into 1½-inch pieces

12 ounces (3¾ cups) 100 percent whole-wheat farfalle

1 ounce Parmesan cheese, grated (½ cup)

1 Heat oil in 12-inch nonstick skillet over medium heat until shimmering. Add sliced fennel, ½ teaspoon salt, and pepper and cook until softened and lightly browned, 8 to 10 minutes.

2 Increase heat to medium-high. Add turkey and cook, breaking up pieces with wooden spoon, until no longer pink and just beginning to brown, 3 to 4 minutes. Stir in ground fennel, thyme, and paprika and cook until fragrant, about 30 seconds.

3 Meanwhile, bring 4 quarts water to boil in large pot. Add broccoli and 1 tablespoon salt and cook, stirring often, until crisp-tender, about 2 minutes. Using slotted spoon, transfer broccoli to skillet with turkey mixture.

4 Return water to boil, add pasta, and cook, stirring often, until al dente. Reserve 1 cup cooking water, then drain pasta and return pasta to pot. Add fennel fronds, turkey-broccoli mixture, ⅓ cup reserved cooking water, Parmesan, and remaining ¼ teaspoon salt and toss to combine. Season with salt and pepper to taste and adjust consistency with remaining ⅔ cup reserved cooking water as needed. Serve.

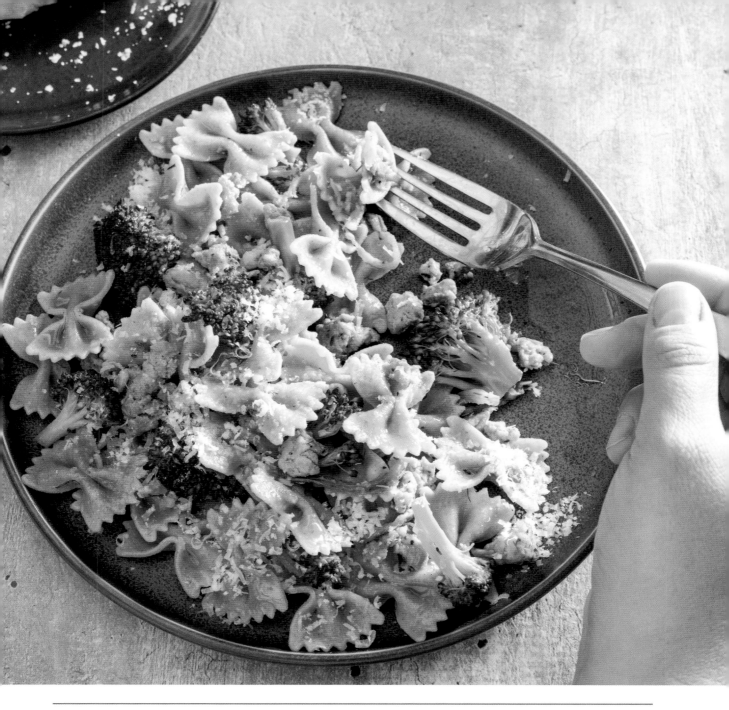

PER SERVING

Dietary Fiber 12g **Cal** 600;
Total Fat 24g, **Sat Fat** 4g;
Chol 30mg; **Sodium** 690mg;
Total Carb 71g, **Total Sugars** 6g,
Added Sugars 0g; **Protein** 32g

LF **MAKE IT LOW FODMAP** Substitute gluten-free pasta (see page 19) for farfalle.

DF **MAKE IT DAIRY FREE** Omit Parmesan cheese.

GF **MAKE IT GLUTEN FREE** Substitute gluten-free pasta (see page 19) for farfalle.

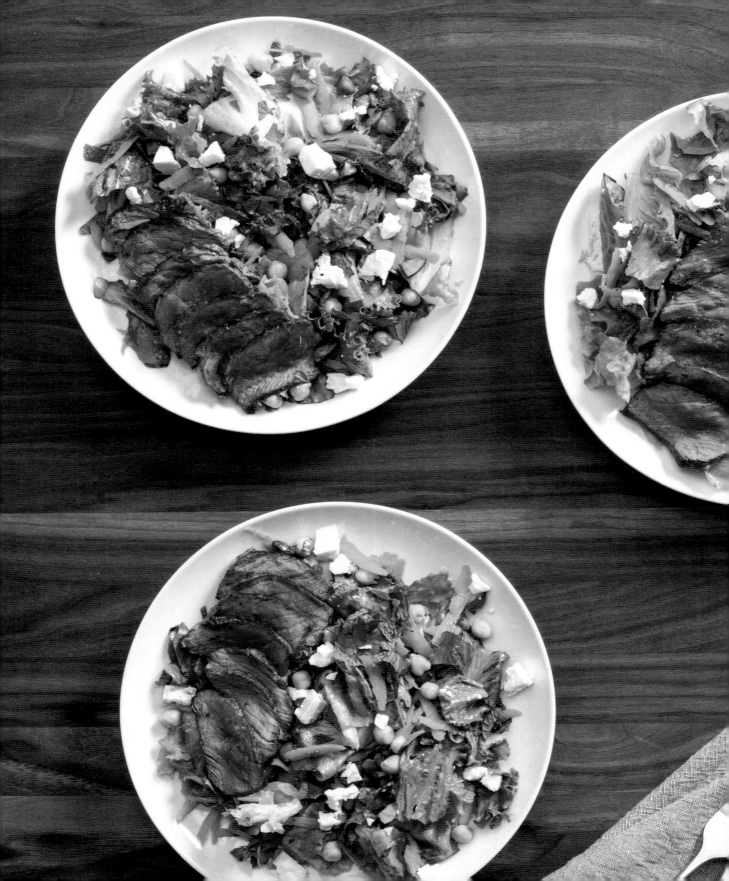

4 Beef & Pork

FLANK STEAK WITH PARSNIPS AND BABY KALE

SERVES 4

WHY THIS RECIPE WORKS A thin cut of juicy steak with a side of crisped potatoes and a zesty horseradish sauce is a comforting bistro dish, and while potatoes are high in fiber, we could go higher: In this nutritious spin we swap in hearty parsnips, a low-FODMAP vegetable that also has a remarkable amount of fiber, contributing to a dish with an impressive 10 grams. We were able to use one pan to cook our flank steak and parsnips, which makes this a weeknight-friendly dish as well. Cooking the steak first allows the savory rendered bits of meat and juices to permeate the sweet parsnips (which we had parcooked in the microwave to hasten the pan cooking). The pan-roasting enhances the parsnips' nutty flavor, and for extra seasoning we add fresh rosemary and garlic oil. Just before serving, we fold in a generous portion of baby kale. We keep the creamy, piquant sauce element—we love how horseradish not only cuts the richness of the steak but offsets the sweetness of the parsnips—but make it deceivingly healthful with Greek yogurt.

¼ cup plain Greek yogurt

1 tablespoon prepared horseradish, drained

1 tablespoon whole-grain mustard

1 teaspoon table salt, divided

¾ teaspoon pepper, divided

2 pounds parsnips, peeled and cut into ½-inch pieces

2 tablespoons water

1 (1-pound) flank steak, trimmed

3 tablespoons garlic oil (see page 20), divided

1 tablespoon minced fresh rosemary

3 ounces (3 cups) baby kale, chopped coarse

1 Whisk yogurt, horseradish, mustard, ¼ teaspoon salt, and ¼ teaspoon pepper together in small bowl; set aside for serving.

2 Microwave parsnips and water in large covered bowl, stirring occasionally, until parsnips are tender, 9 to 14 minutes. Drain parsnips; set aside.

3 Cut steak in half with grain. Pat steaks dry with paper towels, then sprinkle with ¼ teaspoon salt and ¼ teaspoon pepper. Heat 1 tablespoon oil in 12-inch nonstick skillet over medium-high heat until just smoking. Cook steaks until well browned and meat registers 120 to 125 degrees (for medium-rare) or 130 to 135 degrees (for medium), 3 to 6 minutes per side, reducing heat as needed to prevent scorching. Transfer steaks to cutting board, tent with aluminum foil, and let rest while finishing parsnips.

4 Heat 1 tablespoon oil in now-empty skillet over medium-high heat until shimmering. Add parsnips, remaining ½ teaspoon salt, and remaining ¼ teaspoon pepper and cook, stirring occasionally, until parsnips are lightly browned, 8 to 10 minutes.

5 Push parsnips to sides of skillet. Add rosemary and remaining 1 tablespoon oil to center of skillet and cook until fragrant, 15 to 30 seconds. Stir rosemary mixture into parsnips. Stir kale into parsnips, 1 handful at a time, until wilted, about 2 minutes. Season with salt and pepper to taste. Slice steak thin against grain on bias and serve with parsnip mixture and horseradish sauce.

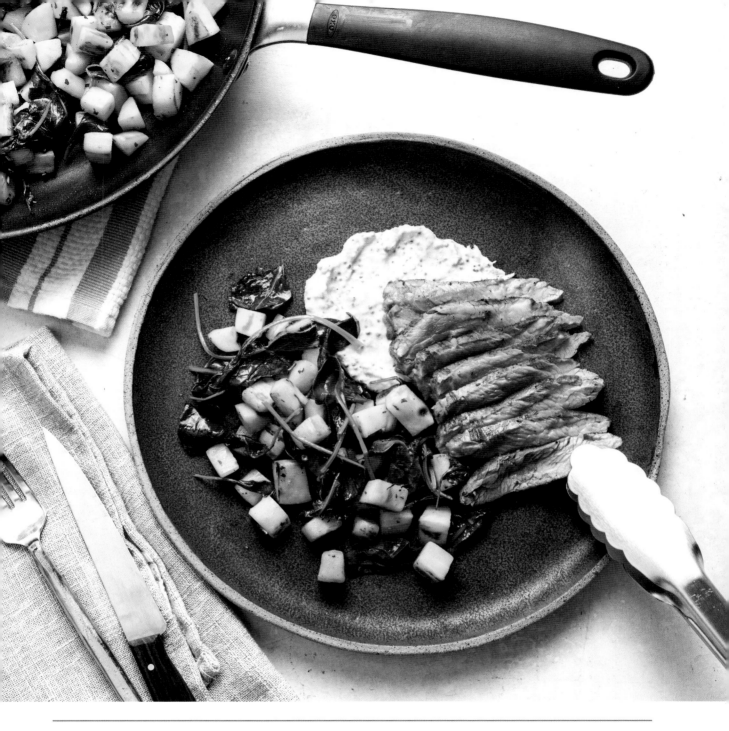

PER SERVING

Dietary Fiber 10g **Cal** 470;
Total Fat 23g, **Sat Fat** 7g;
Chol 80mg; **Sodium** 780mg;
Total Carb 38g, **Total Sugars** 10g,
Added Sugars 0g; **Protein** 28g

 MAKE IT DAIRY FREE Substitute dairy-free yogurt
(see page 19) for Greek yogurt.

PAN-SEARED SIRLOIN STEAK WITH MUSHROOM PAN SAUCE

SERVES 4

WHY THIS RECIPE WORKS Steak, draped in a deeply flavored wine sauce bulked with mushrooms and served with à la carte sides, is a steakhouse classic; when you're at home you can pair a relatively lean cut of steak with something much better for you than what you'd get at a restaurant (see pages 260–303 for ideas) for an elegant treat. There are a few simple keys to getting a steakhouseworthy meal at home. First, you need to take care in choosing the pan itself. A large traditional (not nonstick) skillet will encourage the development of browned bits that, in addition to the full-bodied wine and earthy mushrooms, flavor the pan sauce. But the most important is to get the pan really hot; if the pan isn't properly preheated, the interior of the steak will overcook before it develops a good crust. And finally, to facilitate browning, you need to pat the steak dry before searing, as any moisture would prevent it from browning properly. Side options abound: Swap the tired creamed spinach for Pan-Steamed Kale with Pancetta and Pine Nuts (page 262) or make meat and potatoes with Roasted Red Potatoes with Rosemary (page 276).

STEAK

- 1 (1-pound) boneless beef top sirloin steak, 1 to 1½ inches thick, trimmed
- ¼ teaspoon table salt
- ¼ teaspoon pepper
- 1 tablespoon canola oil

PAN SAUCE

- 1 tablespoon garlic oil (see page 20)
- 8 ounces white mushrooms, sliced thin
- 1 cup dry red wine
- ½ cup chicken broth (see page 18)
- 1 tablespoon balsamic vinegar
- 1 teaspoon Dijon mustard
- 2 tablespoons butter, cut into 4 pieces and chilled
- 1 teaspoon minced fresh thyme

1 **For the steak:** Pat steak dry with paper towels and sprinkle with salt and pepper. Heat oil in 12-inch skillet over medium-high heat until just smoking. Brown steak well on first side, 3 to 5 minutes.

2 Flip steak and continue to cook until meat registers 120 to 125 degrees (for medium-rare) or 130 to 135 degrees (for medium), 5 to 7 minutes, reducing heat as needed to prevent scorching. Transfer steak to cutting board, tent with aluminum foil, and let rest for 5 minutes.

3 **For the pan sauce:** Pour off fat from skillet. Heat oil over medium-high heat until just smoking. Add mushrooms and cook, stirring occasionally, until beginning to brown and liquid has evaporated, about 5 minutes. Increase heat to high; add red wine and broth, scraping up any browned bits. Simmer until liquid and mushrooms are reduced to 1 cup, about 6 minutes. Add vinegar, mustard, and any accumulated steak juices to skillet and cook until thickened, about 1 minute. Off heat, whisk in butter and thyme. Season with salt and pepper to taste. Slice steak thin against grain, spoon sauce over slices, and serve immediately.

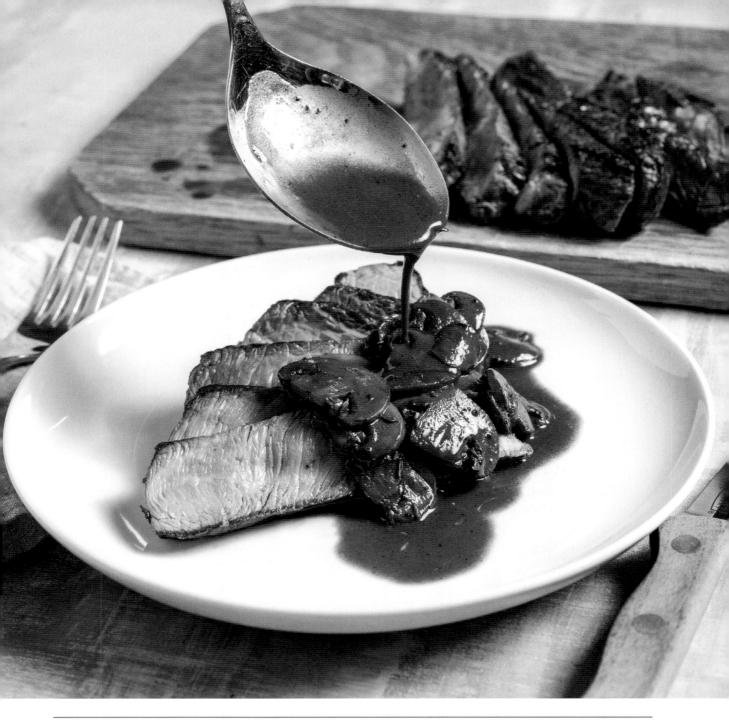

PER SERVING

Dietary Fiber 0g **Cal** 320;
Total Fat 16g, **Sat Fat** 6g;
Chol 85mg; **Sodium** 320mg;
Total Carb 4g, **Total Sugars** 3g,
Added Sugars 0g; **Protein** 26g

LF **MAKE IT LOW FODMAP** Substitute oyster mushrooms for
white mushrooms.

DF **MAKE IT DAIRY FREE** Omit butter.

STEAK TIPS WITH SPICED MILLET AND SPINACH

SERVES 4

WHY THIS RECIPE WORKS Inspired by the warm spices and dried fruit common in Moroccan dishes, we paired spiced steak tips (a good choice, as the sirloin cut is lean but deeply flavored) with a side dish of tender millet (rather than couscous to make the meal gluten-free and low-FODMAP), hearty chickpeas (in a moderate portion), and just enough sunny-sweet golden raisins (for flavor without introducing a hard-to-tolerate amount of fructans). A spice rub of cumin, cinnamon, salt, and pepper thoroughly seasoned the steak tips, which we seared in a hot skillet for flavorful browning. Stirring baby spinach into the millet at the end allowed it to wilt slightly before serving. Sirloin steak tips, also known as flap meat, can be sold as whole steaks, cubes, and strips; we prefer to purchase whole steaks and cut them ourselves. We have found that, unlike other grains, millet can become gluey if allowed to steam off the heat; serve immediately.

1½ teaspoons ground cumin

1 teaspoon ground cinnamon

¾ teaspoon table salt

¼ teaspoon pepper

1 pound sirloin steak tips, trimmed and cut into 2-inch pieces

1 tablespoon vegetable oil

1½ cups water

1 (15-ounce) can chickpeas, rinsed

¾ cup millet, rinsed and dried on dish towel

¼ cup raisins

5 ounces (5 cups) baby spinach, chopped

1 Combine cumin, cinnamon, salt, and pepper in bowl. Pat steak tips dry with paper towels and sprinkle with 1½ teaspoons spice mixture. Heat oil in 12-inch skillet over medium-high heat until just smoking. Add steak and cook until browned on all sides and meat registers 120 to 125 degrees (for medium-rare) or 130 to 135 degrees (for medium), 6 to 10 minutes. Transfer steak tips to plate, tent with aluminum foil, and let rest.

2 Meanwhile, combine water, chickpeas, millet, raisins, and remaining spice mixture in large saucepan and bring to boil over medium-high heat. Reduce heat to low, cover, and simmer until liquid is absorbed, 15 to 20 minutes. Fold in spinach, one handful at a time. Serve with steak tips.

PER SERVING

Dietary Fiber 12g **Cal** 480;
Total Fat 17g, **Sat Fat** 4.5g;
Chol 75mg; **Sodium** 720mg;
Total Carb 49g, **Total Sugars** 7g,
Added Sugars 0g; **Protein** 33g

 MAKE IT LOW FODMAP Omit chickpeas.

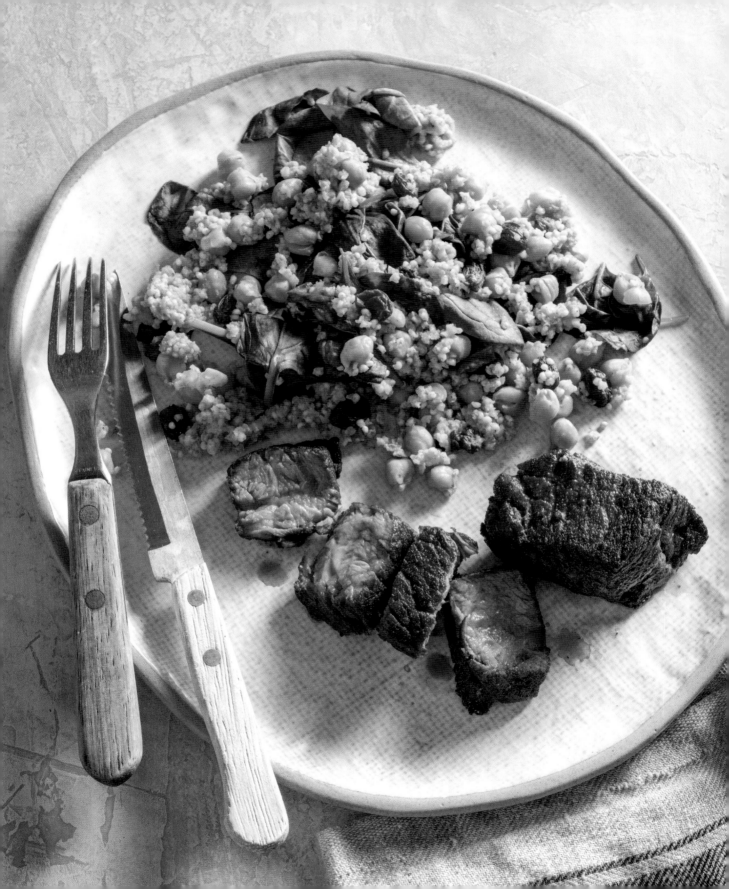

STIR-FRIED BEEF WITH GAI LAN AND OYSTER SAUCE

SERVES 4

DAIRY FREE

WHY THIS RECIPE WORKS Beef and gai lan is a common combination for a stir-fry. For more nutritional value and to up the vegetable quotient, we increase the ratio of gai lan to beef for a pleasing vegetable-forward stir-fry. To ensure properly cooked gai lan, we first blanch it, staggering the cooking time of the stalks and the florets and leaves so they are perfectly crisp-tender. Quarter gai lan stalks that are thicker than 1 inch at base. If you can't find gai lan, broccolini is a good substitute; halve stalks that are thicker than ½ inch. To make slicing the steak easier, freeze for 15 minutes. You will need a 12-inch nonstick skillet or 14-inch flat-bottomed wok for this recipe.

¼ teaspoon baking soda

1 pound flank steak, trimmed

2 tablespoons oyster sauce (see page 18), divided

2 teaspoons cornstarch, divided

1½ tablespoons soy sauce (see page 18)

1 tablespoon packed brown sugar

1 tablespoon toasted sesame oil

2 pounds gai lan, trimmed, florets and leaves chopped, stalks cut into 3-inch lengths and halved lengthwise

3 tablespoons garlic oil (see page 20), divided

1 tablespoon grated fresh ginger

6 scallions, green parts only, cut into 1-inch lengths

1 Combine 1 tablespoon water and baking soda in bowl. Cut beef with grain into 2½- to 3-inch-wide strips, then slice each strip against grain into ⅛-inch-thick slices. Add beef to baking soda mixture and toss to coat; let sit for 5 minutes. Add 1 tablespoon oyster sauce and ½ teaspoon cornstarch and toss until well combined; let sit for 15 minutes.

2 Whisk 3 tablespoons water, remaining 2 tablespoons oyster sauce, soy sauce, sugar, sesame oil, and remaining 1½ teaspoons cornstarch in small bowl until sugar and cornstarch are dissolved; set aside.

3 Bring 4 quarts water to boil in large pot. Add gai lan stalks and 1 tablespoon table salt and cook, stirring often, until crisp-tender, about 3 minutes. Stir in gai lan florets and leaves and cook until wilted, about 1 minute. Drain well and transfer to paper towel–lined plate; set aside.

4 Heat 2 teaspoons garlic oil in 12-inch nonstick skillet or 14-inch flat-bottomed wok over medium-high heat until just smoking. Add half of beef mixture and increase heat to high. Cook, tossing beef slowly but constantly, until exuded juices have evaporated and meat begins to sizzle, 2 to 6 minutes; transfer to large bowl. Repeat with 2 teaspoons oil and remaining beef. Heat 2 teaspoons garlic oil in now-empty pan over high heat until just smoking. Add half of gai lan and cook, tossing slowly but constantly, until dry and beginning to brown, 2 to 3 minutes; transfer to bowl with beef. Repeat with 2 teaspoons garlic oil and remaining gai lan; transfer to bowl.

5 Add remaining 1 teaspoon garlic oil and ginger to again-empty pan and cook over medium-high heat, mashing mixture into pan, until fragrant, about 15 seconds. Whisk soy sauce mixture to recombine and add to pan. Add beef–gai lan mixture and cook, tossing slowly but constantly, until sauce has thickened and beef and gai lan are well coated and heated through, about 1 minute. Stir in scallion greens and serve.

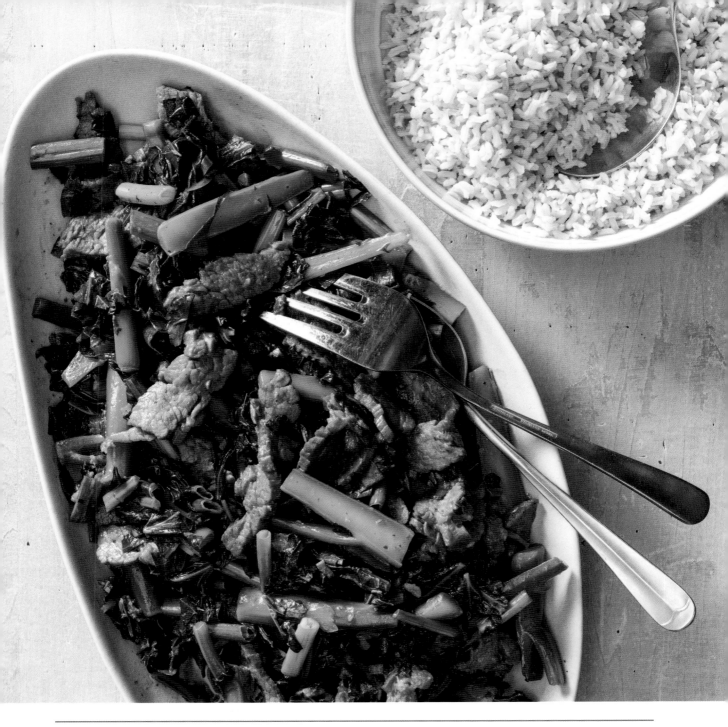

PER SERVING

Dietary Fiber 6g **Cal** 390;
Total Fat 23g, **Sat Fat** 4.5g;
Chol 80mg; **Sodium** 750mg;
Total Carb 17g, **Total Sugars** 6g,
Added Sugars 3g; **Protein** 28g

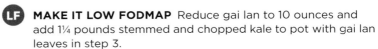

LF **MAKE IT LOW FODMAP** Reduce gai lan to 10 ounces and
add 1¼ pounds stemmed and chopped kale to pot with gai lan
leaves in step 3.

GF **MAKE IT GLUTEN FREE** Substitute gluten-free soy sauce or
tamari (see page 18) for soy sauce.

STEAK TACOS WITH NAPA CABBAGE SLAW

SERVES 4

WHY THIS RECIPE WORKS The garnish for a taco can be an afterthought, playing third fiddle to the meat and to a sauce or salsa you might make. Not here. The slaw in our flank steak tacos is the only topping needed and it's applied liberally. In addition to providing optimal fiber, the slaw makes the tacos more interesting, creating contrasts of rich and fresh, cooked and raw, and soft and crunchy, while the dressing of jalapeño, cilantro, garlic oil, honey, and lime gives the tacos plenty of flavor. Using napa cabbage rather than hardier regular green cabbage means we can toss the slaw together without worrying about a long salting process or refrigerator stay to soften it. The brightness and heat contrast the warmth of steak rubbed with cumin and paprika. With their low-FODMAP and gluten-free status, corn tortillas are flatbreads that are good for nearly anyone.

½ small head napa cabbage, cored and sliced thin (4 cups)

2 carrots, peeled and shredded

1 jalapeño chile, stemmed, seeded, and sliced thin

½ cup chopped fresh cilantro

1 tablespoon plus 2 teaspoons garlic oil (see page 20), divided

1 tablespoon honey

1 teaspoon grated lime zest plus 2 tablespoons juice

¾ teaspoon table salt, divided

1 teaspoon ground cumin

1 teaspoon ground paprika

¼ teaspoon pepper

1 (1-pound) flank steak, trimmed

12 (6-inch) corn tortillas (see page 19), warmed

1 Combine cabbage, carrots, jalapeño, cilantro, 1 tablespoon garlic oil, honey, lime zest and juice, and ½ teaspoon salt in bowl. Cover slaw and refrigerate until ready to serve.

2 Combine cumin, paprika, pepper, and remaining ¼ teaspoon salt in small bowl. Pat steaks dry with paper towels, then sprinkle with spice mixture.

3 Heat remaining 2 teaspoons oil in 12-inch skillet over medium-high heat until just smoking. Cook steak until well browned and meat registers 120 to 125 degrees (for medium-rare) or 130 to 135 degrees (for medium), 3 to 6 minutes per side, reducing heat as needed to prevent scorching. Transfer steaks to cutting board, tent with aluminum foil, and let rest for 5 minutes.

4 Slice steak thin against grain on bias. Toss slaw to recombine and season slaw with salt and pepper to taste. Divide steak evenly among tortillas and top with slaw. Serve.

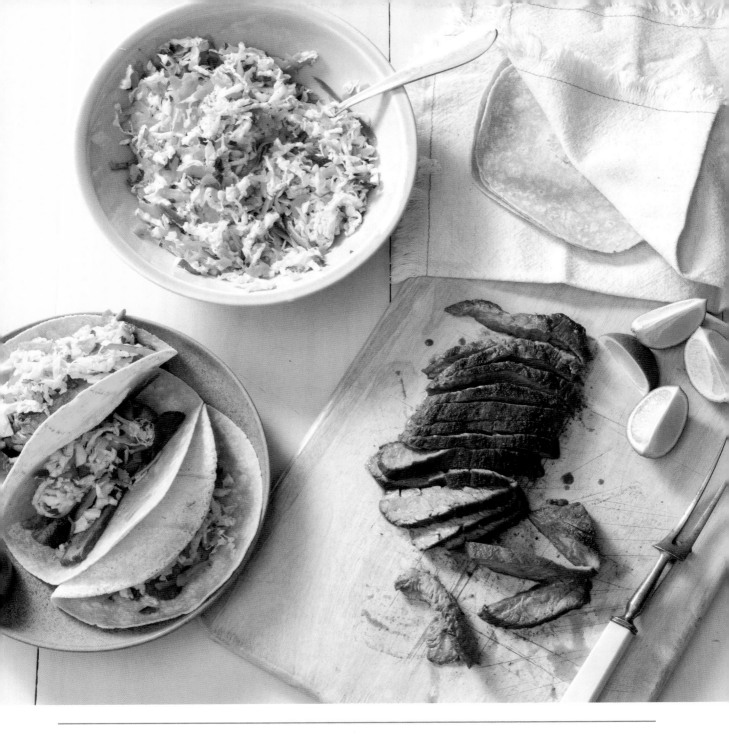

PER SERVING

Dietary Fiber 3g **Cal** 490;
Total Fat 19g, **Sat Fat** 4.5g;
Chol 75mg; **Sodium** 410mg;
Total Carb 52g, **Total Sugars** 12g,
Added Sugars 4g; **Protein** 30g

SIRLOIN STEAK WITH WILTED ESCAROLE AND CHICKPEA SALAD

SERVES 4

WHY THIS RECIPE WORKS For an interesting spin on a simple steak and salad supper, we turned away from basic spinach to escarole, which is beautiful to behold and low FODMAP—but needs some help to balance its bitterness. Our solutions: a warm vinaigrette and the right mix-ins for an incredibly complex-tasting salad that isn't complex to make. A rich, warm mustard-almond vinaigrette, which gets depth from using garlic oil instead of olive oil, serves two purposes: It wilts and softens the hardy escarole just enough to eliminate chewiness, and it balances the leaves' bitterness with sweetness, acidity, and saltiness. Earthy, nutty chickpeas add more fiber to the salad and their creaminess serves the dish well. Shredded carrots provide more welcome sweetness and contrasting color, while mint brings pops of freshness and feta tangy, salty bites. You can substitute chicory for the escarole.

1 (1-pound) boneless beef top sirloin, strip, or rib-eye steak, 1 to 1½ inches thick, trimmed

¼ teaspoon table salt

¼ teaspoon pepper

¼ cup garlic oil (see page 20), divided

¼ cup whole almonds, chopped

¼ cup white wine vinegar

1 tablespoon whole-grain mustard

1 teaspoon sugar

1 head escarole (1 pound), torn into bite-size pieces

1 (15-ounce) can chickpeas, rinsed

3 carrots, peeled and shredded

⅓ cup chopped fresh mint

2 ounces feta cheese, crumbled (½ cup)

1 Pat steak adry with paper towels and sprinkle with salt and pepper. Heat 1 tablespoon oil in 12-inch skillet over medium-high heat until just smoking. Brown steak well on first side, 3 to 5 minutes.

2 Flip steak and continue to cook until meat registers 120 to 125 degrees (for medium-rare) or 130 to 135 degrees (for medium), 5 to 7 minutes, reducing heat as needed to prevent scorching. Transfer steak to cutting board, tent with aluminum foil, and let rest while preparing salad.

3 Heat remaining 3 tablespoons oil in now-empty skillet over medium heat until shimmering. Add almonds and cook, stirring frequently, until toasted and fragrant, 1 to 2 minutes. Off heat, stir in vinegar, mustard, and sugar, scraping up any browned bits. Let vinaigrette sit until heated through, about 30 seconds.

4 Gently toss escarole with warm vinaigrette in large bowl until evenly coated and wilted slightly. Add chickpeas, carrots, and mint and toss to combine. Season with salt and pepper to taste. Sprinkle with feta. Slice steak thin against grain and serve with salad.

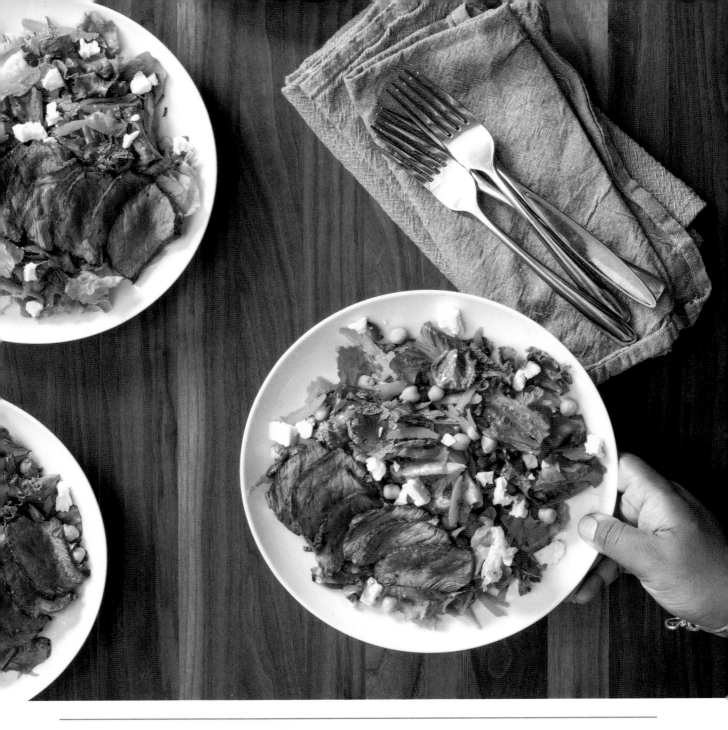

PER SERVING

Dietary Fiber 9g **Cal** 480;
Total Fat 28g, **Sat Fat** 5g;
Chol 80mg; **Sodium** 670mg;
Total Carb 22g, **Total Sugars** 5g,
Added Sugars 1g; **Protein** 34g

DF **MAKE DAIRY FREE** Omit feta cheese.

GRILLED BEEF KEBABS

SERVES 4

WHY THIS RECIPE WORKS Beef kebabs are a grilling favorite and they easily grill next to skewers with plenty of produce for a simple, balanced meal. We like kebabs with a bold-tasting marinade, and steak tips have a beefy flavor to stand up to one. Same goes for meaty eggplant and mushrooms, and sweet cherry tomatoes—all which are high in fiber. We give each their own skewers for control over cooking. Oyster mushrooms, which boast more fiber than others like cremini, are a fun, unexpected addition, their frilly petals charring and crisping up beautifully. Tossing the beef in a mixture of ras el hanout and garlic oil before grilling lets the warm, sweet spices bloom on the grill. Mixing fresh mint and red wine vinegar into a portion of the marinade makes a quick dressing for drizzling. Sirloin steak tips, also known as flap meat, can be sold as whole steaks, cubes, and strips; we prefer to purchase whole steaks and cut them ourselves. If you have long, thin pieces of meat, roll or fold them into approximate 1-inch cubes before skewering. You will need six 12-inch metal skewers for this recipe.

6 tablespoons garlic oil (see page 20), divided

1 tablespoon ras el hanout

1½ teaspoons sugar

1 teaspoon table salt, divided

¾ teaspoon pepper

1 pound sirloin steak tips, trimmed and cut into 1-inch pieces

1 pound oyster mushrooms, trimmed, petals separated

6 ounces cherry tomatoes

1 pound eggplant, sliced into ½-inch-thick rounds

1 tablespoon red wine vinegar

2 tablespoons chopped fresh mint

1 Microwave ¼ cup oil, ras el hanout, sugar, ¾ teaspoon salt, and pepper in large bowl until fragrant, about 30 seconds, stirring once halfway through microwaving. Measure out and reserve 3 tablespoons marinade in small bowl. Add beef to remaining marinade and toss to coat. Thread beef onto two 12-inch metal skewers.

2 Thread mushroom petals through thickest ends onto two 12-inch metal skewers. Thread tomatoes onto two 12-inch skewers. Brush tomatoes, eggplant, and mushrooms with remaining 2 tablespoons oil and sprinkle with remaining ¼ teaspoon salt.

3A For a charcoal grill: Open bottom vent completely. Light large chimney starter mounded with charcoal briquettes (7 quarts). When top coals are partially covered with ash, pour evenly over grill. Set cooking grate in place, cover, and open lid vent completely. Heat grill until hot, about 5 minutes.

3B For a gas grill: Turn all burners to high, cover, and heat grill until hot, about 15 minutes. Leave all burners on high.

4 Clean and oil cooking grate. Place eggplant slices on grill and cook until lightly charred, 2 to 4 minutes per side. Transfer eggplant to serving platter and tent with aluminum foil. Place beef, mushroom, and tomato skewers on grill and cook (covered if using gas), turning as needed, until beef is well browned and registers 120 to 125 degrees (for medium-rare) or 130 to 135 degrees (for medium), and mushrooms and tomatoes are softened and lightly charred, 5 to 15 minutes. Transfer beef and vegetables to platter with eggplant as they finish cooking and tent with aluminum foil.

5 Whisk vinegar and mint into reserved marinade and season with salt and pepper to taste. Using fork, push beef, mushrooms, and tomatoes off skewers onto platter. Drizzle with dressing and serve.

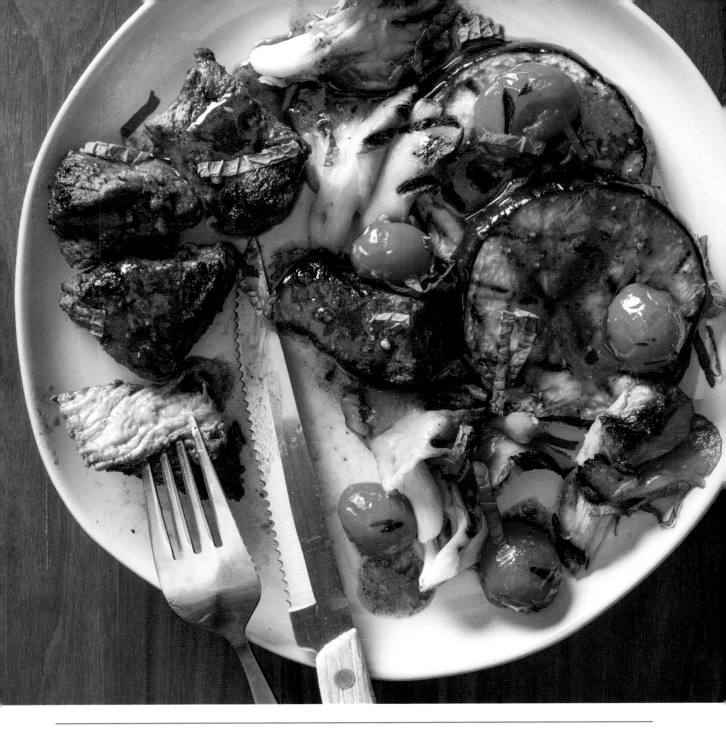

PER SERVING

Dietary Fiber 6g **Cal** 410;
Total Fat 25g, **Sat Fat** 4g;
Chol 55mg; **Sodium** 670mg;
Total Carb 17g, **Total Sugars** 7g,
Added Sugars 2g; **Protein** 30g

 MAKE IT LOW FODMAP Increase mushrooms to 1½ pounds and decrease eggplant to 10 ounces. Thread mushrooms onto 3 skewers.

SPAGHETTI AND MEATBALLS

SERVES 6

WHY THIS RECIPE WORKS Spaghetti and meatballs may seem like a comfort-food classic that might not comfort the gut, but dissect the components, tweak them a bit, and you can have a lean but delicious dish with more fiber than you might expect. First, we make sure to use whole-wheat products: both the spaghetti and the binding bread crumbs. (Although you can use gluten-free pasta and panko if you're following a low-FODMAP or gluten-free diet.) Next, where to get all that allium flavor for the red-sauce favorite? Garlic oil to brown the meatballs does the trick, and oregano and red pepper flakes put in work to scent the sauce. Finally, the meatballs are surprisingly lean; 93 percent lean ground beef, when combined with an egg and a little bit of Parmesan, makes a perfectly good rich-tasting meatball, especially after simmering in the fragrant tomato sauce to cook through. With each bowl of pasta topped with three meatballs, this Sunday supper is just as satisfying as any other—and it happens to nourish your body, not just your soul.

½ cup 100 percent whole-wheat panko bread crumbs

6 tablespoons chopped fresh basil, divided

¼ cup grated Parmesan cheese, plus extra for serving

1 large egg

¼ teaspoon table salt, plus salt for cooking pasta

¼ teaspoon pepper

1½ pounds 93 percent lean ground beef

1 tablespoon garlic oil (see page 20)

½ teaspoon minced fresh oregano or ⅛ teaspoon dried

⅛ teaspoon red pepper flakes (optional)

1 (28-ounce) can crushed tomatoes

1 (14.5-ounce) can diced tomatoes

1 pound 100 percent whole-wheat spaghetti

1 Whisk panko, 3 tablespoons basil, Parmesan, egg, salt, and pepper together in large bowl. Add ground beef and gently knead mixture with your hands until combined. Pinch off and roll mixture into 1½-inch round meatballs (18 meatballs) and place on large plate. Refrigerate until firm, at least 15 minutes or up to 24 hours.

2 Heat oil in 12-inch nonstick skillet over medium heat until just smoking. Brown meatballs on all sides, about 10 minutes. Transfer meatballs to paper towel–lined plate.

3 Add oregano and pepper flakes, if using, to fat left in skillet and cook over medium heat until fragrant, about 30 seconds. Stir in crushed tomatoes and diced tomatoes and their juices. Bring to simmer and cook until sauce has thickened slightly, about 20 minutes.

4 Nestle meatballs into sauce and return to simmer. Cover and cook, turning meatballs occasionally, until cooked through, about 10 minutes.

5 Meanwhile, bring 4 quarts water to boil in large pot. Add pasta and 1 tablespoon salt and cook, stirring often, until al dente. Reserve ½ cup cooking water, then drain pasta and return to pot.

6 Add remaining 3 tablespoons basil and several large spoonfuls of sauce (without meatballs) to the pasta and toss to combine. Adjust consistency with reserved cooking water as needed. Divide pasta evenly among 6 serving bowls and top with 3 meatballs each and additional sauce. Serve, passing extra Parmesan separately.

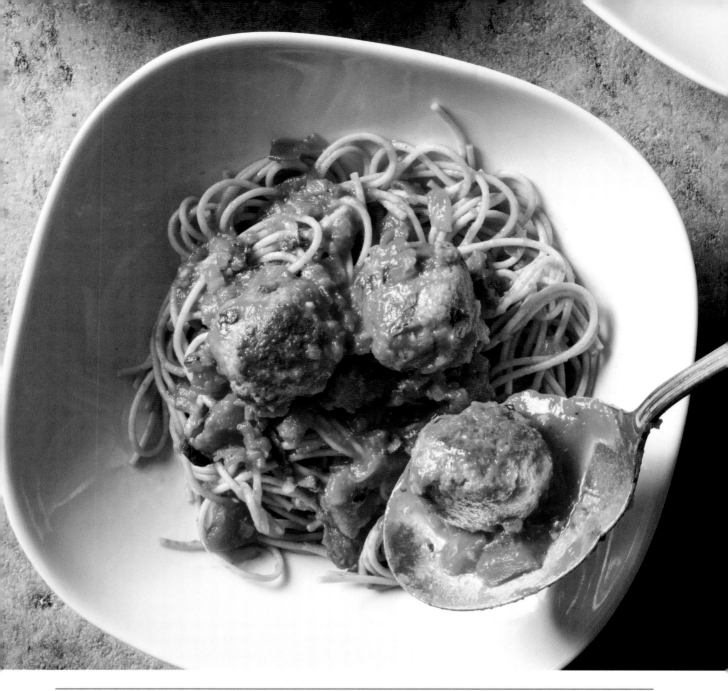

PER SERVING

Dietary Fiber 12g **Cal** 530;
Total Fat 14g, **Sat Fat** 4g;
Chol 105mg; **Sodium** 790mg;
Total Carb 65g, **Total Sugars** 9g,
Added Sugars 0g; **Protein** 39g

LF **MAKE IT LOW FODMAP** Substitute gluten-free panko bread crumbs for whole-wheat crumbs and gluten-free pasta (see page 19) for whole-wheat spaghetti.

DF **MAKE IT DAIRY FREE** Omit Parmesan.

GF **MAKE IT GLUTEN FREE** Substitute gluten-free panko bread crumbs for whole-wheat crumbs and gluten-free pasta (see page 19) for whole-wheat spaghetti.

BEEF AND SPINACH LASAGNA

SERVES 12

WHY THIS RECIPE WORKS Lasagna is often layered high with meat and served in overly generous digestion-slowing squares. With our version, you can still enjoy this ultimate casserole while keeping the health of your gut in mind. We didn't need to be sneaky to add fiber: Using whole-wheat noodles and stirring a pound of frozen spinach into the meat sauce were delicious recipe edits that helped make a smaller serving more filling. It's not lasagna without cheese, so we didn't compromise on a cheese layer, sticking with tradition and combining ricotta, Parmesan, and fresh basil with an egg to help thicken and bind the mixture. As for the tomatoey sauce, we used lean ground beef (93 percent lean) instead of 80 or 85 percent lean—grease isn't an essential lasagna ingredient. This more-healthful lasagna comes out of the oven bubbling, with a beautifully browned cheese topping.

1 pound (2 cups) whole-milk ricotta cheese

12 ounces whole-milk mozzarella cheese, shredded (3 cups), divided

1 ounce Parmesan cheese, grated (½ cup)

1 cup chopped fresh basil, divided

1 large egg, lightly beaten

½ teaspoon table salt, divided, plus salt for cooking pasta

½ teaspoon pepper

1 tablespoon garlic oil

¼ teaspoon dried oregano

⅛ teaspoon red pepper flakes (optional)

1 pound 93 percent lean ground beef

1 (28-ounce) can crushed tomatoes

1 (28-ounce) can diced tomatoes

1 pound frozen spinach, thawed, squeezed dry, and chopped coarse

16 100 percent whole-wheat lasagna noodles

1 Mix ricotta, 2 cups mozzarella, Parmesan, ½ cup basil, egg, ¼ teaspoon salt, and pepper in bowl until well combined; cover and refrigerate until needed.

2 Cook oil, oregano, and red pepper flakes, if using, in Dutch oven over medium heat until fragrant, about 30 seconds. Add ground beef and cook, breaking up meat with wooden spoon, until no longer pink, about 5 minutes. Stir in crushed tomatoes and diced tomatoes with their juices and remaining ¼ teaspoon salt and bring to simmer. Cook, stirring occasionally, until sauce has thickened slightly, about 15 minutes. Off heat, stir in spinach and remaining ½ cup basil, cover, and set aside.

3 Adjust oven rack to middle position and heat oven to 375 degrees. Lightly coat 13 by 9-inch baking dish with canola oil spray. Bring 4 quarts water to boil in large pot. Add noodles and 1 tablespoon salt and cook, stirring often, until almost al dente. Drain and rinse noodles under cold water until cool. Lay pasta out on clean dish towels.

4 Spread 1½ cups meat sauce over bottom of prepared dish. Place 4 noodles on top of sauce (noodles may overlap) and spread ¼ cup ricotta mixture evenly down center of each noodle. Spoon 1½ cups more sauce evenly over ricotta. Repeat layering two more times.

5 For final layer, place remaining 4 noodles on top and spread remaining sauce over noodles. Sprinkle with remaining 1 cup mozzarella. Spray large sheet of aluminum foil lightly with canola oil spray, then cover lasagna.

6 Place lasagna on foil-lined rimmed baking sheet and bake until sauce is bubbling, 40 to 45 minutes. Uncover lasagna and continue to bake until cheese is melted and beginning to brown, about 20 minutes. Let cool for 10 to 20 minutes before serving.

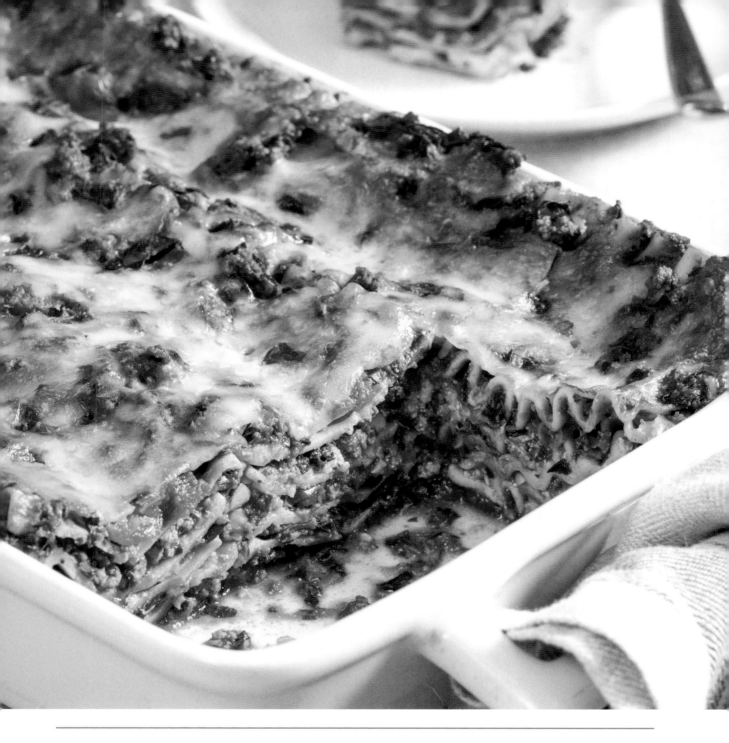

PER 3¼ BY 3-INCH SERVING

Dietary Fiber 6g Cal 370;
Total Fat 17g, Sat Fat 9g;
Chol 75mg; Sodium 480mg;
Total Carb 32g, Total Sugars 6g,
Added Sugars 0g; Protein 27g

MEATLOAF WITH ROASTED POTATOES AND GREEN BEANS

SERVES 6

WHY THIS RECIPE WORKS The secret to this dish with meat in the name is actually mushrooms. A large batch marries with lean ground beef to provide extra moisture and deep—yes, meatier—flavor to the loaf. Potatoes and green beans make it a meal. Use small red potatoes measuring 1 to 2 inches in diameter; if your potatoes are larger, cut them into 1-inch pieces.

¼ cup garlic oil
(see page 20), divided

20 ounces cremini mushrooms, trimmed and sliced thin, divided

1½ teaspoons minced fresh thyme, divided

½ cup 100 percent whole-wheat panko bread crumbs

1 large egg

3 tablespoons minced fresh parsley, divided

4 teaspoons soy sauce, divided

1 tablespoon Dijon mustard

¾ teaspoon pepper, divided

1½ pounds 93 percent lean ground beef

2 pounds small red potatoes, unpeeled, halved

½ teaspoon table salt, divided

1 pound green beans, trimmed and halved crosswise

¼ ounce dried porcini mushrooms, rinsed and minced

2 tablespoons all-purpose flour

2 cups beef broth

1 Adjust oven rack to lower-middle position and heat oven to 400 degrees. Spray rimmed baking sheet with canola oil spray. Heat 1 tablespoon oil in 12-inch nonstick skillet over medium heat until shimmering. Add half of cremini mushrooms and cook until they have released their liquid and are lightly browned, about 10 minutes. Stir in 1 teaspoon thyme and cook until fragrant, about 30 seconds. Transfer to food processor and let cool for 5 minutes. Add panko and process until mixture forms fine paste, about 25 seconds, scraping down sides of bowl as needed.

2 Whisk egg, 2 tablespoons parsley, 1 tablespoon soy sauce, mustard, and ½ teaspoon pepper together in large bowl. Add mushroom mixture and beef and gently knead mixture with your hands until combined. Transfer meatloaf mixture to center of prepared sheet. Using your wet hands, shape into 9 by 5-inch rectangle; top should be flat and meatloaf should be an even 1½ inches thick.

3 Toss potatoes with 1 tablespoon oil, ¼ teaspoon salt, and remaining ¼ teaspoon pepper in bowl. Place potatoes cut side down on sheet around meatloaf and roast for 20 minutes. Toss green beans with 1 tablespoon oil and remaining ¼ teaspoon salt. Arrange green beans on top of potatoes and roast until meatloaf registers 160 degrees and vegetables are tender, 15 to 25 minutes, rotating sheet halfway through baking.

4 Meanwhile, heat remaining 1 tablespoon oil in now-empty skillet over medium heat until shimmering. Add porcini mushrooms and remaining cremini mushrooms and cook until they have released their liquid and are lightly browned, about 10 minutes. Stir in remaining ½ teaspoon thyme and cook until fragrant, about 30 seconds. Add flour and cook, stirring frequently, until golden, about 2 minutes. Slowly whisk in broth and remaining 1 teaspoon soy sauce, scraping up any browned bits. Bring to simmer and cook, whisking occasionally, until thickened, 8 to 10 minutes. Cover gravy to keep warm.

5 Transfer meatloaf to cutting board, tent with foil, and let rest for 10 minutes. Stir remaining 1 tablespoon parsley into gravy and season with pepper to taste. Slice meatloaf and serve with potatoes, green beans, and gravy.

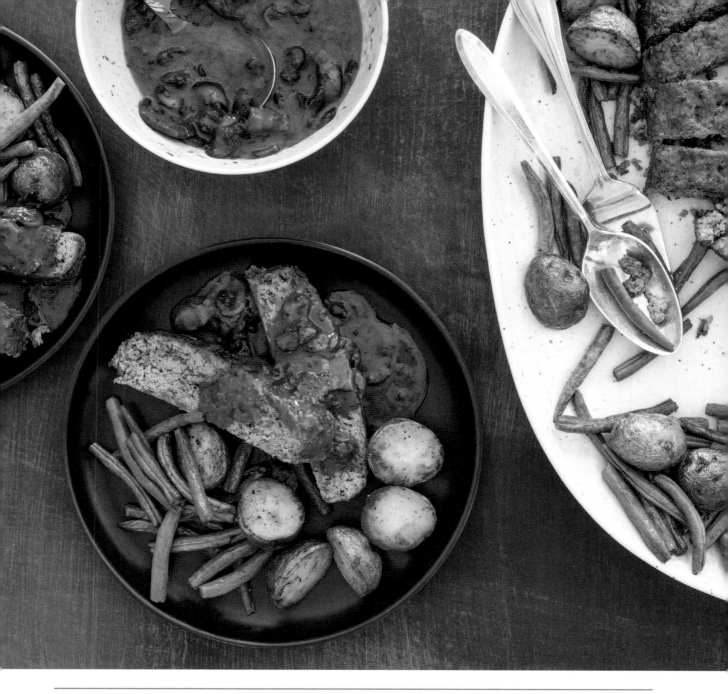

PER SERVING

Dietary Fiber 6g **Cal** 460;
Total Fat 19g, **Sat Fat** 4.5g;
Chol 100mg; **Sodium** 750mg;
Total Carb 40g, **Total Sugars** 6g,
Added Sugars 0g; **Protein** 34g

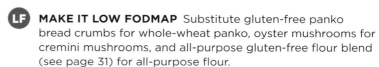

LF **MAKE IT LOW FODMAP** Substitute gluten-free panko bread crumbs for whole-wheat panko, oyster mushrooms for cremini mushrooms, and all-purpose gluten-free flour blend (see page 31) for all-purpose flour.

GF **MAKE IT GLUTEN FREE** Substitute gluten-free panko bread crumbs for whole-wheat panko, gluten-free soy sauce or tamari (see page 18) for soy sauce, and all-purpose gluten-free flour blend (see page 31) for all-purpose flour.

ROASTED PORK CHOPS AND VEGETABLES WITH PARSLEY VINAIGRETTE

SERVES 4

WHY THIS RECIPE WORKS We know pairing ample vegetables with a protein is important for gut health, and combining the two on one pan is the ideal streamlined way to do it. Thick-cut bone-in pork rib chops deliver the succulence of a larger pork roast but cook in just 10 to 15 minutes, making them a perfect weeknight choice for a smaller group. They stand up to high heat and bold flavors, so we pair them with root vegetables and season everything with a parsley vinaigrette. We partially roast our rustic mix of thick-sliced Yukon Gold potatoes, carrots, and parsnips to give them a head start. We often toss root vegetables with shallots or add garlic cloves before roasting; instead, here we coat them with minced fresh rosemary and garlic oil, which perfume the whole dish through cooking—without the allium. Once the vegetables soften and take on some color, we add our pork chops, which we seasoned with a bold rub of pepper, salt, paprika, and coriander for a deeply flavored crust. Drizzling a parsley vinaigrette over the pork ensures our meal ends on a high note.

1 pound Yukon Gold potatoes, unpeeled

1 pound carrots, peeled

1 pound parsnips, peeled

3 tablespoons plus 1 teaspoon garlic oil (see page 20), divided

2 teaspoons minced fresh rosemary

1½ teaspoons pepper, divided

1 teaspoon table salt, divided

1 teaspoon paprika

1 teaspoon ground coriander

2 (12-ounce) bone-in pork rib chops, 1 to 1½ inches thick, trimmed

4 teaspoons red wine vinegar

3 tablespoons chopped fresh parsley

1 Adjust oven rack to upper-middle position and heat oven to 450 degrees. Halve potatoes lengthwise and slice them ½ inch thick. Cut carrots and parsnips into 3-inch lengths (quarter thick ends lengthwise). Toss potatoes, parsnips, and carrots with 1 tablespoon oil, rosemary, ¼ teaspoon pepper, and ¼ teaspoon salt together in bowl. Spread vegetables into single layer on rimmed baking sheet. Roast until beginning to soften, about 25 minutes.

2 Combine 1 teaspoon oil, paprika, coriander, 1 teaspoon pepper, and ½ teaspoon salt in bowl. Pat pork dry with paper towels, then rub with spice mixture. Lay chops on top of vegetables and continue to roast until pork registers 145 degrees and vegetables are tender, 10 to 15 minutes, rotating sheet halfway through roasting.

3 Remove sheet from oven, tent with aluminum foil, and let rest for 5 minutes. Whisk remaining 2 tablespoons oil, remaining ¼ teaspoon pepper, remaining ¼ teaspoon salt, vinegar, and parsley together in bowl. Transfer chops to carving board, carve meat from bones, and slice ½ inch thick. Drizzle vinaigrette over pork before serving with vegetables.

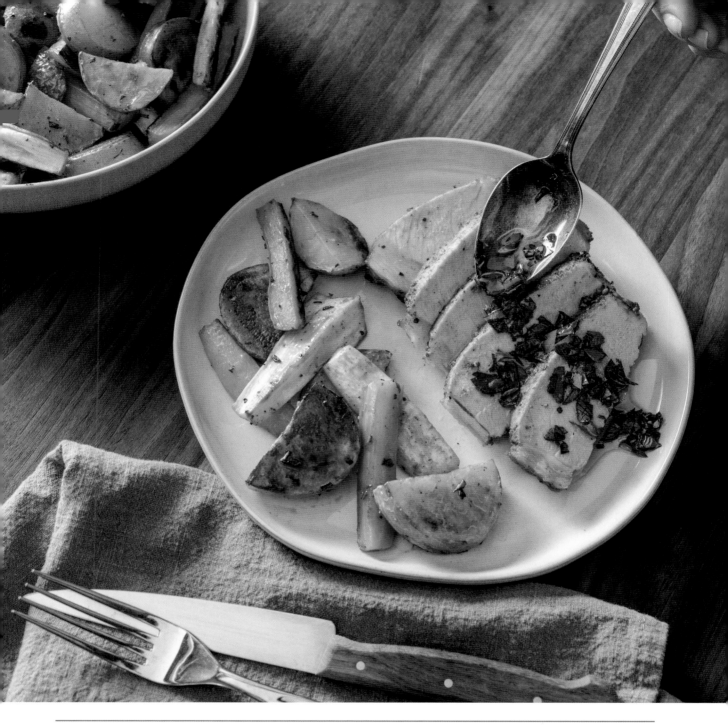

PER SERVING

Dietary Fiber 10g **Cal** 450;
Total Fat 17g, **Sat Fat** 3.5g;
Chol 55mg; **Sodium** 730mg;
Total Carb 47g, **Total Sugars** 11g,
Added Sugars 0g; **Protein** 26g

GRILLED PORK CHOPS WITH SWEET POTATO SALAD

SERVES 4

WHY THIS RECIPE WORKS Grill, pork chops, and potato salad are a winning trio of summer staples. Pairing potatoes is a smart low-FODMAP trick: Red potatoes are free from FODMAPs, while nutritious sweet potatoes pack fiber. Combining the two gives you a high-fiber and low-FODMAP side—and contributes to a harmony of sweet and savory. To up the complexity more, we dress the salad with bright chermoula rather than mayo. Steaming the potatoes with the sauce in a disposable pan before charring them cooks them through and seasons them. We quickly sear the chops on the grate after the potatoes. Buy potatoes measuring 2 to 3 inches in diameter; they fit neatly in the pan.

½ cup fresh cilantro leaves

¼ cup garlic oil (see page 20)

2 tablespoon lemon juice, plus lemon wedges for serving

1 teaspoon ground coriander, divided

1 teaspoon paprika, divided

¾ teaspoon table salt, divided

Pinch cayenne pepper (optional)

1¼ pounds red potatoes, unpeeled and sliced ½ inch thick

12 ounces sweet potatoes, peeled and sliced ½ inch thick

1 (13 by 9-inch) disposable aluminum pan

1 tablespoon packed brown sugar

4 (6- to 8-ounce) bone-in pork rib or center-cut chops, ½ inch thick, trimmed

1½ ounces feta cheese, crumbled (⅓ cup)

4 scallions, greens parts only, sliced thin

1 Process cilantro, oil, lemon juice, ½ teaspoon coriander, ½ teaspoon paprika, ¼ teaspoon salt, and cayenne, if using, in food processor until smooth, about 1 minute, scraping down sides of bowl as needed. Measure out and reserve ¼ cup chermoula. Toss red potatoes and sweet potatoes with remaining chermoula in large bowl. Layer potatoes in disposable pan, then pour any remaining chermoula from bowl over top. Cover tightly with aluminum foil.

2 Combine sugar, remaining ½ teaspoon coriander, remaining ½ teaspoon paprika, and remaining ½ teaspoon salt in bowl. Pat pork chops dry with paper towels and sprinkle with spice mixture; set aside.

3A For a charcoal grill: Open bottom vent completely. Light large chimney starter filled with charcoal briquettes (6 quarts). When top coals are partially covered with ash, pour evenly over grill. Set cooking grate in place, cover, and open lid vent completely. Heat grill until hot, about 5 minutes.

3B For a gas grill: Turn all burners to high, cover, and heat grill until hot, about 15 minutes. Turn all burners to medium. Adjust burners as needed to maintain grill temperature around 400 degrees.

4 Clean and oil cooking grate. Place disposable pan on grill. Cover grill and cook until potatoes are tender, 20 to 25 minutes, shaking pan halfway through cooking to redistribute potatoes. Remove pan from grill. Place potatoes directly on cooking grate. Cook (covered if using gas) until lightly charred and tender, 3 to 6 minutes per side. Transfer potatoes to large bowl as they finish cooking. Add feta, scallion greens, and reserved chermoula to potatoes and toss to coat. Season potato salad with salt and pepper to taste.

5 Place chops on grill. Cook until chops are browned and register 140 degrees, 2 to 3 minutes per side. Transfer chops to serving platter, tent with aluminum foil, and let rest for 5 minutes before serving with potato salad and lemon wedges.

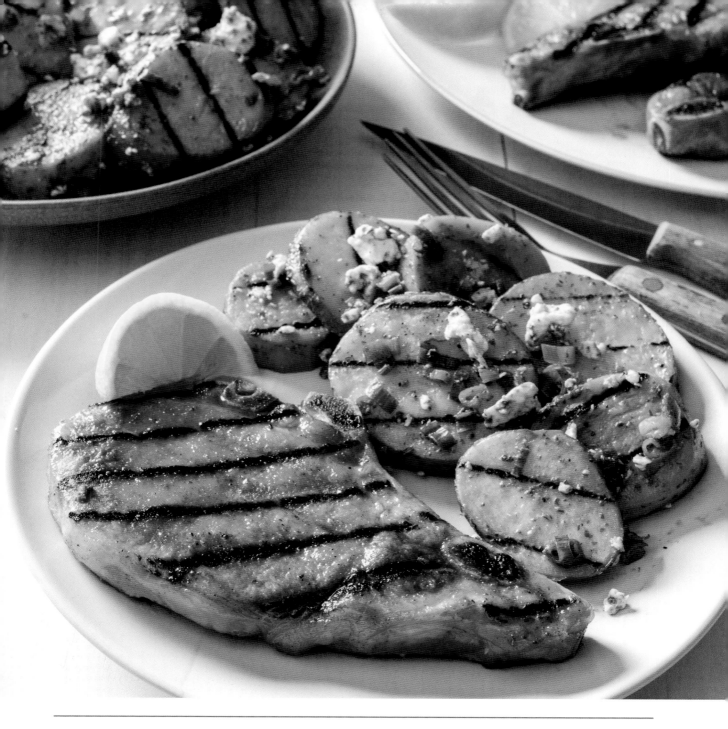

PER SERVING

Dietary Fiber 6g **Cal** 470;
Total Fat 22g, **Sat Fat** 5g;
Chol 65mg; **Sodium** 670mg;
Total Carb 40g, **Total Sugars** 7g,
Added Sugars 0g; **Protein** 28g

DF **MAKE IT DAIRY FREE** Omit feta cheese.

CHIPOTLE-BRAISED PORK AND RICE

SERVES 6

WHY THIS RECIPE WORKS Rich, stewy pork butt spiced with chipotle chile powder and bathed in a tomatoey sauce sounds more indulgent than healthful, but often the key to eating rich meat is balancing portions. Here, rather than spooning loads of braised pork onto tortillas, we cook a smaller amount and serve it with fiberful brown rice to absorb the sauce's flavors in a one-pot meal. We build upon the fond from browning the pork by adding bell peppers and chipotle chile powder. To provide this rice dish with extra substance still, we add low-FODMAP canned lentils, which combine seamlessly with the rice. We finish our dish with green: scallions and cilantro. Pork butt roast is often labeled Boston butt in the supermarket; you can substitute boneless country-style pork ribs. You will need a Dutch oven with a tight-fitting lid for this recipe.

1 tablespoon garlic oil (see page 20), plus extra for serving

2 red bell peppers, chopped

¼ teaspoon table salt

2 teaspoons minced fresh oregano or ½ teaspoon dried

1 teaspoon chipotle chile powder

1 teaspoon minced fresh thyme or ¼ teaspoon dried

2½ cups chicken broth (see page 18)

1 (8-ounce) can tomato sauce (see page 18)

1½ pounds boneless pork butt roast, trimmed and cut into 1-inch pieces

1 cup long-grain brown rice, rinsed

1 (15-ounce) can lentils, rinsed

½ cup chopped fresh cilantro, divided

4 scallions, green parts only, sliced thin

1 tablespoon lime juice

1 Adjust oven rack to lower-middle position and heat oven to 300 degrees. Heat oil in Dutch oven over medium heat until shimmering. Add bell peppers and salt and cook until softened, about 5 minutes. Stir in oregano, chipotle, and thyme and cook until fragrant, about 30 seconds. Stir in broth and tomato sauce, scraping up any browned bits, and bring to simmer. Stir in pork, cover, and transfer pot to oven. Cook until pork is just tender, 1 to 1¼ hours.

2 Remove pot from oven and increase oven temperature to 350 degrees. Stir in rice, cover, and return pot to oven. Cook until rice is tender, about 1 hour, gently stirring rice from bottom of pot to top halfway through cooking.

3 Remove pot from oven. Gently fold in lentils and let sit, covered, until heated through, about 5 minutes. Fold in ¼ cup cilantro, scallions, and lime juice. Season with salt and pepper to taste. Sprinkle with remaining ¼ cup cilantro and drizzle with extra oil. Serve.

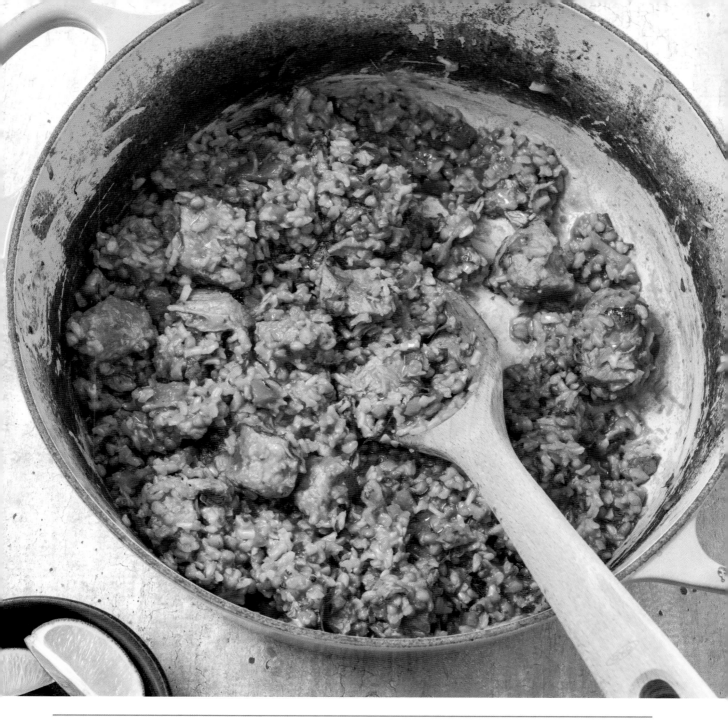

PER SERVING

Dietary Fiber 7g **Cal** 390;
Total Fat 12g, **Sat Fat** 3.5g;
Chol 75mg; **Sodium** 720mg;
Total Carb 39g, **Total Sugars** 5g,
Added Sugars 0g; **Protein** 30g

MAPLE-GINGER ROASTED PORK TENDERLOIN WITH SWISS CHARD AND CARROTS

SERVES 4

WHY THIS RECIPE WORKS Pork tenderloin is the leanest part of the pig, so it cooks much more quickly than other pork roasts and makes a great everyday meal. Its leanness also means it benefits from a stellar side—and that's where the fiber comes in. This combination couldn't be simpler. We pan-sear and then roast the tenderloin in a skillet and then sauté a colorful medley of sweet carrots and earthy Swiss chard in the same pan. And we don't just use the chard leaves. You can quickly boost fiber in a recipe by saving the stems: We slice them thin on the bias and sauté them first with the carrots over relatively high heat to achieve the desirable tender-crisp texture. In addition, the lightly caramelized stems act as a foil to the tender leaves, which we add later in separate handfuls. What makes the complete dish extra special is a whisk-together maple, ginger, and soy glaze: We brush a portion over the tenderloin, toss a portion into the vegetable side, and pour the remainder elegantly over the slices of perfectly cooked pork.

3 tablespoons maple syrup

3 tablespoons garlic oil (see page 20), divided

1 tablespoon soy sauce (see page 18)

1 tablespoon rice vinegar

2 teaspoons grated fresh ginger

1 teaspoon toasted sesame oil

1 (1-pound) pork tenderloin, trimmed

⅛ teaspoon pepper

2 pounds Swiss chard, stems sliced ¼ inch thick on bias, leaves chopped

4 carrots, peeled and sliced ¼ inch thick on bias

1 tablespoon sesame seeds, toasted

1 Adjust oven rack to middle position and heat oven to 400 degrees. Whisk maple syrup, 2 tablespoons garlic oil, soy sauce, vinegar, ginger, and sesame oil in bowl until smooth; set glaze aside.

2 Pat tenderloin dry with paper towels and sprinkle with pepper. Heat remaining 1 tablespoon garlic oil in 12-inch ovensafe skillet over medium-high heat until just smoking. Brown tenderloin on all sides, 5 to 7 minutes. Transfer skillet to oven and roast until pork registers 140 degrees, 10 to 15 minutes, rotating tenderloin halfway through roasting.

3 Using pot holder, remove skillet from oven. Transfer tenderloin to carving board, tent with aluminum foil, and let rest while preparing vegetables.

4 Being careful of hot skillet handle, add chard stems and carrots to fat left in skillet and cook over medium-high heat, stirring occasionally, until crisp-tender, 8 to 10 minutes. Add chard leaves, one handful at a time, and cook until tender, about 5 minutes. Increase heat to high and cook until liquid has evaporated, about 5 minutes. Off heat, stir in half of maple mixture until vegetables are well coated, then transfer to serving platter.

5 Slice tenderloin ½ inch thick and shingle over vegetables. Drizzle remaining maple glaze over pork and sprinkle with sesame seeds. Serve.

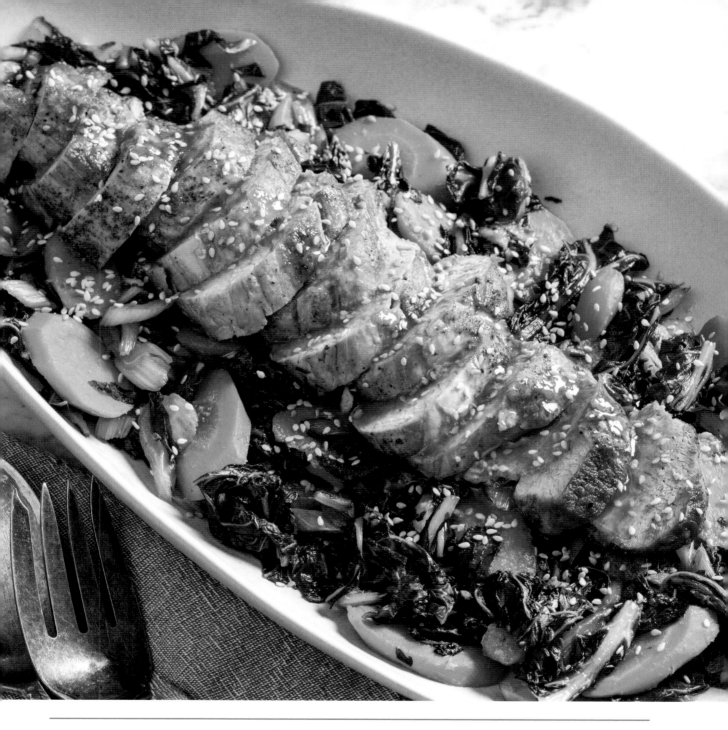

PER SERVING

Dietary Fiber 6g **Cal** 350;
Total Fat 16g, **Sat Fat** 2g;
Chol 75mg; **Sodium** 790mg;
Total Carb 25g, **Total Sugars** 15g,
Added Sugars 9g; **Protein** 29g

 MAKE IT GLUTEN FREE Substitute gluten-free soy sauce or tamari (see page 18) for soy sauce.

CARAWAY-CRUSTED PORK TENDERLOIN WITH SAUERKRAUT AND APPLES

SERVES 4

WHY THIS RECIPE WORKS In this recipe, we pack the winning combination of pork and cabbage with elevated punches that happen to be great for the gut. First, the cabbage is in the form of sauerkraut, giving us an opportunity to cook with the fermented vegetable that we always keep around to eat raw for its beneficial probiotics (see page 5). Pairing it with apples in a sweet-tart side dish, balanced with a little brown sugar, makes it extra special. And a caraway crust on the pork adds crunchy texture and aromatic flavor to the lean pork in the absence of allium. We soften the side in the same skillet used to brown the tenderloin and then finish roasting the tenderloin on top of it to meld the flavors. To ensure that the tenderloins don't curl during cooking, be sure to remove the silverskin from the meat. There's no need to peel the apples. We prefer red-skinned Fujis or Galas to give the dish more color, but any sweet apple will do.

2 (12-ounce) pork tenderloins, trimmed

1 tablespoon caraway seeds

½ teaspoon table salt

½ teaspoon plus ⅛ teaspoon pepper, divided

2 tablespoons garlic oil (see page 20), divided

3 apples, cored, halved, and cut into ¼-inch-thick slices

1 pound sauerkraut, rinsed and squeezed dry

2 tablespoons packed light brown sugar

2 tablespoons minced fresh dill

1 Adjust oven rack to middle position and heat oven to 400 degrees. Pat tenderloins dry with paper towels and sprinkle with caraway seeds, salt, and ½ teaspoon pepper, pressing lightly to adhere. Heat 1 tablespoon oil in 12-inch ovensafe skillet over medium-high heat until just smoking. Brown tenderloins on all sides, 5 to 7 minutes; transfer to plate.

2 Add remaining 1 tablespoon oil, apples, and remaining ⅛ teaspoon pepper to now-empty skillet and cook over medium heat until softened, about 5 minutes, scraping up any browned bits. Stir in sauerkraut and sugar. Place tenderloins on top of sauerkraut mixture. Transfer skillet to oven and roast until pork registers 140 degrees, 10 to 15 minutes.

3 Using potholder, remove skillet from oven and transfer tenderloins to carving board, tent with aluminum foil, and let rest for 5 minutes. Slice tenderloins ½ inch thick. Being careful of hot skillet handle, stir dill into sauerkraut mixture and serve with pork.

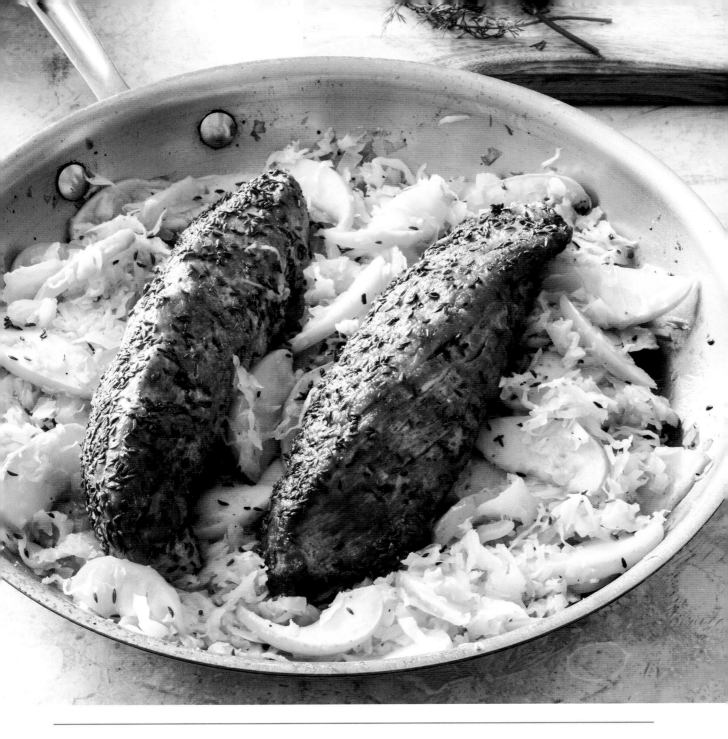

PER SERVING

Dietary Fiber 7g **Cal** 380;
Total Fat 11g, **Sat Fat** 2g;
Chol 105mg; **Sodium** 820mg;
Total Carb 34g, **Total Sugars** 24g,
Added Sugars 7g; **Protein** 35g

GRILLED PORK TENDERLOIN WITH PINEAPPLE-LENTIL SALAD

SERVES 4

WHY THIS RECIPE WORKS Salsa doesn't have to be just a chip dip or light garnish to a dish—in fact, you can bulk up the vegetables (or in this case, fruit) with legumes for a bright, spicy salad that contributes to the heft of the dish. Here we pair a smoky, perfectly grilled pork tenderloin, made ultrasavory with a cumin and chile powder rub, with a bright, sweet pineapple salsa fortified big time with a can of low-FODMAP lentils. To make the most of the fire, we grill the pineapple and a poblano chile and then combine the two with a raw serrano chile (for fresh heat), plus cilantro, lime juice, a bit of reserved spice mixture, and the satisfying lentils.

PORK

- ½ teaspoon table salt
- ¾ teaspoon sugar
- ¼ teaspoon ground cumin
- ¼ teaspoon chipotle chile powder
- 1 (1-pound) pork tenderloin, trimmed

SALAD

- ½ pineapple, peeled, cored, and cut lengthwise into 6 wedges
- 1 poblano chile, stemmed, seeded, and quartered
- 2 tablespoons garlic oil (see page 20), divided
- 1 (15-ounce) can lentils, rinsed
- ½ cup fresh cilantro leaves
- 2 tablespoons lime juice, plus lime wedges for serving
- ¼ cup pepitas, toasted

1 **For the pork:** Combine salt, sugar, cumin, and chile powder in small bowl. Reserve ½ teaspoon spice mixture for the salad. Pat tenderloin dry with paper towels. Rub remaining spice mixture evenly over surface of tenderloin. Refrigerate while preparing grill.

2A **For a charcoal grill:** Open bottom vent completely. Light large chimney starter filled with charcoal briquettes (6 quarts). When top coals are partially covered with ash, pour evenly over half of grill. Set cooking grate in place, cover, and open lid vent completely. Heat grill until hot, about 5 minutes.

2B **For a gas grill:** Turn all burners to high, cover, and heat grill until hot, about 15 minutes. Leave primary burner on high and turn off other burner(s).

3 Clean and oil cooking grate. Place tenderloin on hotter side of grill. Cover and cook, turning tenderloin every 2 minutes, until well browned on all sides, about 8 minutes.

4 **For the salad:** Brush pineapple and poblano with 1 tablespoon oil. Move tenderloin to cooler side of grill (6 to 8 inches from heat source) and place pineapple and poblano on hotter side of grill. Cover and cook until charred on both sides and softened, 8 to 10 minutes, and until pork registers 140 degrees, 12 to 17 minutes, turning tenderloin every 5 minutes. Transfer pineapple and poblano to plate and transfer tenderloin to cutting board. Tent tenderloin with aluminum foil and let rest for 5 minutes.

5 Chop pineapple and poblano. Transfer to large bowl and add remaining 1 tablespoon oil, lentils, cilantro, lime juice, and reserved spice mixture and toss gently to combine. Season with salt and pepper to taste. Sprinkle with pepitas. Slice tenderloin ½ inch thick and serve with salad and lime wedges.

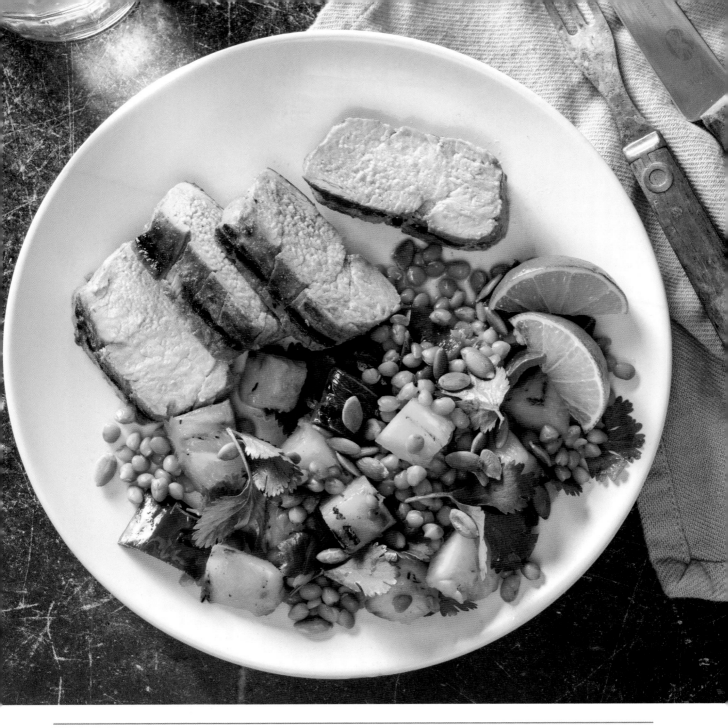

PER SERVING

Dietary Fiber 8g **Cal** 350;
Total Fat 14g, **Sat Fat** 2g;
Chol 70mg; **Sodium** 430mg;
Total Carb 28g, **Total Sugars** 14g,
Added Sugars 1g; **Protein** 30g

ROASTED PORK LOIN WITH BUTTERNUT AND BRUSSELS SPROUTS

SERVES 6 TO 8

WHY THIS RECIPE WORKS This impressive yet simple dinner of warmly spiced pork with hearty roasted butternut squash and Brussels sprouts is ideal for entertaining (or when you're looking to cook for leftovers) on a crisp autumn day—and ideal for getting two good sources of fiber on the plate. Since we wanted to take steps to make this meal special, we rubbed the pork loin with a salt-sugar mixture and let it sit before cooking so that it could retain moisture and caramelize. Starting the pork ahead of the vegetables ensured perfectly cooked meat and tender (not mushy) vegetables. The vegetables simply roast around the partially cooked pork in the pan and then get some more time in the oven to finish while the roast rests. Look for a pork roast that is 7 to 8 inches long and 4 to 5 inches wide. We like to leave a ¼-inch-thick layer of fat on top of the roast; if your roast has a thicker fat cap, trim it back to be about ¼ inch thick. Use Brussels sprouts no bigger than golf balls, as larger ones are often tough and woody. If the pork is enhanced (injected with a salt solution), do not add salt in step 1.

2 tablespoons plus 1 teaspoon packed brown sugar, divided

2 tablespoons kosher salt, divided

1 (2½- to 3-pound) boneless pork loin roast, trimmed

1 teaspoon pepper, divided

4 pounds butternut squash, peeled, seeded, and cut into 1-inch pieces

2 pounds Brussels sprouts, trimmed and halved

½ cup garlic oil (see page 20), divided

½ cup chopped fresh parsley

¼ tablespoon cider vinegar

1 tablespoon Dijon mustard

1 Combine 2 tablespoons sugar and 1 tablespoon salt in bowl. Rub pork with sugar mixture, wrap in plastic wrap, and refrigerate for at least 1 hour or up to 24 hours.

2 Adjust oven rack to middle position, place 16 by 12-inch roasting pan on rack, and heat oven to 400 degrees. Pat pork dry with paper towels, sprinkle with ½ teaspoon pepper, and tie at 1½-inch intervals with kitchen twine. Arrange pork fat side down in center of hot pan and roast for 30 minutes.

3 Meanwhile, toss squash and Brussels sprouts with ¼ cup oil and 2 teaspoons salt in bowl. Arrange squash mixture in pan around pork. Roast until pork registers 135 degrees, 30 to 40 minutes longer.

4 Remove pan from oven. Transfer roast to carving board, tent with aluminum foil, and let rest for 15 minutes. Meanwhile, gently stir squash mixture and continue to roast until tender, 5 to 10 minutes.

5 Whisk remaining ¼ cup oil, parsley, vinegar, mustard, remaining 1 teaspoon sugar, remaining 1 teaspoon salt, and remaining ½ teaspoon pepper together in bowl. Season with salt and pepper to taste. Slice pork ½ inch thick and serve with vegetables, drizzling each individual portion with 2 tablespoons vinaigrette.

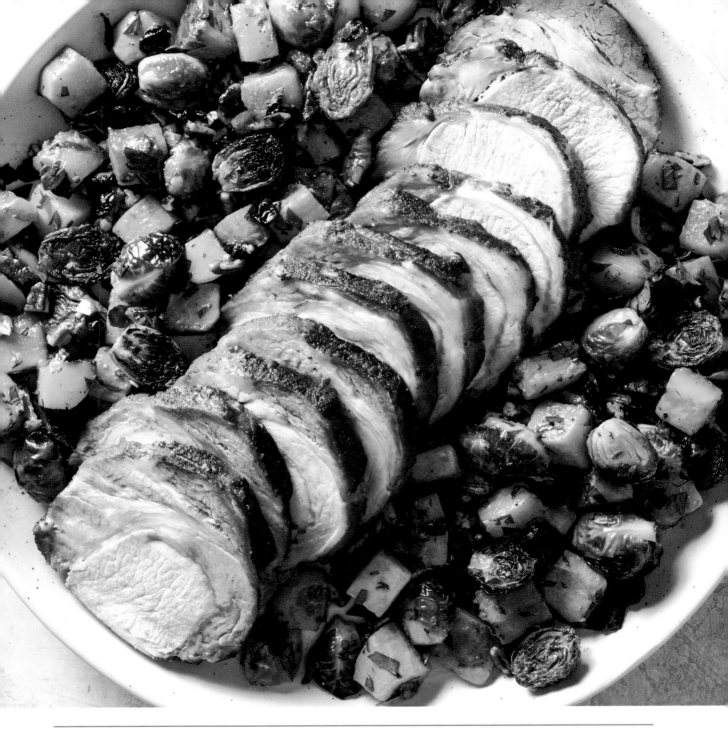

PER SERVING

Dietary Fiber 9g **Cal** 480;
Total Fat 21g, **Sat Fat** 4g;
Chol 90mg; **Sodium** 710mg;
Total Carb 39g, **Total Sugars** 9g,
Added Sugars 9g; **Protein** 38g

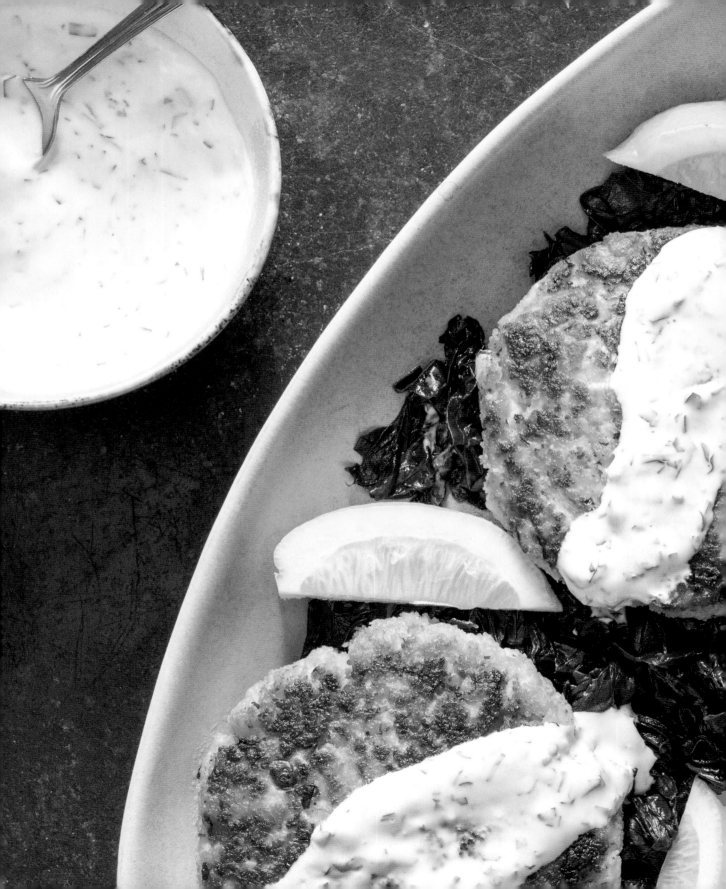

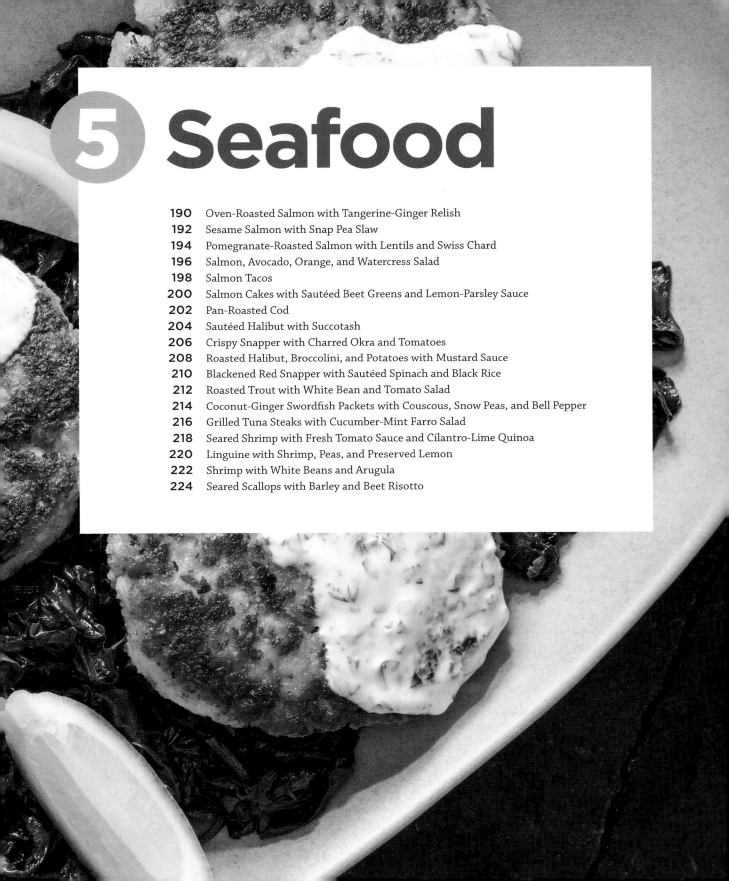

5 Seafood

OVEN-ROASTED SALMON WITH TANGERINE-GINGER RELISH

SERVES 4

WHY THIS RECIPE WORKS Salmon fillets are one of the top cuts of fish to cook and, luckily, they're also great for general health, packed with beneficial omega-3 fatty acids (the very good fat). This salmon gets a lively low-FODMAP tangerine-ginger topping and pairs well with nearly any good-for-you side. To get dinner on the table with ease, we turn to a dual-temperature oven roasting technique; it's a hands-off way to serve up perfectly cooked fish. We preheat a baking sheet in a 500-degree oven and then drop the temperature to 275 degrees just before placing the fillets on the hot pan and into the oven. The initial contact with the hot pan crisps the skin (as searing would), and the heat of the gradually cooling oven cooks the fillets gently, ensuring silky fish. The process frees your burners for dishes like Skillet-Roasted Broccoli (page 270) or Curried Millet with Almonds and Raisins (page 290). It is important to keep the skin on during cooking; remove it afterward if desired. You can substitute arctic char or wild salmon for farmed salmon; cook those fillets to 120 degrees (for medium-rare).

RELISH

- 4 tangerines, rind and pith removed and segments cut into ½-inch pieces (about 1 cup)
- 1 scallion, green part only, sliced thin
- 2 teaspoons lemon juice
- 2 teaspoons extra-virgin olive oil
- 1½ teaspoons grated fresh ginger

SALMON

- 4 (4- to 6-ounce) skin-on salmon fillets, 1 inch thick
- 2 teaspoons canola oil
- ½ teaspoon table salt
- ¼ teaspoon pepper

1 **For the relish:** Place tangerines in fine-mesh strainer set over bowl and let drain for 15 minutes.

2 Pour off all but 1 tablespoon tangerine juice from bowl; whisk in scallion, lemon juice, oil, and ginger. Stir in tangerines and season with salt and pepper to taste.

3 **For the salmon:** Adjust oven rack to lowest position, place aluminum foil–lined rimmed baking sheet on rack, and heat oven to 500 degrees. Make 4 or 5 shallow slashes, about 1 inch apart, on skin side of each fillet, being careful not to cut into flesh. Pat salmon dry with paper towels, rub with oil, and sprinkle with salt and pepper.

4 Reduce oven temperature to 275 degrees and remove sheet from oven. Carefully place salmon skin side down on hot sheet. Roast until center is still translucent when checked with tip of paring knife and registers 125 degrees (for medium-rare), 8 to 12 minutes. Transfer salmon to individual plates or serving platter. Serve.

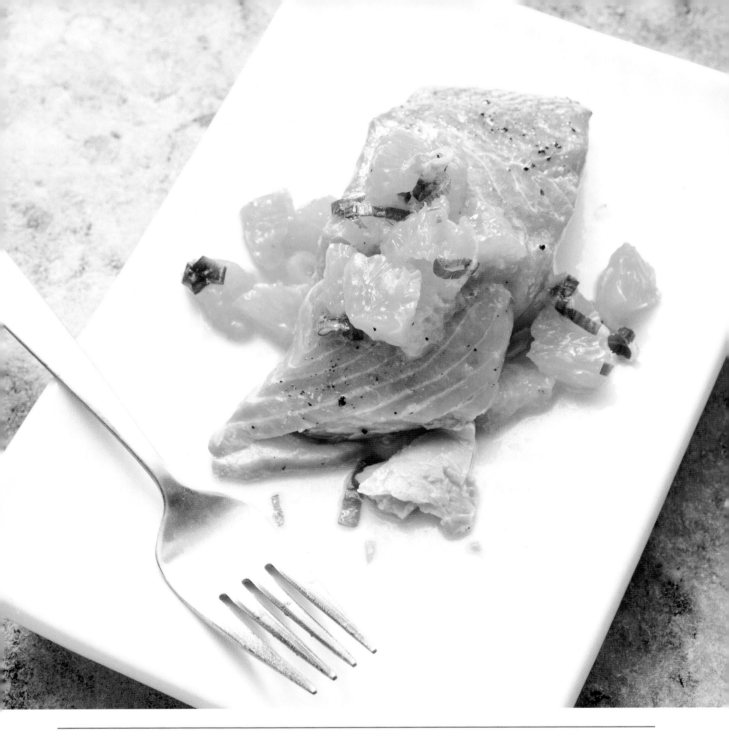

PER SERVING

Dietary Fiber 2g **Cal** 330;
Total Fat 20g, **Sat Fat** 4g;
Chol 60mg; **Sodium** 360mg;
Total Carb 12g, **Total Sugars** 9g,
Added Sugars 0g; **Protein** 24g

SESAME SALMON WITH SNAP PEA SLAW

SERVES 4

GLUTEN FREE

WHY THIS RECIPE WORKS Achieving an interesting salmon dinner with a lively high-fiber side doesn't have to mean multicomponent cooking. We serve this salmon, coated with crunchy sesame seeds, with a cool, complex slaw of sugar snap peas, edamame, cucumber, and radishes that continues the crunch without cooking. We smartly utilize a bold, bright tahini-ginger-lemon paste to adhere the coating of crunchy sesame seeds to the fish. The matching slaw, made creamy with a combo of mayonnaise and tangy yogurt, requires just a whisk of the dressing and a toss of the vegetables. You can substitute arctic char or wild salmon for farmed salmon; cook fillets to 120 degrees (for medium-rare).

3 scallions, green parts only, sliced thin

2 tablespoons plain yogurt

2 tablespoons mayonnaise

3½ teaspoons grated lemon zest plus 5 teaspoons juice, divided

¾ teaspoon table salt, divided

12 ounces sugar snap peas, strings removed, sliced thin on bias

2 cups frozen edamame, thawed

1 English cucumber, halved lengthwise, seeded, and sliced thin

6 radishes, trimmed, halved lengthwise, and sliced thin

4 teaspoons tahini

2 teaspoons grated fresh ginger

⅓ cup toasted sesame seeds

4 (4- to 6-ounce) skinless salmon fillets, 1 inch thick

¼ teaspoon pepper

1 teaspoon garlic oil (see page 20), plus extra for drizzling

1 Whisk scallions, yogurt, mayonnaise, ½ teaspoon lemon zest and 1 tablespoon juice, and ½ teaspoon salt together in large bowl. Add snap peas, edamame, cucumber, and radishes and stir to coat. Season with salt and pepper to taste; set slaw aside.

2 Adjust oven rack to middle position and heat oven to 325 degrees. Combine tahini, ginger, and remaining 1 tablespoon lemon zest and 2 teaspoons juice in bowl. Spread sesame seeds in shallow dish. Pat salmon dry with paper towels and sprinkle with remaining ¼ teaspoon salt and pepper.

3 Spread half of tahini paste over skinned side of fillets. Press coated sides of fillets into seeds and transfer, seed side down, to large plate. Spread remaining paste over tops of fillets, then press coated side of fillets in remaining seeds.

4 Heat oil in 12-inch ovensafe nonstick skillet over medium heat until shimmering. Place fillets skinned side up in skillet and reduce heat to medium-low. Cook until seeds begin to brown, 1 to 4 minutes. Off heat, flip fillets with 2 spatulas, then transfer skillet to oven. Bake until center of salmon is still translucent when checked with tip of paring knife and registers 125 degrees (for medium-rare), 7 to 12 minutes. Serve salmon with slaw, drizzling individual portions with extra oil, if desired.

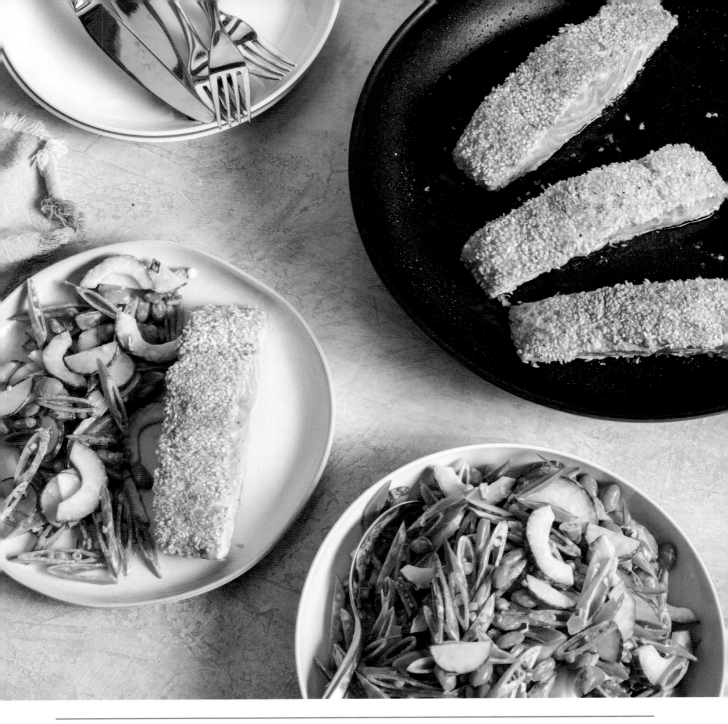

PER SERVING

Dietary Fiber 9g **Cal** 540;
Total Fat 34g, **Sat Fat** 6g;
Chol 65mg; **Sodium** 570mg;
Total Carb 22g, **Total Sugars** 8g,
Added Sugars 0g; **Protein** 39g

LF **MAKE IT LOW FODMAP** Omit snap peas and increase radishes to 12. Substitute dairy-free or lactose-free yogurt (see page 19) for plain yogurt.

DF **MAKE IT DAIRY FREE** Substitute dairy-free yogurt (see page 19) for plain yogurt.

POMEGRANATE-ROASTED SALMON WITH LENTILS AND SWISS CHARD

SERVES 4

WHY THIS RECIPE WORKS We love using lentils to add fiber to meals, and salmon and lentils are a popular combination: Here, a sweet-tart, modest pomegranate glaze brightens the flavors of the rich salmon and earthy lentils, and Swiss chard adds even more nutrition. We keep the flavorful, fiberful chard stems and soften them in garlic oil before simmering with our lentils and then stirring in the leaves. A little bit of time and a final drizzle of garlic oil are all that's needed to add a heady aroma from the jump. Fresh pomegranate seeds tie the molasses-painted salmon components to the savory side. If your knife is not sharp enough to easily cut through the salmon skin, try a serrated knife. It is important to keep the skin on during cooking; remove it afterward if desired. You can substitute arctic char or wild salmon for farmed salmon; cook those fillets to 120 degrees (for medium-rare).

2 tablespoons plus 1 teaspoon garlic oil (see page 20), divided

12 ounces Swiss chard, stemmed, ½ cup stems chopped fine, leaves chopped

2 teaspoons minced fresh thyme or ¾ teaspoon dried

½ teaspoon table salt, divided

1 (15-ounce) can lentils, rinsed

½ cup chicken or vegetable broth (see page 18)

4 (4- to 6-ounce) skin-on salmon fillets, 1 inch thick

2 tablespoons pomegranate molasses, divided

¼ teaspoon pepper

½ cup pomegranate seeds

1 Adjust oven rack to lowest position, place aluminum foil–lined rimmed baking sheet on rack, and heat oven to 500 degrees. Heat 1 tablespoon oil in large saucepan over medium-high heat until shimmering. Add chard stems, thyme, and ¼ teaspoon salt and cook until softened, about 5 minutes.

2 Stir in lentils and broth and bring to simmer. Reduce heat to medium. Add chard leaves, one handful at a time, and cook, stirring occasionally, until wilted and tender, about 4 minutes. Off heat, stir in 1 tablespoon oil and season with salt and pepper to taste; cover to keep warm.

3 Meanwhile, make 4 or 5 shallow slashes, about 1 inch apart, on skin side of each fillet, being careful not to cut into flesh. Pat salmon dry with paper towels. Brush with remaining 1 teaspoon oil, then brush with 1 tablespoon pomegranate molasses and sprinkle with pepper and remaining ¼ teaspoon salt. Reduce oven temperature to 275 degrees and remove sheet from oven. Carefully place salmon skin side down on hot sheet. Roast until center is still translucent when checked with tip of paring knife and registers 125 degrees (for medium-rare), 8 to 12 minutes.

4 Stir pomegranate seeds into lentil mixture. Brush salmon with remaining 1 tablespoon pomegranate molasses and serve with lentils.

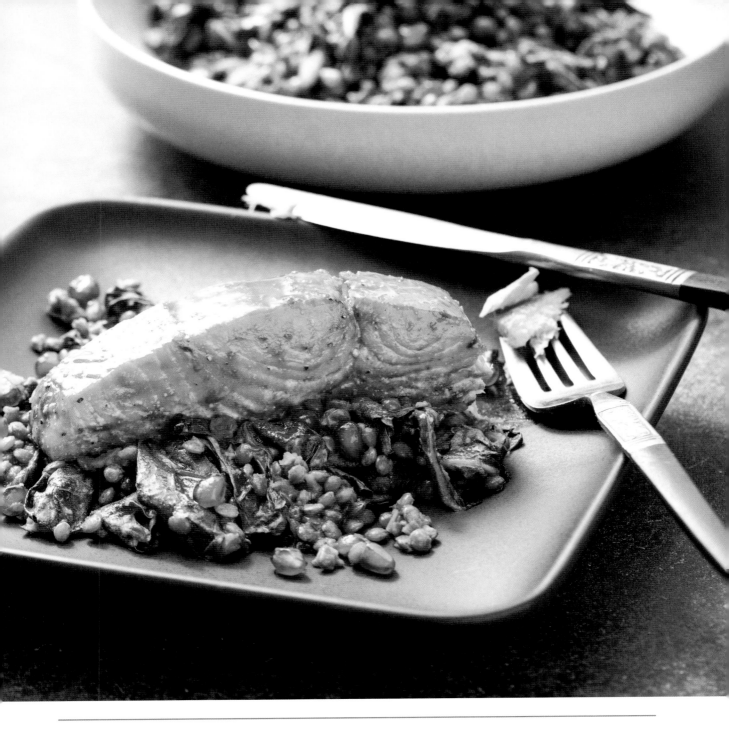

PER SERVING

Dietary Fiber 8g **Cal** 450;
Total Fat 24g, **Sat Fat** 4.5g;
Chol 60mg; **Sodium** 680mg;
Total Carb 26g, **Total Sugars** 9g,
Added Sugars 0g; **Protein** 32g

 MAKE IT LOW FODMAP Substitute 2 tablespoons maple syrup for pomegranate molasses.

SALMON, AVOCADO, ORANGE, AND WATERCRESS SALAD

SERVES 4

WHY THIS RECIPE WORKS A lively salad is a great way to get your greens—but too often, the expected option for turning it into a complete meal is to add a tired grilled chicken breast. But we favor seafood as a great choice for creating a main dish–worthy salad for a change. Our simple salad showcases ingredients that brighten up lunch or dinner: Salmon and avocado both bring richness and make the meal filling and satisfying. For a sweet-tart contrast and vibrant color, we cut up three oranges and reserve some of the orange juice to whisk up a simple citrus vinaigrette that is brought into focus with a little white wine vinegar and Dijon mustard. Watercress is just the right green: It balances the sweetness and richness with its peppery punch. Finally, we add a sprinkle of crunchy toasted hazelnuts and torn mint leaves for complexity. If your knife is not sharp enough to easily cut through the salmon skin, try a serrated knife. It is important to keep the skin on during cooking. You can substitute arctic char or wild salmon for farmed salmon; cook those fillets to 120 degrees (for medium-rare).

2 (6- to 8-ounce) skin-on salmon fillets, 1 inch thick

3 tablespoons plus 1 teaspoon extra-virgin olive oil, divided

¾ teaspoon table salt, divided

⅛ teaspoon pepper

3 oranges

1 teaspoon white wine vinegar

1 teaspoon Dijon mustard

4 ounces (4 cups) watercress, torn into bite-size pieces

1 avocado, halved, pitted, and sliced thin

¼ cup fresh mint leaves, torn

¼ cup hazelnuts, toasted and chopped

1 Adjust oven rack to lowest position, place aluminum foil–lined rimmed baking sheet on rack, and heat oven to 500 degrees. Make 4 or 5 shallow slashes, about 1 inch apart, on skin side of each fillet, being careful not to cut into flesh. Pat salmon dry with paper towels, rub with 1 teaspoon oil, and sprinkle with ¼ teaspoon salt and pepper.

2 Reduce oven temperature to 275 degrees and remove sheet from oven. Carefully place salmon skin side down on hot sheet. Roast until center is still translucent when checked with tip of paring knife and registers 125 degrees (for medium-rare), 8 to 12 minutes. Transfer salmon to plate. Let cool completely, about 20 minutes. Using 2 forks, flake salmon into rough 2-inch pieces; discard skin.

3 Meanwhile, cut away peel and pith from oranges. Holding fruit over bowl, use paring knife to slice between membranes to release segments. Measure out 2 tablespoons orange juice and transfer to separate bowl.

4 Add vinegar, mustard, remaining 3 tablespoons oil, and remaining ½ teaspoon salt to bowl with orange juice and whisk until smooth. Arrange watercress in even layer on serving platter. Top with salmon pieces, orange segments, and avocado. Drizzle vinaigrette over top, then sprinkle with mint and hazelnuts. Serve.

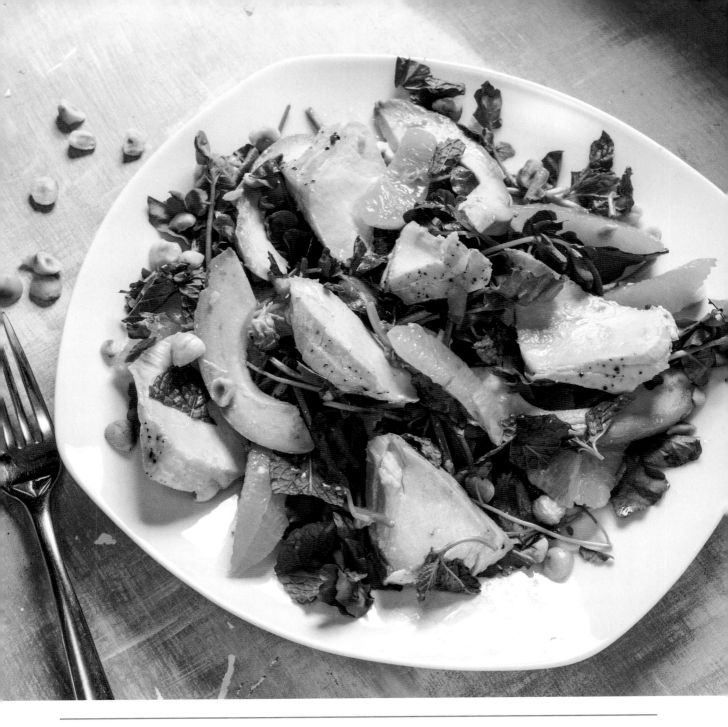

PER SERVING

Dietary Fiber 9g **Cal** 280;
Total Fat 18g, **Sat Fat** 2.5g;
Chol 30mg; **Sodium** 650mg;
Total Carb 17g, **Total Sugars** 10g,
Added Sugars 0g; **Protein** 14g

 MAKE IT LOW FODMAP Reduce avocado to ½ avocado (4 ounces).

SALMON TACOS

SERVES 6

WHY THIS RECIPE WORKS California-style fish tacos generally feature deep-fried fish, a tangy cabbage slaw, and avocado, but they're not the only way to taco. We wanted to boost the nutritional value of each element for a supercharged take on fish tacos. Since we were forgoing the frying, we opted for salmon, which carries more flavor than the typically used cod or other white fish. A flavorful spice rub gave the fillets a nice crust. For a slaw that would stand up to the salmon, we wondered if we could incorporate nutrient-rich dark leafy greens, and collards proved just the ticket. When thinly sliced, they required no precooking. Combined with cilantro and lime, they perfectly complemented the rich fish and, along with crunchy radish and cooling jícama, gave these tacos the fiber boost we envisioned. You can substitute 2 cups thinly sliced cabbage for the collard greens. You can substitute arctic char or wild salmon for farmed salmon; cook those fillets to 120 degrees (for medium-rare).

¼ teaspoon grated lime zest and 2 tablespoons juice, plus lime wedges for serving

1 teaspoon table salt, divided

4 ounces collard greens, stemmed and sliced thin (2 cups)

4 ounces jícama, peeled and cut into 2-inch-long matchsticks

4 radishes, trimmed and cut into 1-inch-long matchsticks

¼ cup fresh cilantro leaves

1½ teaspoons chipotle chile powder

¼ teaspoon pepper

4 (6- to 8-ounce) skin-on salmon fillets, 1 inch thick

2 teaspoons canola oil

2 avocados, halved, pitted, and cut into ½-inch pieces

12 (6-inch) corn tortillas (see page 19), warmed

1 Whisk lime zest and juice and ¼ teaspoon salt together in large bowl. Add collard greens, jícama, radishes, and cilantro leaves and toss to combine; set slaw aside.

2 Combine chile powder, pepper, and remaining ¾ teaspoon salt in small bowl. Pat salmon dry with paper towels and sprinkle evenly with spice mixture. Heat oil in 12-inch nonstick skillet over medium-high heat until shimmering. Cook salmon skin side up until well browned, 3 to 5 minutes. Gently flip salmon using 2 spatulas and cook until salmon is still translucent when checked with tip of paring knife and registers 125 degrees (for medium-rare), 3 to 5 minutes. Transfer salmon to plate and let cool slightly, about 2 minutes. Using 2 forks, flake fish into rough 2-inch pieces; discard skin.

3 Divide fish, collard slaw, and avocado evenly among tortillas. Serve.

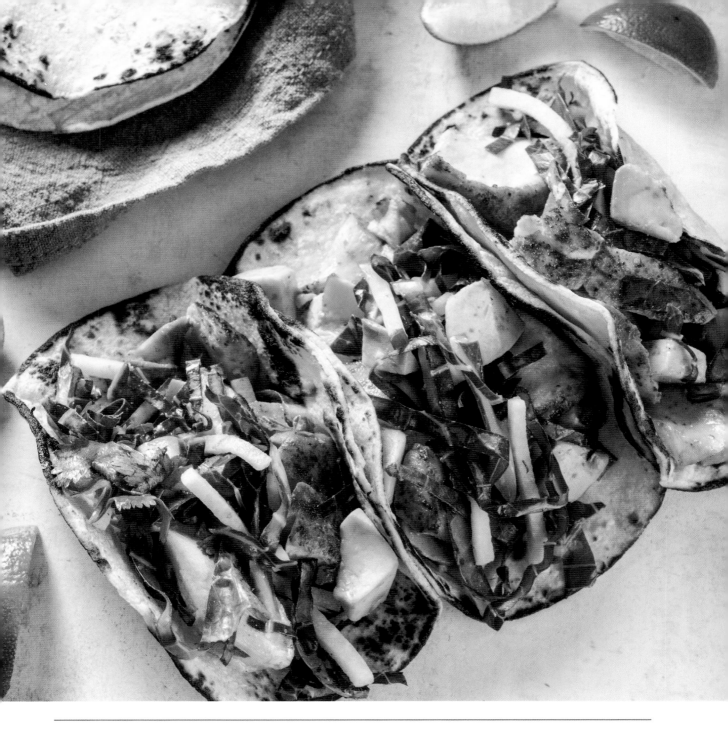

PER SERVING

Dietary Fiber 8g **Cal** 480;
Total Fat 28g, **Sat Fat** 5g;
Chol 60mg; **Sodium** 490mg;
Total Carb 31g, **Total Sugars** 1g,
Added Sugars 0g; **Protein** 27g

LF **MAKE IT LOW FODMAP** Omit avocado.

SALMON CAKES WITH SAUTÉED BEET GREENS AND LEMON-PARSLEY SAUCE

SERVES 4

WHY THIS RECIPE WORKS We love fish cakes because they can transcend appetizer, becoming a creative way to enjoy a healthful protein and complementary side (and, of course, a creamy sauce) as a main meal. We wanted to pair ultraflavorful salmon cakes with a mild but hardy green, so we sautéed nutritious, delicious beet greens, still wet from washing, in some garlic oil while the cakes kept warm in the oven after cooking. For the cakes, we knew they should deliver rich flavor and tender texture without flavor-muting binders. We used a food processor to coarsely chop salmon so that it wasn't overly dense. Whole-wheat panko bread crumbs provided enough binding without compromising flavor, although you can use gluten-free panko if that's best for you. A combination of parsley, mustard, and capers added fresh, tangy complexity; a bit of yogurt ensured our patties would stay moist. Some of these ingredients then became the quick bright, creamy sauce to drizzle over the cakes and greens. Be sure to use raw salmon here; do not substitute cooked or canned salmon. You can substitute arctic char or wild salmon for farmed salmon. Don't overprocess salmon in step 2 or cakes will have a pasty texture. You can substitute Swiss chard for the beet greens.

¼ cup plain yogurt, divided

3 tablespoons minced fresh parsley, divided

2 tablespoons mayonnaise

2 teaspoons lemon juice, plus lemon wedges for serving

1 tablespoon Dijon mustard

2 teaspoons capers, rinsed and minced

¼ teaspoon table salt, divided

¼ teaspoon pepper, divided

1 pound skinless salmon fillets, cut into 1-inch pieces

¾ cup 100 percent whole-wheat panko bread crumbs

2 pounds beet greens, stemmed and chopped

5 teaspoons garlic oil (see page 20), divided

1 Combine 2 tablespoons yogurt, 1 tablespoon parsley, mayonnaise, and lemon juice in small bowl. Cover sauce and refrigerate until ready to serve. Whisk remaining 2 tablespoons yogurt, remaining 2 tablespoons parsley, mustard, capers, ⅛ teaspoon salt, and ⅛ teaspoon pepper together in large bowl.

2 Working in 2 batches, pulse salmon in food processor until coarsely ground, about 4 pulses; transfer to large bowl with yogurt mixture. Gently fold in panko until well combined. Using your lightly moistened hands, divide salmon mixture into 4 equal portions, then gently shape each portion into 4-inch-wide cake. (Shaped salmon cakes can be refrigerated for up to 24 hours.)

3 Wash and drain beet greens, leaving greens slightly wet; set aside. Heat 2 teaspoons oil in 12-inch nonstick skillet over medium heat until shimmering. Cook cakes until well browned, 3 to 4 minutes per side. Transfer cakes to serving platter and tent with aluminum foil.

4 Heat remaining 1 tablespoon oil in now-empty skillet over medium-high heat until shimmering. Add drained greens, remaining ⅛ teaspoon salt, and remaining ⅛ teaspoon pepper. Cover and cook, stirring occasionally, until greens are wilted but still bright green, about 3 minutes. Increase heat to high and cook, uncovered, until liquid evaporates, 2 to 3 minutes. Serve salmon cakes with beet greens, lemon-parsley sauce, and lemon wedges.

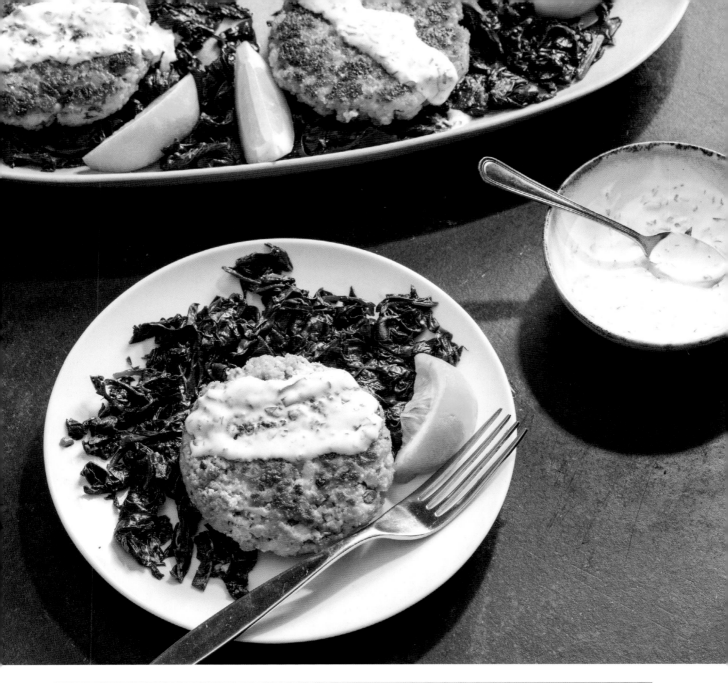

PER SERVING

Dietary Fiber 6g **Cal** 400;
Total Fat 27g, **Sat Fat** 5g;
Chol 65mg; **Sodium** 710mg;
Total Carb 12g, **Total Sugars** 2g,
Added Sugars 0g; **Protein** 28g

LF **MAKE IT LOW FODMAP** Substitute dairy-free or lactose-free yogurt (see page 19) for plain yogurt. Substitute gluten-free panko bread crumbs for whole-wheat crumbs.

DF **MAKE IT DAIRY FREE** Substitute dairy-free yogurt (see page 19) for plain yogurt.

GF **MAKE IT GLUTEN FREE** Substitute gluten-free panko bread crumbs for whole-wheat crumbs.

PAN-ROASTED COD

SERVES 4

WHY THIS RECIPE WORKS There are not many things that are more pristine than a perfectly portioned, moist white fish fillet sporting a chestnut-brown crust with some crispness—and nothing more convenient than the lean fish's minutes-long cooking time so you can focus your energy on complementary sides (see pages 260–303). For a cooking method that reliably turns out delicious flaky white fish fillets, we use a common technique borrowed from professional kitchens: Sear the fillets in a hot pan, flip, then transfer to the oven to continue cooking rather than finishing on the stove. This ensures the lean flesh stays moist. With a tiny sprinkle of sugar, a well-browned crust appears in around a minute, giving the interior time to turn succulent in the oven. Carry the beautiful browning over to a vegetable side dish with also-low-FODMAP Sautéed Radishes with Curry Powder and Almonds (page 264), or keep things cool with an elegant Chickpea Salad with Orange and Celery (page 302). You can substitute black sea bass, haddock, hake, or pollack for cod. Serve with one of the sauces on pages 21–25.

4 **(4- to 6-ounce) skinless cod fillets, 1 inch thick**

½ **teaspoon table salt**

¼ **teaspoon pepper**

½ **teaspoon sugar**

1 **tablespoon canola oil**

1 Adjust oven rack to middle position and heat oven to 425 degrees. Pat cod dry with paper towels, sprinkle with salt and pepper, and then sprinkle sugar lightly over 1 side of each fillet.

2 Heat oil in 12-inch ovensafe nonstick skillet over medium-high heat until just smoking. Place fillets sugared side down in skillet and, using spatula, lightly press fillets for 20 to 30 seconds to ensure even contact with skillet. Cook until browned on first side, 1 to 2 minutes.

3 Using 2 spatulas, flip fillets, then transfer skillet to oven. Roast until fish flakes apart when gently prodded with paring knife and registers 135 degrees, 6 to 8 minutes. Serve.

PER SERVING

Dietary Fiber 0g **Cal** 130;
Total Fat 4.5g, **Sat Fat** 0g;
Chol 50mg; **Sodium** 350mg;
Total Carb 1g, **Total Sugars** 1g,
Added Sugars 1g; **Protein** 20g

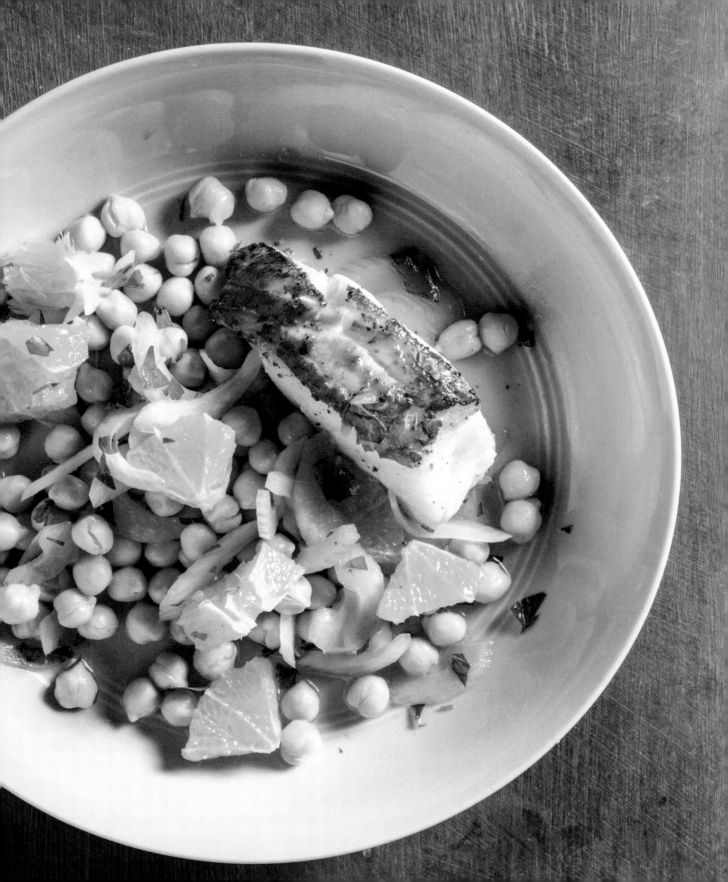

SAUTÉED HALIBUT WITH SUCCOTASH

SERVES 4

GLUTEN FREE

WHY THIS RECIPE WORKS If there were a great American side dish designed for fiber consumption, it would be succotash, that summertime confection of lima beans and fresh sweet corn, often with other vegetables thrown into the mix. The medley stands somewhere between a salad and a light vegetable stew, making it a thoroughly flexible accompaniment; here it plays well with perfectly cooked fillets of meaty halibut. To keep the succotash bright and summery, we forgo any cream in favor of a little butter for some richness without heaviness. Frozen, canned, and dried lima beans all have comparable fiber contents, but we find frozen to be the freshest in flavor and most vividly green in color. Some acidic lemon juice balances the sweetness of the corn. Fresh tarragon sprinkled over the dish adds the perfect aroma to complement the sweetness. You can substitute 3 cups thawed frozen corn for fresh corn. You can substitute red snapper, mahi-mahi, striped bass, or swordfish for halibut.

2 tablespoons unsalted butter

1 red bell pepper, stemmed, seeded, and chopped

¾ teaspoon table salt, divided

Pinch cayenne pepper (optional)

4 ears corn, kernels cut from cobs

3 cups frozen lima beans, thawed

3 tablespoons water

2 tablespoons garlic oil (see page 20), divided

2 tablespoons chopped fresh tarragon, divided

2 teaspoons lemon juice

¼ teaspoon pepper

4 (4- to 6-ounce) skinless halibut fillets

1 Melt butter in 12-inch nonstick skillet over medium-high heat. Add bell pepper and ¼ teaspoon salt and cook until softened and lightly browned, 5 to 7 minutes. Stir in cayenne, if using, and cook until fragrant, about 10 seconds.

2 Reduce heat to medium. Add corn and beans and cook, stirring occasionally, until corn and beans have cooked through, about 4 minutes. Add water and cook, stirring constantly, for 1 minute. Off heat, stir in 1 tablespoon oil, 1 tablespoon tarragon, lemon juice, and pepper. Season with salt and pepper to taste. Transfer succotash to serving dish and cover to keep warm. Wipe skillet clean with paper towels.

3 Pat halibut dry with paper towels and sprinkle with remaining ½ teaspoon salt. Heat remaining 1 tablespoon oil in now-empty skillet over medium-high heat until shimmering. Cook halibut, flipping every 2 minutes, until golden brown and registers 130 degrees, 6 to 9 minutes. Sprinkle succotash with remaining 1 tablespoon tarragon and serve with halibut.

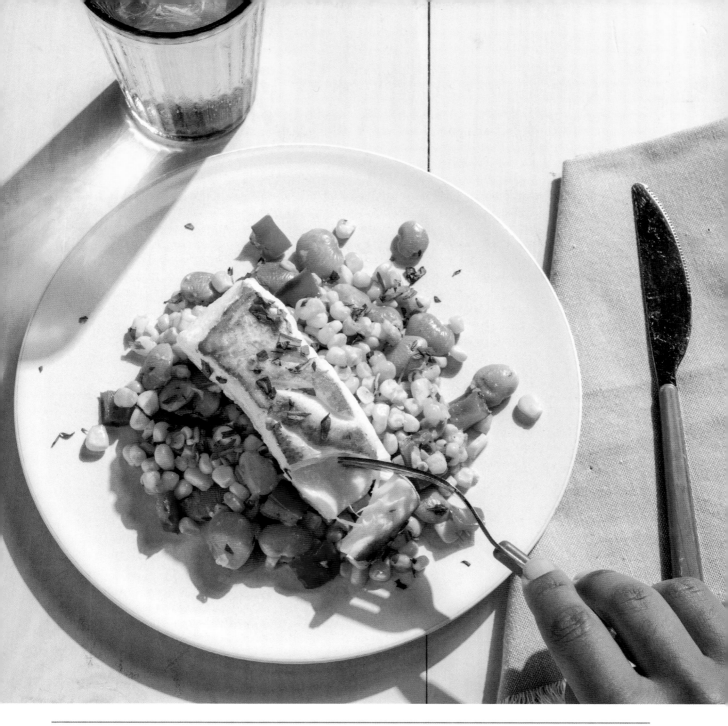

PER SERVING

Dietary Fiber 10g **Cal** 480;
Total Fat 17g, **Sat Fat** 4.5g;
Chol 70mg; **Sodium** 580mg;
Total Carb 51g, **Total Sugars** 6g,
Added Sugars 0g; **Protein** 35g

LF **MAKE IT LOW FODMAP** Reduce corn to 2 ears and lima beans to 1 cup. Stir 8 ounces cherry tomatoes, halved, into succotash with oil.

DF **MAKE IT DAIRY FREE** You can substitute 2 tablespoons extra-virgin olive oil for butter.

CRISPY SNAPPER WITH CHARRED OKRA AND TOMATOES

SERVES 4

WHY THIS RECIPE WORKS We've learned that pairing vegetables for a cohesive side on a low-FODMAP diet can require a bit of finesse since most vegetables contain a bit of FODMAPs and you don't want the offenders to stack. In this snapper and vegetable dish, okra, which does have some fructans in large portion sizes, is the surprise star of the show. Often maligned for its sliminess, okra, when cooked well, is a fantastic ingredient: It takes on char beautifully and has a sturdy, satisfying texture. Searing the okra first over high heat dramatically improves its texture so that it can be stewed in a mix of additional vegetables: FODMAP-free plum tomatoes and red peppers, with ginger and cayenne for warmth. Meanwhile, salting the skin of the snapper and letting it sit helps pull out moisture and allows for a crisp, well-rendered skin to contrast the stew. You can substitute black sea bass, arctic char, or salmon for snapper. Do not use fillets thicker than 1 inch for this recipe. Look for okra pods that are less than 3 inches in length; they will be the most tender. Do not substitute frozen okra here.

- **4** (4- to 6-ounce) skin-on red snapper fillets, 1 inch thick
- **¾** teaspoon plus ⅛ teaspoon table salt, divided
- **3** tablespoons garlic oil (see page 20), divided, plus extra for drizzling
- **12** ounces okra, trimmed
- **2** red bell peppers, stemmed, seeded, and chopped
- **2** teaspoons grated fresh ginger
- **1¼** teaspoons ground coriander
- **¼** teaspoon cayenne pepper (optional)
- **1** pound plum tomatoes, cored and cut into ½-inch pieces
- **½** cup water
- **½** cup fresh cilantro leaves, divided
- **1** teaspoon red wine vinegar
- **⅓** cup toasted sliced almonds

1 Using sharp knife, score snapper skin lengthwise at ½-inch intervals, making ¼-inch-deep cuts, stopping ½ inch from top and bottom of fillet. Sprinkle skin side of fillets with ⅛ teaspoon salt and flesh side of fillets with ¼ teaspoon salt. Transfer fillets skin side up to plate and refrigerate, uncovered, until needed.

2 Heat 1 teaspoon oil in 12-inch nonstick skillet over high heat until just smoking. Add okra and cook until well charred, 6 to 8 minutes, stirring halfway through cooking; transfer to bowl.

3 Heat 2 teaspoons oil in large saucepan over medium-high heat until shimmering. Add bell peppers and cook until softened and lightly browned, 5 to 7 minutes. Stir in ginger, coriander, and cayenne, if using, and cook until fragrant, about 30 seconds. Stir in tomatoes, water, and remaining ½ teaspoon salt and bring to simmer. Stir in okra, reduce heat to medium-low, and simmer gently until okra is tender and tomatoes have begun to break down, 15 to 20 minutes. Off heat, stir in ¼ cup cilantro, 1 tablespoon oil, and vinegar. Season with salt and pepper to taste; cover to keep warm.

4 Pat fillets dry with paper towels. Heat remaining 1 tablespoon oil in now-empty skillet over high heat until just smoking. Place fillets skin side down in skillet. Immediately reduce heat to medium-low and cook until skin is well browned and flesh is opaque except for top ¼ inch, 5 to 8 minutes.

5 Off heat, flip fillets with 2 spatulas and continue to cook using residual heat of skillet until snapper registers 135 degrees, 30 seconds to 1 minute. Divide okra mixture among individual plates and arrange snapper skin side up on top. Sprinkle with almonds and remaining ¼ cup cilantro and drizzle with extra oil. Serve.

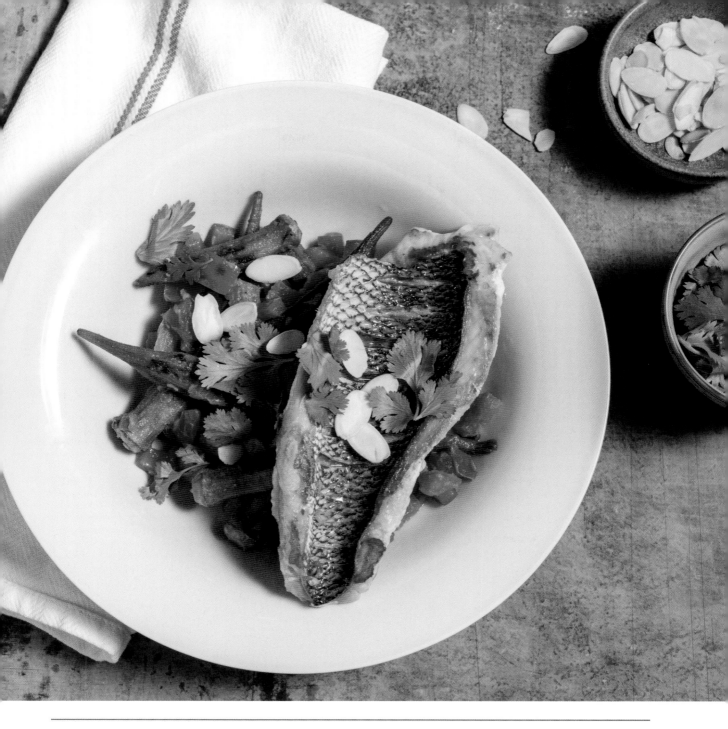

PER SERVING

Dietary Fiber 6g **Cal** 310;
Total Fat 16g, **Sat Fat** 1.5g;
Chol 40mg; **Sodium** 600mg;
Total Carb 15g, **Total Sugars** 7g,
Added Sugars 0g; **Protein** 28g

ROASTED HALIBUT, BROCCOLINI, AND POTATOES WITH MUSTARD SAUCE

SERVES 4

WHY THIS RECIPE WORKS Looking for a from-the-sea swap for typical meat and potatoes? Try this one-pan meal of hearty halibut, golden potatoes, and charred broccolini (a fiber bonus in the equation), plus an intensely flavorful stir-together mustard sauce. We start by roasting the potatoes and broccolini on separate sides of a baking sheet. We remove the broccolini once it's attractively charred, then add our fish to the freed-up side of the sheet and drop the oven temperature to allow the fish to cook gently. A paprika-honey mixture brushed on the fillets before roasting pairs beautifully with the bright sauce of mustard and gut-friendly chives. Use small red potatoes measuring 1 to 2 inches in diameter. Look for broccolini that is approximately ½ inch thick at its base; larger broccolini should be halved lengthwise after peeling. You can substitute mahi-mahi, striped bass, swordfish, or red snapper for halibut.

5 tablespoons plus
2 teaspoons extra-virgin
olive oil, divided

¼ cup minced fresh chives

2 tablespoons whole-grain
mustard

1 teaspoon grated lemon
zest plus 2 teaspoons juice

1 tablespoon honey, divided

1¼ pounds small red potatoes,
unpeeled, halved

½ teaspoon table salt,
divided

½ teaspoon pepper, divided

1¼ pounds broccolini, trimmed

½ teaspoon paprika

4 (4- to 6-ounce) skinless
halibut fillets, 1 to
1½ inches thick

1 Adjust oven rack to lowest position and heat oven to 500 degrees. Combine 2 tablespoons oil, chives, mustard, lemon juice, and 1 teaspoon honey in bowl. Season with salt and pepper to taste; set sauce aside for serving. Brush rimmed baking sheet with 1 tablespoon oil.

2 Toss potatoes with 1 tablespoon oil, ⅛ teaspoon salt, and ⅛ teaspoon pepper in bowl. Place potatoes cut side down on one half of sheet. Peel bottom halves of broccolini spears until white flesh is exposed. In now-empty bowl, toss broccolini with 1 tablespoon oil, ⅛ teaspoon salt, and ⅛ teaspoon pepper. Arrange half of broccolini on empty side of sheet with tops pointed in one direction; arrange remaining spears on top of first layer with tops pointed in opposite direction. Roast until potatoes are golden brown and broccolini is spotty brown, 12 to 14 minutes, tossing broccolini and rotating sheet halfway through roasting.

3 Meanwhile, combine 1 teaspoon oil, lemon zest, paprika, remaining 2 teaspoons honey, remaining ¼ teaspoon salt, and remaining ¼ teaspoon pepper in small bowl; microwave until bubbling, 10 to 15 seconds. Pat halibut dry with paper towels, brush skinned side with remaining 1 teaspoon oil, then brush tops with honey mixture.

4 Remove sheet from oven and reduce oven temperature to 275 degrees. Transfer broccolini to serving platter and tent with aluminum foil to keep warm. Place halibut skinned side down on now-empty side of sheet and continue to roast until fish flakes apart when gently prodded with paring knife and registers 130 degrees, 6 to 8 minutes, rotating sheet halfway through roasting. Transfer potatoes and halibut to platter with broccolini. Serve with sauce.

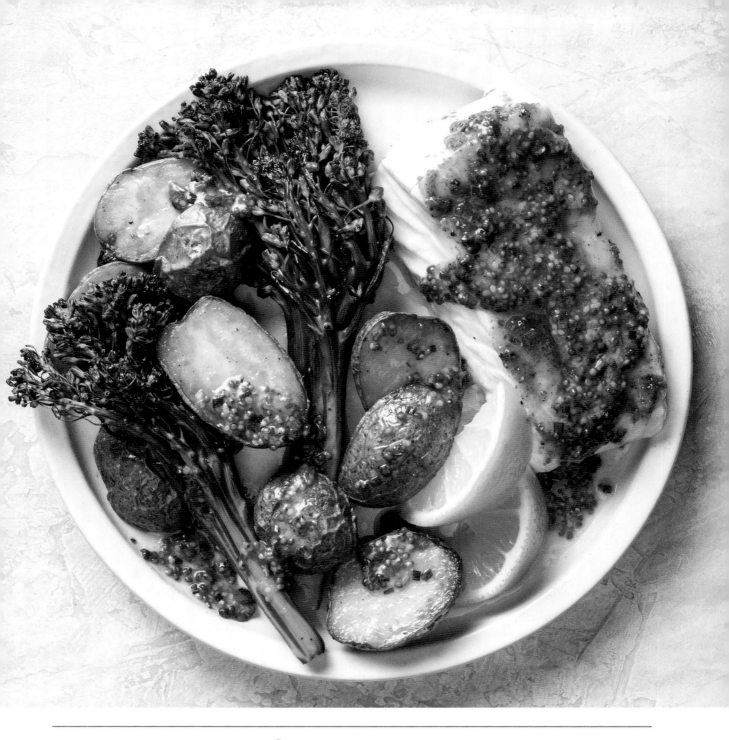

PER SERVING

Dietary Fiber 6g **Cal** 450;
Total Fat 22g, **Sat Fat** 3g;
Chol 55mg; **Sodium** 610mg;
Total Carb 35g, **Total Sugars** 8g,
Added Sugars 4g; **Protein** 28g

 MAKE IT LOW FODMAP Decrease broccolini to 12 ounces and increase potatoes to 1½ pounds.

BLACKENED RED SNAPPER WITH SAUTÉED SPINACH AND BLACK RICE

SERVES 4

WHY THIS RECIPE WORKS Blackening fish is a scorching-hot situation and it's therefore easy to pay little attention to what you serve with it. Here we skip the stovetop smoke, cooking snapper under the broiler; with the fish under better control, we prepare some fiber-rich sautéed spinach and nutty black rice. Yogurt sauce provides cooling contrast to the spiced fish and extra flavor to its worthy pairings. If you can't find black rice, you can use brown rice, although it may need a few extra minutes of cooking. You can substitute halibut, mahi-mahi, striped bass, or swordfish for red snapper. If you don't have a large microwave-safe bowl, microwave the spinach in two batches; reduce the water to 2 tablespoons per batch and cook each for about 1½ minutes.

1½ cups black rice

¾ teaspoon table salt, divided, plus salt for cooking rice

½ cup plain yogurt

2 teaspoons grated lemon zest plus 1 teaspoon juice

3 tablespoons garlic oil (see page 20), divided

1½ teaspoons smoked paprika

½ teaspoon ground coriander

½ teaspoon ground fennel

¼ teaspoon cayenne pepper

⅛ teaspoon ground cloves

¼ teaspoon pepper

18 ounces (18 cups) baby spinach

4 (4- to 6-ounce) skin-on red snapper fillets, ¾ to 1 inch thick

1 Bring 4 quarts water to boil in Dutch oven over medium-high heat. Add rice and 1 teaspoon salt and cook until rice is tender, 20 to 25 minutes. Drain rice, transfer to bowl, and season with salt and pepper to taste; cover to keep warm.

2 Meanwhile, combine yogurt and lemon zest and juice in bowl and season with salt and pepper to taste; refrigerate until ready to serve. Microwave 1 tablespoon oil, paprika, coriander, fennel, cayenne, cloves, pepper, and ½ teaspoon salt in small bowl until fragrant, about 30 seconds; set aside to cool slightly.

3 Microwave spinach and ¼ cup water in large covered bowl until spinach is wilted and decreased in volume by half, 3 to 4 minutes. Remove bowl from microwave and keep covered for 1 minute. Carefully remove cover and transfer spinach to colander. Using back of rubber spatula, gently press spinach against colander to release excess liquid.

4 Adjust oven rack 4 inches from broiler element and heat broiler. Line rimmed baking sheet with aluminum foil. Pat red snapper dry with paper towels and brush flesh side evenly with spice mixture. Arrange snapper skin side down on prepared sheet. Broil until snapper flakes apart when gently prodded with paring knife and registers 130 degrees, 4 to 6 minutes. Transfer snapper to individual plates or serving platter.

5 Meanwhile, heat remaining 2 tablespoons oil in 12-inch skillet over medium heat until shimmering. Add spinach and toss to coat. Season with remaining ¼ teaspoon salt and continue stirring with tongs until spinach is glossy green, about 2 minutes. Season with salt and pepper to taste. Serve with snapper, rice, and yogurt sauce.

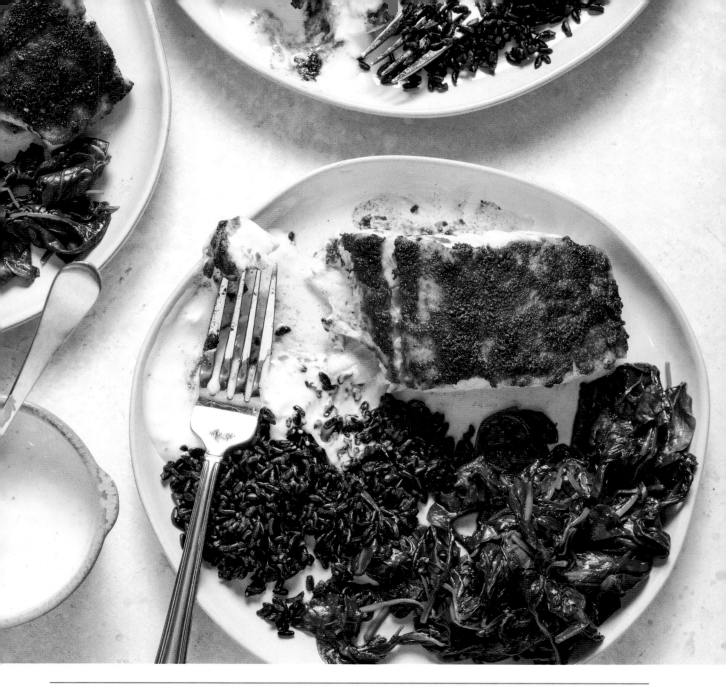

PER SERVING

Dietary Fiber 8g **Cal** 480;
Total Fat 16g, **Sat Fat** 2.5g;
Chol 45mg; **Sodium** 710mg;
Total Carb 57g, **Total Sugars** 2g,
Added Sugars 0g; **Protein** 33g

LF **MAKE IT LOW FODMAP** Decrease spinach to 6 ounces. Substitute dairy-free or lactose-free yogurt (see page 19) for plain yogurt.

DF **MAKE IT DAIRY FREE** Substitute dairy-free yogurt (see page 19) for plain yogurt.

ROASTED TROUT WITH WHITE BEAN AND TOMATO SALAD

SERVES 4

WHY THIS RECIPE WORKS Since whole trout have already been boned and butterflied, you can easily roast this rich, flavorful fish (just throw it on a hot greased baking sheet) and also focus on creating an attractive complementary and fiber-rich side dish. Roasting the trout on the preheated baking sheet ensures that it develops a nice, crisp skin with no effort. Since the roasting time is quick, we partner the trout with an equally quick accompaniment: a salad of creamy cannellini beans and bright tomatoes tossed with the appealing aromatic flavors of fresh parsley, tangy lemon juice, briny capers, woodsy rosemary, and our go-to garlic oil. Spooned over the roasted butterflied fillets, the salad makes a beautiful presentation and a hearty dish. We like cannellini beans for this salad, but any canned small white beans will work.

5 tablespoons garlic oil
   (see page 20), divided

4 teaspoons minced
   fresh rosemary

2 tablespoons capers,
   rinsed and minced

¼ cup lemon juice
   (2 lemons), plus lemon
   wedges for serving

2 (15-ounce) cans cannellini
   beans, rinsed

12 ounces cherry
   tomatoes, halved

¼ cup chopped fresh parsley

2 (10- to 12-ounce) boneless,
   butterflied whole trout,
   halved between fillets

¼ teaspoon table salt

¼ teaspoon pepper

1 Adjust oven rack to middle position, place rimmed baking sheet on rack, and heat oven to 450 degrees. Whisk 3 tablespoons oil, rosemary, capers, and lemon juice together in large bowl. Add beans, tomatoes, and parsley and toss to coat. Season with salt and pepper to taste; set salad aside.

2 Add remaining 2 tablespoons oil to preheated sheet, tilting to coat evenly, and return to oven for 4 minutes. Pat trout dry with paper towels and sprinkle with salt and pepper.

3 Carefully place trout skin side down on hot sheet. Roast until trout flakes apart when gently prodded with paring knife, 4 to 6 minutes. Serve trout with bean salad and lemon wedges.

PER SERVING
Dietary Fiber 8g **Cal** 470;
Total Fat 25g, **Sat Fat** 4g;
Chol 65mg; **Sodium** 680mg;
Total Carb 27g, **Total Sugars** 5g,
Added Sugars 0g; **Protein** 33g

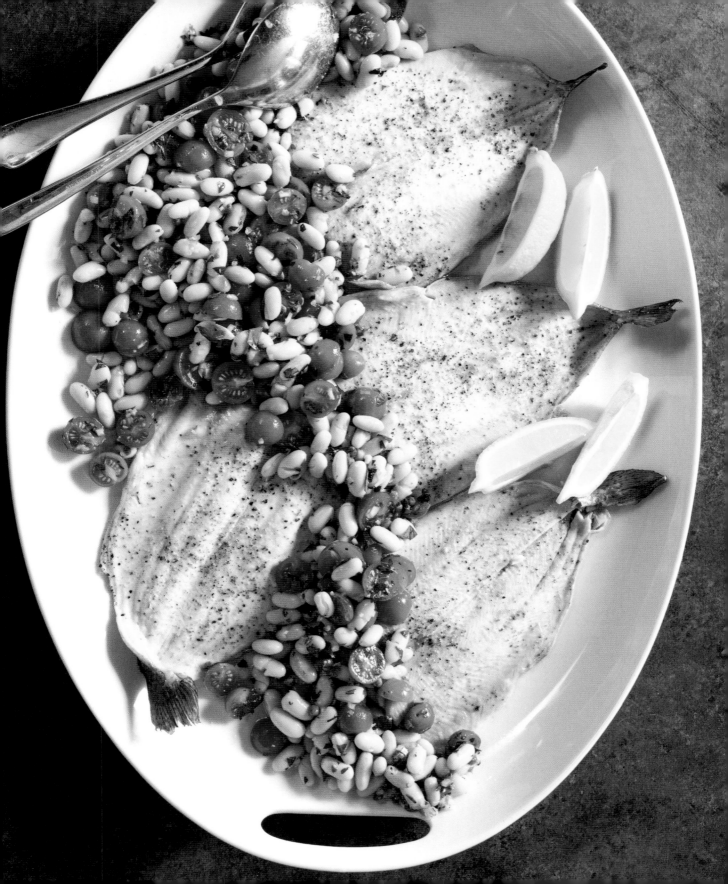

COCONUT-GINGER SWORDFISH PACKETS WITH COUSCOUS, SNOW PEAS, AND BELL PEPPER

SERVES 4

WHY THIS RECIPE WORKS For a spin on the delicate French technique of cooking fish in a packet, or en papillote, we wanted to cook swordfish steaks on a grain and chose a bed of fluffy whole-wheat couscous (it's super-quick-cooking) with a zesty sauce. We mixed coconut milk, ginger, garlic oil, fish sauce, cilantro, and red pepper flakes together for a bold sauce that transformed the couscous into a rich and creamy side and infused the fish with flavor. If we used too much sauce during cooking, the couscous soaked up all of the liquid and ended up gummy while the fish tasted bland, so we reserved some for drizzling. You can substitute halibut, mahi-mahi, red snapper, or striped bass for swordfish. For an accurate measurement of boiling water, bring a full kettle of water to a boil and then measure out the desired amount. To test for doneness without opening the foil packets, use a permanent marker to mark an "X" on the outside of the foil where the fish fillet is the thickest, then insert an instant-read thermometer through the "X" into the fish to measure its internal temperature.

1½ **cups 100 percent whole-wheat couscous**

½ **teaspoon table salt, divided**

1½ **cups boiling water**

½ **cup canned coconut milk**

2 **tablespoons minced fresh cilantro**

1 **tablespoon garlic oil (see page 20)**

2 **teaspoons fish sauce**

2 **teaspoons grated fresh ginger**

1 **teaspoon lime zest plus ½ teaspoon juice**

⅛ **teaspoon red pepper flakes (optional)**

8 **ounces snow peas, strings removed**

1 **red bell pepper, stemmed, seeded, and sliced thin**

4 **(4- to 6-ounce) skinless swordfish steaks, ¾ to 1 inch thick**

1 Adjust oven rack to middle position and heat oven to 400 degrees. Combine couscous, ¼ teaspoon salt, and boiling water in bowl, cover, and let sit until liquid is absorbed and couscous is tender, about 5 minutes. Fluff couscous with fork. Combine coconut milk, cilantro, oil, fish sauce, ginger, lime zest, and pepper flakes, if using, in small bowl.

2 Lay four 16 by 12-inch rectangles of aluminum foil on counter with short sides parallel to counter edge. Divide couscous evenly among foil rectangles, arranging in center of lower half of each sheet of foil, and top with snow peas and bell pepper. Pat swordfish dry with paper towels and sprinkle with remaining ¼ teaspoon salt. Place on top of vegetables and spoon 2 tablespoons coconut sauce over top of each steak; reserve remaining coconut sauce for serving. Fold top half of foil over fish and couscous, then tightly crimp edges into rough 9 by 6-inch packets.

3 Place packets on rimmed baking sheet (they may overlap slightly) and bake until fish registers 130 degrees, 20 to 25 minutes. Carefully open packets, allowing steam to escape away from you, then let swordfish rest in packets for 10 minutes.

4 Microwave reserved coconut sauce until warmed through, about 30 seconds, then stir in lime juice. Using thin metal spatula, gently slide swordfish and couscous onto individual plates, drizzle with sauce, and serve.

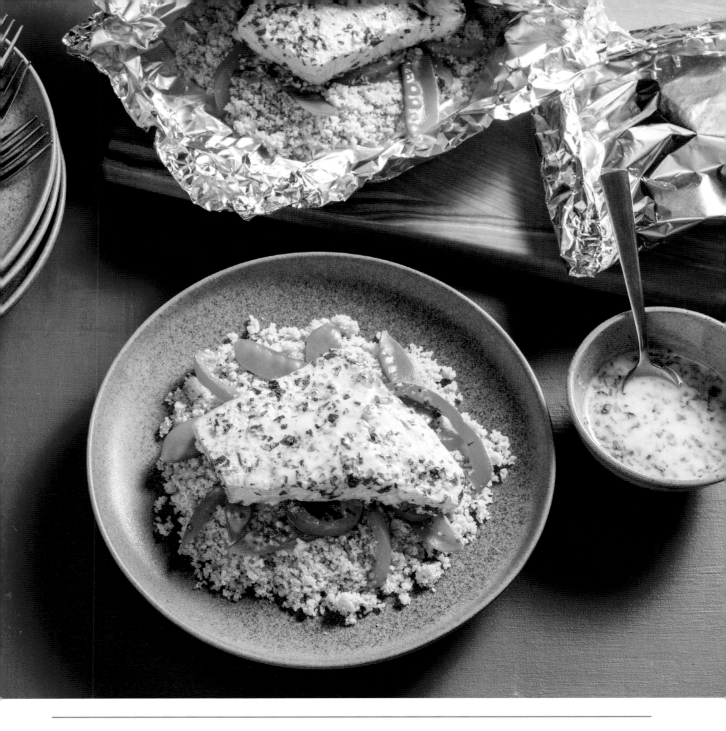

PER SERVING

Dietary Fiber 10g **Cal** 530;
Total Fat 18g, **Sat Fat** 7g;
Chol 75mg; **Sodium** 630mg;
Total Carb 57g, **Total Sugars** 8g,
Added Sugars 0g; **Protein** 34g

GRILLED TUNA STEAKS WITH CUCUMBER-MINT FARRO SALAD

SERVES 4

WHY THIS RECIPE WORKS Farro is a perfect whole grain for salad because of its pleasantly chewy texture, here interrupted by crisp, refreshing cucumbers. A creamy yogurt dressing makes the salad a cooling side to grilled tuna. We prefer the flavor and texture of whole farro; pearled farro can be used, but the texture may be softer. Do not use quick-cooking or presteamed farro. The cooking time for farro can vary greatly across brands, so we recommend beginning to check for doneness after 10 minutes. We prefer our tuna served rare or medium-rare. If you like your tuna cooked medium, observe the timing for medium-rare, then tent the steaks with foil for 5 minutes.

1½ cups whole farro

1 teaspoon table salt, divided, plus salt for cooking farro

6 tablespoons extra-virgin olive oil, divided

2 tablespoons lemon juice

2 tablespoons plain Greek yogurt

¼ teaspoon pepper, divided

1 English cucumber, halved lengthwise, seeded, and cut into ¼-inch pieces

6 ounces cherry tomatoes, halved

2 ounces (2 cups) baby arugula

3 tablespoons chopped fresh mint

2 teaspoons honey

1 teaspoon water

2 (8- to 12-ounce) skinless tuna steaks, 1 inch thick, halved crosswise

1 Bring 4 quarts water to boil in Dutch oven. Add farro and 1 tablespoon salt and cook until grains are tender with slight chew, 15 to 30 minutes. Drain farro, spread evenly on rimmed baking sheet, and let cool completely, about 15 minutes.

2 Whisk 3 tablespoons oil, lemon juice, yogurt, ½ teaspoon salt, and ⅛ teaspoon pepper together in large bowl. Add drained farro, cucumber, tomatoes, arugula, and mint and toss gently to combine. Season with salt and pepper to taste; set aside. Whisk remaining 3 tablespoons oil, honey, water, remaining ½ teaspoon salt, and remaining ⅛ teaspoon pepper together in bowl. Pat tuna dry with paper towels and generously brush with oil-honey mixture.

3A For a charcoal grill: Open bottom vent completely. Light large chimney starter filled with charcoal briquettes (6 quarts). When top coals are partially covered with ash, pour evenly over half of grill. Set cooking grate in place, cover, and open lid vent completely. Heat grill until hot, about 5 minutes.

3B For a gas grill: Turn all burners to high, cover, and heat grill until hot, about 15 minutes. Leave all burners on high.

4 Fold paper towels into compact wad. Holding paper towels with tongs, dip in oil, then wipe grate. Dip paper towels in oil again and wipe grate for second time. Cover grill and heat for 5 minutes. Uncover and wipe grate twice more with oiled paper towels.

5 Place tuna on grill (on hotter side if using charcoal) and cook (covered if using gas) until grill marks form and bottom is opaque, 1 to 3 minutes. Flip tuna and cook until center is translucent red when checked with tip of paring knife and registers 110 degrees (for rare), about 1½ minutes; or until opaque at perimeter and reddish pink at center and registers 125 degrees (for medium-rare), about 3 minutes. Serve tuna with farro salad.

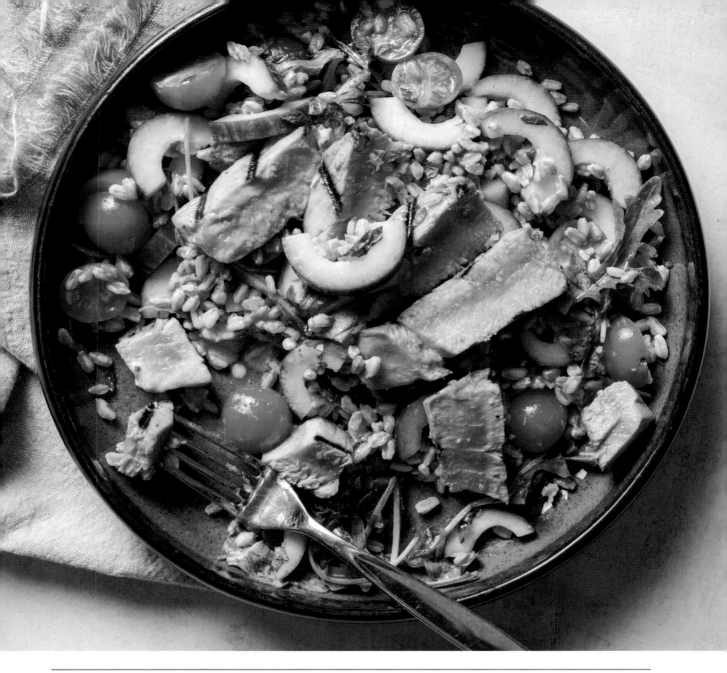

PER SERVING

Dietary Fiber 8g **Cal** 620;
Total Fat 25g, **Sat Fat** 4g;
Chol 45mg; **Sodium** 790mg;
Total Carb 63g, **Total Sugars** 9g,
Added Sugars 3g; **Protein** 39g

LF **MAKE IT LOW FODMAP** Substitute 1 cup oat berries
(groats) for farro and cook for 45 to 50 minutes. Increase
arugula to 4 ounces. Substitute dairy-free or lactose-free
yogurt (see page 19) for plain yogurt.

DF **MAKE IT DAIRY FREE** Substitute dairy-free yogurt
(see page 19) for plain yogurt.

GF **MAKE IT GLUTEN FREE** Substitute 1 cup oat berries (groats)
(see page 18) for farro and cook for 45 to 50 minutes.

SEARED SHRIMP WITH FRESH TOMATO SAUCE AND CILANTRO-LIME QUINOA

SERVES 4

WHY THIS RECIPE WORKS If you like shrimp over pasta, rice, or grits, try this healthful approach, which pairs seared shrimp in a zesty tomato sauce with quinoa, the quick-cooking super grain. We add freshness to the quinoa with lime zest, juice, and cilantro and then sear chipotle chile powder–dusted shrimp (in two batches to ensure that they brown, rather than steam). We remove the shrimp from the skillet and quickly cook a fresh tomato sauce for tossing the smoky shrimp back into, then serve it all with the nutty quinoa. Creamy avocado tops things off with richness. We like the convenience of prewashed quinoa; rinsing removes the quinoa's bitter protective coating (called saponin). If you buy unwashed quinoa, rinse it and then spread it out on a clean dish towel to dry for 15 minutes.

1½ cups prewashed white quinoa

1¾ cups water

1⅛ teaspoons table salt, divided

¼ teaspoon grated lime zest plus 2 tablespoons juice, plus lime wedges for serving

½ cup chopped fresh cilantro, divided

1 pound extra-large shrimp (21 to 25 per pound), peeled, deveined, and tails removed

½ teaspoon chipotle chile powder

¼ teaspoon pepper

2 tablespoons garlic oil (see page 20), divided

1 pound tomatoes, cored and cut into ½-inch pieces

2 avocados, halved, pitted, and cut into ½-inch pieces

1 Toast quinoa in medium saucepan over medium-high heat, stirring frequently, until quinoa is very fragrant and makes continuous popping sound, 5 to 7 minutes. Stir in water and ½ teaspoon salt and bring to simmer. Cover, reduce heat to low, and simmer until quinoa is tender and liquid is absorbed, 18 to 22 minutes, stirring once halfway through cooking.

2 Remove quinoa from heat and let sit, covered, for 10 minutes. Fluff quinoa with fork, then stir in lime zest, 1 tablespoon lime juice, and ¼ cup cilantro. Season with salt and pepper to taste; cover to keep warm.

3 Pat shrimp dry with paper towels, then toss with chile powder, pepper, and ½ teaspoon salt in bowl. Heat 1 tablespoon oil in 12-inch nonstick skillet over medium-high heat until just smoking. Add half of shrimp in single layer and cook, without stirring, until spotty brown and edges turn pink on bottom side, about 1 minute. Flip shrimp and continue to cook until all but very center is opaque, about 30 seconds. Transfer shrimp to large plate. Repeat with remaining 1 tablespoon oil and remaining shrimp; transfer to plate.

4 Return now-empty skillet to medium-high heat. Add tomatoes, remaining 1 tablespoon lime juice, remaining ⅛ teaspoon salt, and remaining ¼ cup cilantro. Cook until tomatoes are just softened, about 1 minute. Stir in shrimp and cook until shrimp are opaque throughout, about 1 minute. Season with salt and pepper to taste. Transfer shrimp and tomatoes to individual plates and top with avocado. Serve with quinoa and lime wedges.

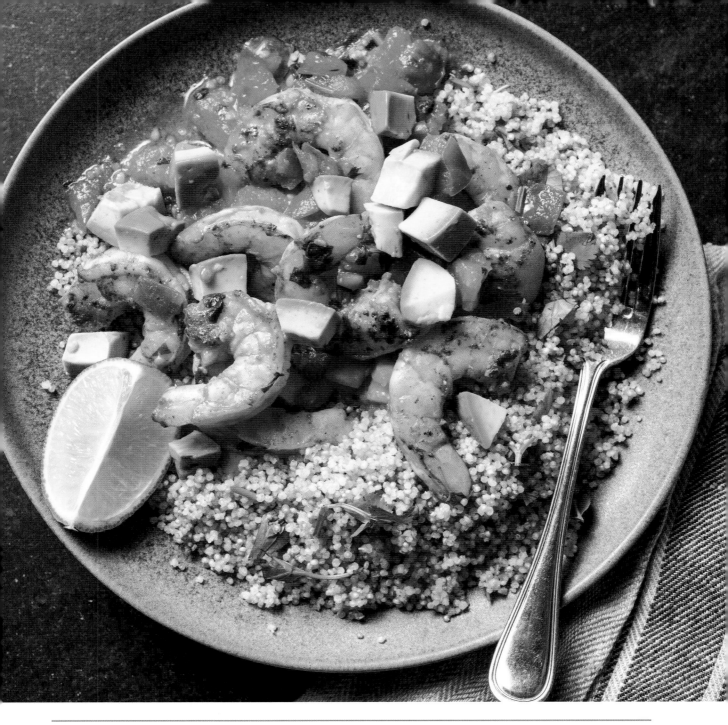

PER SERVING

Dietary Fiber 13g **Cal** 560;
Total Fat 27g, **Sat Fat** 3.5g;
Chol 145mg; **Sodium** 770mg;
Total Carb 55g, **Total Sugars** 5g,
Added Sugars 0g; **Protein** 27g

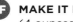 **MAKE IT LOW FODMAP** Reduce avocado to ½ avocado (4 ounces).

LINGUINE WITH SHRIMP, PEAS, AND PRESERVED LEMON

SERVES 4

WHY THIS RECIPE WORKS Shrimp pasta dishes of many flavor profiles are popular for good reason: They're super quick and provide a lot of meal for not much effort. The combination of shrimp, lemon, and garlic is a heady one that we thought we could make friendly to most guts simply by replacing the garlic with garlic oil. But without the pungency of fresh garlic found in common iterations of this dish, it fell flat. We changed tack and instead focused on pointing up what we didn't need a replacement for: natural shrimp flavor. Poaching the shrimp in just a little water, some garlic oil, and tart-savory preserved lemon not only coaxed out the shrimp's delicate flavor but produced nicely cooked shrimp that wasn't dried out. Adding some frozen peas with the shrimp fortified the sweetness—but with fiber and freshness. We reinforced the spring theme with fresh mint and pea tendrils. If preserved lemon is unavailable, substitute 1 tablespoon grated lemon zest for the preserved lemon, increase salt to ½ teaspoon in step 1, and serve the shrimp with lemon wedges. Arugula or watercress can be substituted for the pea tendrils.

1 pound large shrimp (26 to 30 per pound), peeled, deveined, and tails removed

¼ teaspoon table salt, plus salt for cooking pasta

2 tablespoons garlic oil (see page 20), divided, plus extra for drizzling

1½ teaspoons ground coriander

¾ preserved lemon, pulp and white pith removed, rind rinsed and minced (3 tablespoons), divided

1 cup frozen peas

2 tablespoons unsalted butter

12 ounces 100 percent whole-wheat linguine

¼ cup chopped fresh mint

2 ounces (2 cups) pea tendrils

1 Toss shrimp with salt in bowl. Heat 1 tablespoon oil and coriander in 12-inch skillet over medium-high heat until fragrant, 1 to 2 minutes. Stir in ¼ cup water and 2 tablespoons preserved lemon and bring to simmer. Add shrimp and peas, cover, and cook, stirring occasionally, until shrimp are just opaque, 2 to 4 minutes. Off heat, stir in remaining 1 tablespoon preserved lemon, butter, and remaining 1 tablespoon oil.

2 Meanwhile, bring 4 quarts water to boil in large pot. Add pasta and 1 tablespoon salt and cook, stirring often, until al dente. Reserve ½ cup cooking water, then drain pasta and return it to pot. Add shrimp mixture and mint and toss to coat. Adjust consistency with reserved cooking water as needed. Season with salt and pepper to taste. Divide pasta among serving bowls, top with pea tendrils, and drizzle with extra oil. Serve.

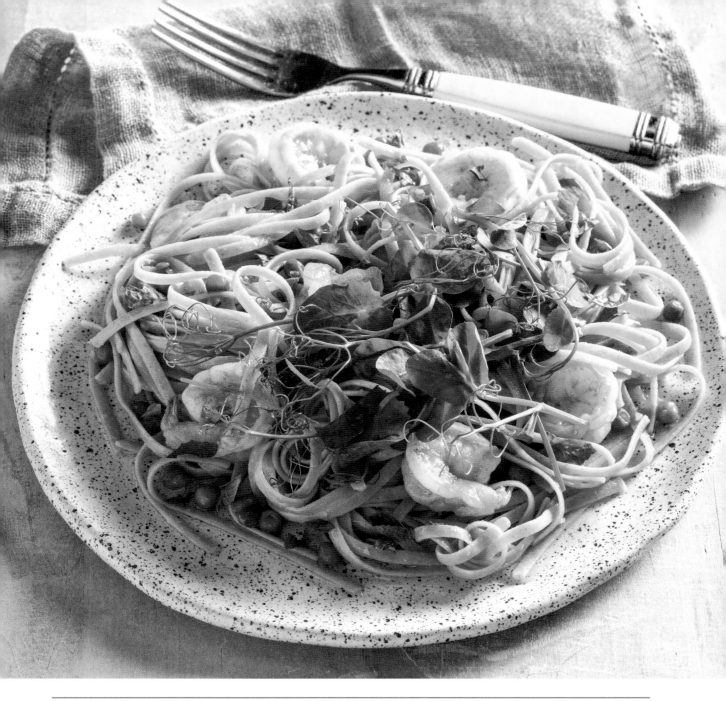

PER SERVING

Dietary Fiber 12g **Cal** 480;
Total Fat 16g, **Sat Fat** 4.5g;
Chol 120mg; **Sodium** 670mg;
Total Carb 61g, **Total Sugars** 4g,
Added Sugars 0g; **Protein** 25g

LF **MAKE IT LOW FODMAP** Substitute gluten-free pasta (see page 19) for whole-wheat linguine.

DF **MAKE IT GLUTEN FREE** Substitute gluten-free pasta (see page 19) for whole-wheat linguine.

GF **MAKE IT DAIRY FREE** Substitute 2 tablespoons extra-virgin olive oil for butter.

SHRIMP WITH WHITE BEANS AND ARUGULA

SERVES 4

WHY THIS RECIPE WORKS Pairing shrimp and white beans is a great idea: The sweetness of mild, creamy beans is the perfect foil to briny, chewy shrimp. What is it also great for? Your gut, because of the beans' abundant fiber. Canned beans at the heart of this dish passed muster—they guarantee creaminess. We also briefly soften a red bell pepper, which keeps its flavor fresh and its texture appealingly crunchy, for another fiber boost to the beans. And the peppery bite of arugula successfully interweaves all the other ingredients. Although we prefer this dish warm, with bread (gluten-free if needed), it can also be served chilled as a salad or antipasto.

1 pound extra-large shrimp (21 to 25 per pound), peeled and deveined

¼ teaspoon table salt, divided

⅛ teaspoon pepper

Pinch sugar

5 tablespoons garlic oil (see page 20), divided

1 red bell pepper, stemmed, seeded, and chopped fine

¼ teaspoon red pepper flakes (optional)

2 (15-ounce) cans cannellini beans, rinsed

2 ounces (2 cups) baby arugula, chopped coarse

2 tablespoons lemon juice

1 Pat shrimp dry with paper towels and sprinkle with ⅛ teaspoon salt, pepper, and sugar. Heat 1 tablespoon oil in 12-inch nonstick skillet over high heat until just smoking. Add shrimp to skillet in single layer and cook, without stirring, until spotty brown and edges turn pink on first side, about 1 minute. Off heat, flip shrimp and let sit until opaque throughout, about 30 seconds. Transfer shrimp to bowl and cover to keep warm.

2 Heat remaining ¼ cup oil in now-empty skillet over medium heat until shimmering. Add bell pepper and remaining ⅛ teaspoon salt and cook until softened, about 5 minutes. Stir in pepper flakes, if using, and cook until fragrant, about 30 seconds. Stir in beans and cook until heated through, about 5 minutes.

3 Add arugula and shrimp, along with any accumulated juices, and gently toss until arugula is wilted, about 1 minute. Stir in lemon juice and season with salt and pepper to taste. Serve.

PER SERVING

Dietary Fiber 7g **Cal** 370;
Total Fat 19g, **Sat Fat** 3g;
Chol 145mg; **Sodium** 690mg;
Total Carb 26g, **Total Sugars** 4g,
Added Sugars 0g; **Protein** 21g

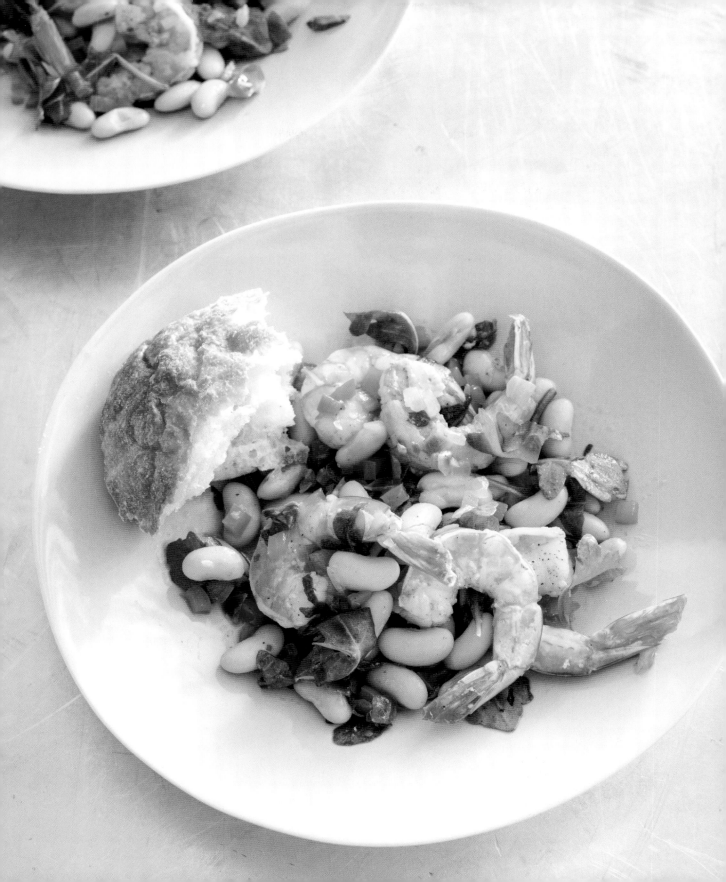

SEARED SCALLOPS WITH BARLEY AND BEET RISOTTO

SERVES 4

WHY THIS RECIPE WORKS Scallops are a lean protein source that feel rich and luxurious, and we especially like the tender morsels with a creamy side dish—here a risotto-style dish made with barley and beets. How do we beet up the barley? We use grated raw beets—stirring half into the barley at the start of cooking for a base of flavor, and half at the end for freshness. We incorporate the beet greens as well for an even more vegetable-packed risotto to prop up our perfect scallops. If you can't find beets with greens attached, use 10 ounces of beets and 2 cups stemmed and chopped Swiss chard. We recommend buying "dry" scallops, which don't have chemical additives and taste better than "wet." Dry scallops look ivory or pinkish; wet scallops are bright white. Use the large holes of a box grater or a food processor fitted with a shredding disk to shred the beets. Do not substitute hulled, hull-less, quick-cooking, or presteamed barley (read the ingredient list on the package to determine this).

2 cups vegetable broth (see page 19)

4 cups water

2 tablespoons garlic oil (see page 20), divided

1 pound beets with greens attached, beets trimmed, peeled, and shredded, divided; greens stemmed and chopped (2 cups)

1½ cups pearl barley, rinsed

1 teaspoon minced fresh thyme or ¼ teaspoon dried

1 cup dry white wine

¼ cup grated Parmesan cheese

1 pound large sea scallops, tendons removed

⅛ teaspoon table salt

⅛ teaspoon pepper

1 Bring broth and water to simmer in medium saucepan. Reduce heat to lowest setting and cover to keep warm. Heat 1 tablespoon oil in large saucepan over medium heat until shimmering. Add half of shredded beets and cook until softened, 5 to 7 minutes. Stir in barley and cook, stirring often, until fragrant, about 4 minutes. Stir in thyme and cook until fragrant, about 30 seconds. Stir in wine and cook until fully absorbed, about 2 minutes.

2 Stir in 3 cups warm broth mixture and bring to simmer. Reduce heat to medium-low and simmer, stirring occasionally, until liquid is absorbed and bottom of pan is dry, 22 to 25 minutes. Stir in 2 cups warm broth and simmer, stirring occasionally, until liquid is absorbed and bottom of pan is dry, 15 to 18 minutes. Stir in beet greens and continue to cook, stirring often and adding remaining broth as needed to prevent pan bottom from becoming dry, until greens are tender and barley is cooked through but still somewhat firm in center, 5 to 10 minutes. Off heat, stir in remaining shredded beets and Parmesan. Season with salt and pepper to taste; cover to keep warm.

3 Meanwhile, place scallops on rimmed baking sheet lined with clean kitchen towel. Place second clean kitchen towel on top of scallops and press gently on towel to blot liquid. Let scallops sit at room temperature, covered with towel, for 10 minutes. Sprinkle scallops with salt and pepper.

4 Heat remaining 1 tablespoon oil in 12-inch nonstick skillet over medium heat until just smoking. Add scallops and cook, without moving, until well browned on first side, about 1½ minutes. Flip scallops and continue to cook, without moving, until well browned on second side, sides are firm, and centers are opaque, about 1½ minutes. Serve scallops with beet risotto.

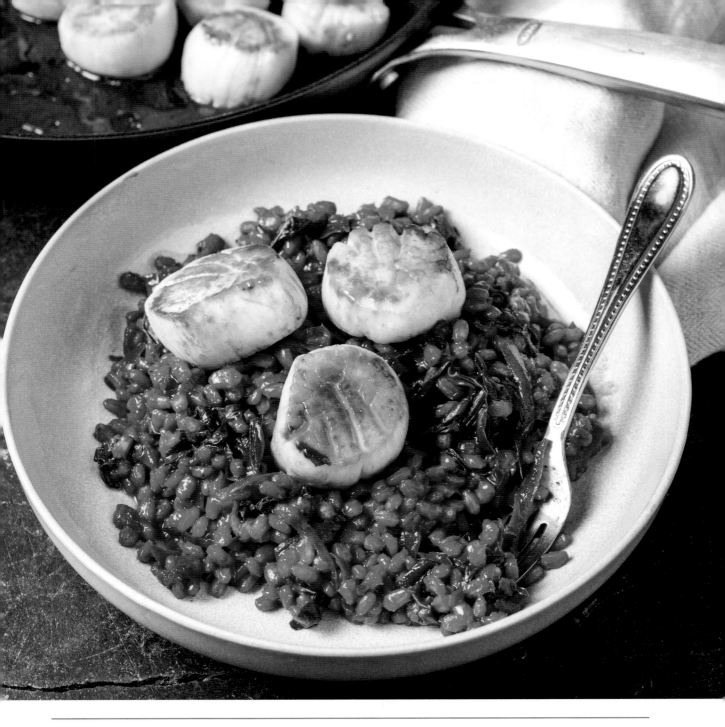

PER SERVING

Dietary Fiber 14g **Cal** 520;
Total Fat 10g, **Sat Fat** 1g;
Chol 30mg; **Sodium** 760mg;
Total Carb 73g, **Total Sugars** 6g,
Added Sugars 0g; **Protein** 24g

 MAKE IT DAIRY FREE Omit Parmesan cheese.

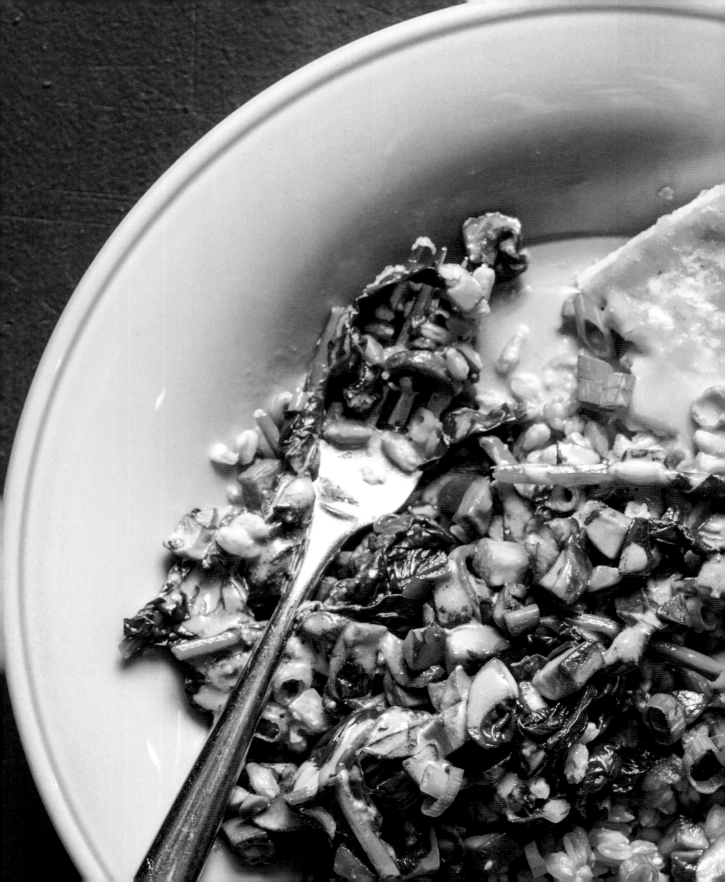

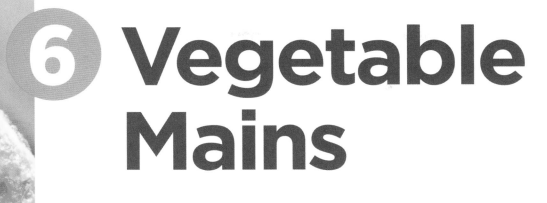

6 Vegetable Mains

RAINBOW SALAD WITH CRISPY TEMPEH

SERVES 4

DAIRY FREE

WHY THIS RECIPE WORKS We think tempeh is a perfect plant-based protein to eat for your gut. It's lean, high in fiber (it's not often that you can have your fiber and eat your protein too in one ingredient), low in FODMAPs, and fermented to boot! Here it gets crumbled and pan-fried for some crunch to top a stunning salad featuring a rainbow of fruits and vegetables on a bed of greens. Just before frying we boil the tempeh in a soy sauce mixture, which makes each crumble an umami bomb, perfect for contrasting orange-dressed beets (roasted to bring out their natural sweetness) and cherry tomatoes in this salad with deep savor. Buttery avocado and peppery, crisp radishes add balance, and a refreshing dressing with orange juice and ginger brings everything together. Look for beets measuring approximately 3 inches in diameter.

1 pound beets, trimmed

3 tablespoons soy sauce (see page 18)

8 ounces tempeh, crumbled into ¼-inch pieces

1 cup peanut or canola oil, for frying

2 oranges

3 tablespoons garlic oil (see page 20)

2 tablespoons white wine vinegar

½ teaspoon table salt

10 ounces (10 cups) baby arugula

8 ounces cherry tomatoes, halved

1 ripe avocado, halved, pitted, and cut into ½-inch pieces

8 radishes, trimmed and sliced thin

1 Adjust oven rack to middle position and heat oven to 400 degrees. Wrap beets individually in aluminum foil and place on rimmed baking sheet. Roast until beets can be pierced easily with paring knife, 45 minutes to 1 hour, removing beets individually from oven as they finish cooking.

2 Open foil packets to allow steam to escape and let cool slightly. Once beets are cool enough to handle, rub off skins using paper towels. Cut beets into ¾-inch pieces and set aside to cool. (Beets can be refrigerated for up to 1 week; bring to room temperature before using.)

3 Meanwhile, bring 4 cups water and soy sauce to boil in large saucepan. Add tempeh, return to boil, and cook for 10 minutes. Drain tempeh well and wipe saucepan dry with paper towels.

4 Set wire rack in rimmed baking sheet and line with triple layer of paper towels. Heat peanut oil in now-empty dry saucepan over medium-high heat until shimmering. Add tempeh and cook until golden brown and crisp, about 12 minutes, adjusting heat as needed if tempeh begins to scorch. Using wire skimmer or slotted spoon, transfer tempeh to prepared sheet to drain, then season with salt and pepper to taste; set aside.

5 Grate 1 teaspoon zest from 1 orange. Cut away peel and pith from oranges. Holding fruit over bowl, use paring knife to slice between membranes to release segments. Whisk orange zest, garlic oil, vinegar, salt, and any accumulated orange juice in second bowl until combined. Toss arugula with 2 tablespoons vinaigrette and season with salt and pepper to taste. Divide arugula evenly among individual serving bowls, then top with beets, orange segments, tomatoes, avocado, and radishes. Drizzle each salad evenly with remaining vinaigrette and sprinkle with tempeh. Serve.

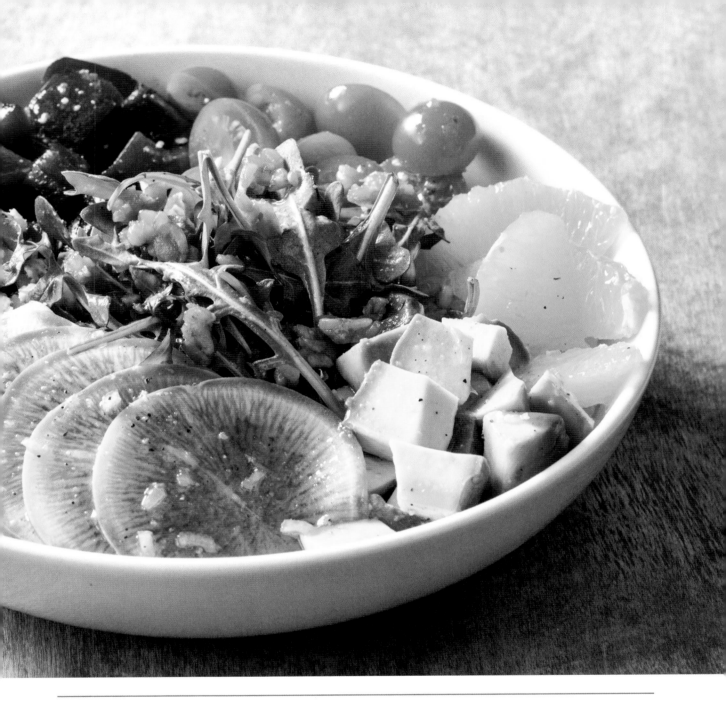

PER SERVING

Dietary Fiber 10g **Cal** 390;
Total Fat 24g, **Sat Fat** 3g;
Chol 0mg; **Sodium** 480mg;
Total Carb 34g, **Total Sugars** 15g,
Added Sugars 0g; **Protein** 13g

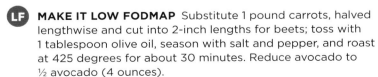

LF **MAKE IT LOW FODMAP** Substitute 1 pound carrots, halved lengthwise and cut into 2-inch lengths for beets; toss with 1 tablespoon olive oil, season with salt and pepper, and roast at 425 degrees for about 30 minutes. Reduce avocado to ½ avocado (4 ounces).

GF **MAKE IT GLUTEN FREE** Substitute gluten-free soy sauce or tamari (see page 18) for soy sauce.

FATTOUSH WITH ESCAROLE

SERVES 4

DAIRY FREE

WHY THIS RECIPE WORKS Crisp cucumbers and sweet-savory tomatoes may not make a meal unless you're talking fattoush, an eastern Mediterranean bread salad. Here, cucumbers and tomatoes share the stage with toasted pita and light greens to create the most texturally pleasing of salads. Ours is heartier than most, as we use escarole rather than romaine or arugula. A defining flavor of the salad is bright, tangy sumac. We use an ample amount of ground sumac in the dressing and as a garnish for the finished salad. Many recipes call for eliminating excess moisture from the salad by taking the time-consuming step of seeding and salting the cucumbers and tomatoes; we skip this in order to preserve the crisp texture of the cucumber and the flavorful seeds and juice of the tomatoes. Instead, we make the pita pieces more resilient by brushing them with plenty of olive oil before baking, which prevents them from becoming soggy in the dressing. Whole-wheat pita, a detour from tradition, makes this fresh salad fiberful too. The success of this recipe depends on ripe, in-season tomatoes.

2 (8-inch) 100 percent whole-wheat pita breads

7 tablespoons extra-virgin olive oil, divided

¾ teaspoon table salt, divided

⅛ teaspoon pepper

3 tablespoons lemon juice

4 teaspoons ground sumac, plus extra for serving

1 head escarole (1 pound), trimmed and cut into 1-inch pieces

1 pound ripe tomatoes, cored and cut into ¾-inch pieces

1 English cucumber, sliced ⅛ inch thick

½ cup chopped fresh cilantro

½ cup chopped fresh mint

4 scallions, green parts only, sliced thin

1 Adjust oven rack to middle position and heat oven to 375 degrees. Using kitchen shears, cut around perimeter of each pita and separate into 2 thin rounds. Cut each round in half. Place pitas smooth side down on wire rack set in rimmed baking sheet. Brush 3 tablespoons oil on surface of pitas and sprinkle with ¼ teaspoon salt and pepper. (Pitas do not need to be uniformly coated; oil will spread during baking.) Bake until pitas are crisp and golden brown, 10 to 14 minutes. Let cool completely on wire rack, about 15 minutes, then break toasted pitas into ½-inch pieces.

2 Whisk lemon juice, sumac, remaining ¼ cup oil, and remaining ½ teaspoon salt together in large bowl until smooth. Add escarole, tomatoes, cucumber, cilantro, mint, scallions, and toasted pita pieces and toss gently to combine. Season with salt and pepper to taste. Serve, sprinkling individual portions with extra sumac.

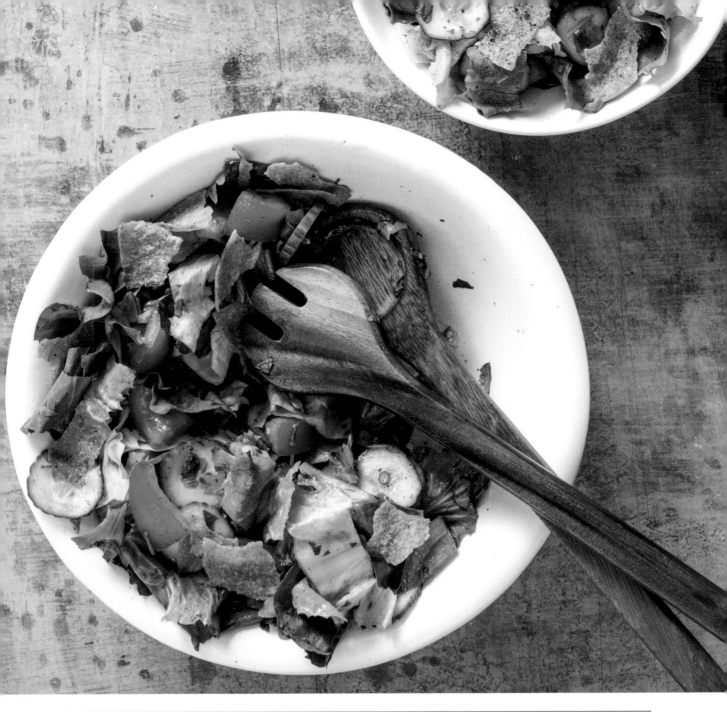

PER SERVING

Dietary Fiber 8g **Cal** 360;
Total Fat 26g, **Sat Fat** 3.5g;
Chol 0mg; **Sodium** 710mg;
Total Carb 30g, **Total Sugars** 5g,
Added Sugars 0g; **Protein** 6g

LF **MAKE IT LOW FODMAP** Omit pita breads and skip step 1.
Substitute 3½ cups crumbled gluten-free flatbread crackers or
gluten-free pita chips for toasted pita pieces.

GF **MAKE IT GLUTEN FREE** Omit pita breads and skip step 1.
Substitute 3½ cups crumbled gluten-free flatbread crackers or
gluten-free pita chips for toasted pita pieces.

QUINOA TACO SALAD

SERVES 4

GLUTEN FREE

WHY THIS RECIPE WORKS De-shell tacos and you have taco salad, a lighter version of the Tuesday hardshell special. "Lighter" isn't necessarily so much better for you, however—fiber and nutrients are required to actually make a salad healthful. Here we replace the greasy ground meat with seasoned quinoa. Don't knock it: This high-fiber source of protein is a great stand-in for ground meat, as it's chewy and absorbs flavors well. Toasted and simmered in vegetable broth with tomato paste, chipotle chile powder, and cumin, it acquires a rich, spiced, meaty flavor. We substitute hardier escarole for lettuce; cut back on cheese, opting for low-lactose queso fresco; and add lots of fresh cilantro. Cherry tomatoes and avocado complete the updated gut-healthy profile. We like the convenience of prewashed quinoa. If you buy unwashed quinoa (or if you are unsure whether it's washed), rinse it before cooking to remove its bitter protective coating (called saponin). Serve with your favorite taco toppings, if desired.

¾ cup prewashed white quinoa

3 tablespoons garlic oil (see page 20), divided

2 teaspoons tomato paste

½ teaspoon chipotle chile powder

½ teaspoon ground cumin

1 cup vegetable broth (see page 18)

¾ teaspoon table salt, divided

2 tablespoons lime juice

1 head escarole (1 pound), trimmed and sliced thin

½ cup chopped fresh cilantro, divided

8 ounces cherry or grape tomatoes, quartered

1 ripe avocado, halved, pitted, and chopped

2 ounces queso fresco, crumbled (½ cup)

1 Toast quinoa in medium saucepan over medium-high heat, stirring frequently, until quinoa is very fragrant and makes continuous popping sound, 5 to 7 minutes; transfer to bowl.

2 Cook 1 tablespoon oil, tomato paste, chipotle, and cumin in now-empty saucepan over medium heat until fragrant, about 1 minute. Stir in quinoa, broth, and ¼ teaspoon salt and bring to simmer. Cover, reduce heat to low, and cook until quinoa is tender and liquid has been absorbed, 18 to 22 minutes, stirring once halfway through cooking. Remove saucepan from heat and let sit, covered, for 10 minutes. Spread quinoa onto large plate and let cool for 20 minutes.

3 Whisk remaining 2 tablespoons oil, remaining ½ teaspoon salt, and lime juice in large bowl. Add escarole and ¼ cup cilantro and toss to combine. Gently fold in tomatoes and avocado. Transfer to serving platter and top with quinoa, queso fresco, and remaining ¼ cup cilantro. Serve.

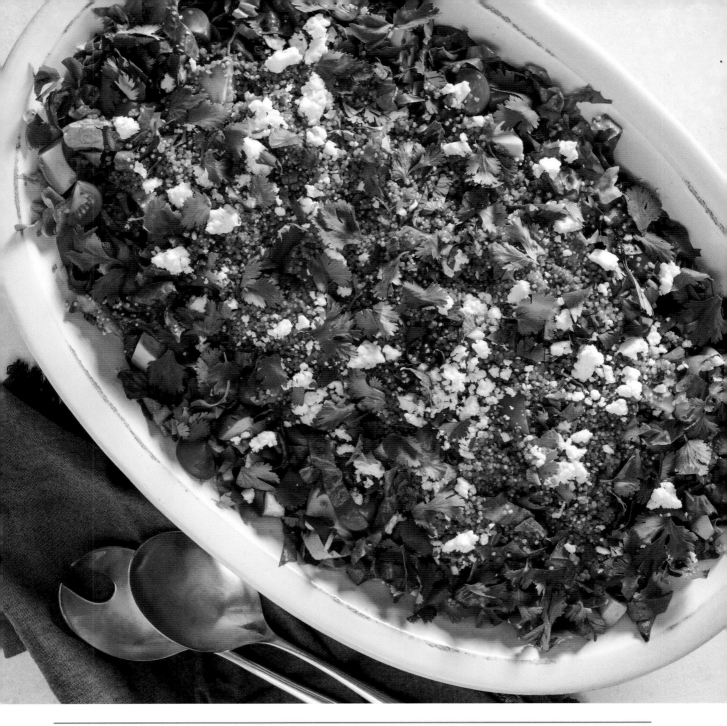

PER SERVING

Dietary Fiber 10g **Cal** 350;
Total Fat 21g, **Sat Fat** 3g;
Chol 5mg; **Sodium** 710mg;
Total Carb 34g, **Total Sugars** 3g,
Added Sugars 0g; **Protein** 9g

LF **MAKE IT LOW FODMAP** Decrease avocado to ½ avocado (4 ounces) and increase tomatoes to 10 ounces.

DF **MAKE IT DAIRY FREE** Omit queso fresco.

FREEKEH SALAD WITH SWEET POTATOES, WALNUTS, AND RAISINS

SERVES 4

WHY THIS RECIPE WORKS High-fiber freekeh is a wheat-based grain commonly used across the eastern Mediterranean and North Africa. It deserves a spot on your pantry shelf (if you eat wheat), not just for its fiber but also for its unique grassy, slightly smoky flavor that's absent from other whole-wheat products. That profile works perfectly when paired with caramel-flavored roasted sweet potatoes for a hearty lunch or light dinner. To give the potatoes more dimension, we season them with fenugreek, a slightly sweet and nutty seed with a unique maple-like flavor. To bring all the elements together, we stir in a rich yet bright tahini-lemon dressing. Chopped walnuts offer complementary crunch and raisins amplify the sweetness in pops. We prefer the texture of whole, uncracked freekeh; cracked freekeh can be substituted, but you will need to decrease the cooking time in step 1.

1½ cups freekeh

¾ teaspoon table salt, divided, plus salt for cooking freekeh

12 ounces sweet potato, peeled and cut into 1-inch pieces

¼ cup extra-virgin olive oil, divided

½ teaspoon ground fenugreek

¼ teaspoon pepper, divided

2½ tablespoons lemon juice

2 tablespoons tahini

1 tablespoon water

2 cups fresh cilantro leaves

⅓ cup walnuts, toasted and chopped

¼ cup golden raisins

1 Adjust oven rack to lowest position and heat oven to 450 degrees. Bring 4 quarts water to boil in large pot. Add freekeh and 1 tablespoon salt and cook until grains are tender, 30 to 45 minutes. Drain freekeh, spread over rimmed baking sheet, and let cool completely, about 15 minutes.

2 Meanwhile, toss sweet potato with 1 tablespoon oil, fenugreek, ¼ teaspoon salt, and ⅛ teaspoon pepper. Spread over second rimmed baking sheet and roast until well browned and tender, 20 to 25 minutes, stirring halfway through roasting. Let cool completely on sheet, about 15 minutes.

3 Whisk lemon juice, tahini, water, remaining ½ teaspoon salt, remaining ⅛ teaspoon pepper, and remaining 3 tablespoons oil together in large bowl until smooth. Add freekeh, potatoes, cilantro, walnuts, and raisins and toss to combine. Season with salt and pepper to taste. Serve.

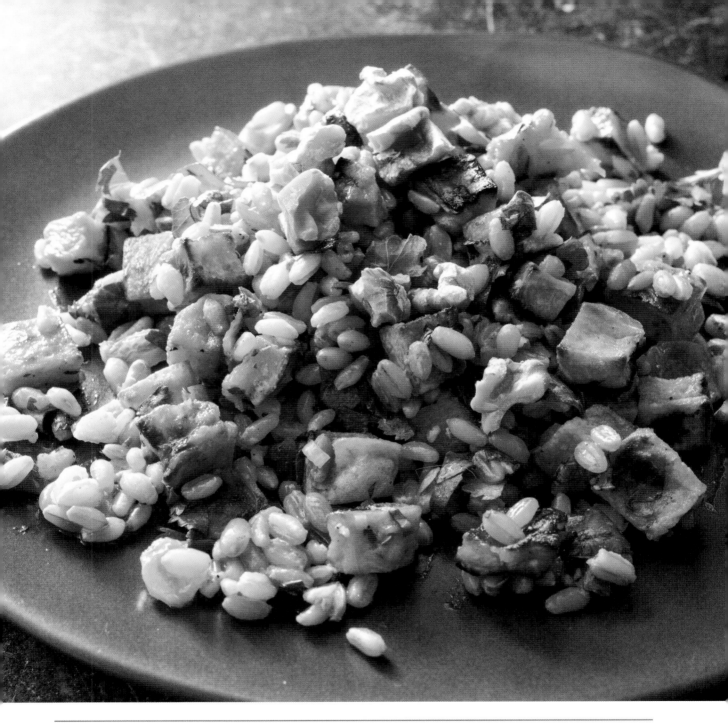

PER SERVING

Dietary Fiber 14g **Cal** 570;
Total Fat 26g, **Sat Fat** 3g;
Chol 0mg; **Sodium** 520mg;
Total Carb 72g, **Total Sugars** 10g,
Added Sugars 0g; **Protein** 13g

 MAKE IT LOW FODMAP Substitute brown rice for freekeh and decrease cooking time to 22 to 25 minutes.

 MAKE IT GLUTEN FREE Substitute brown rice for freekeh and decrease cooking time to 22 to 25 minutes.

GREEN RICE AND VEGETABLE BOWLS WITH FRIED EGGS

SERVES 4

WHY THIS RECIPE WORKS Good-for-you brown rice is a great foundational ingredient for a meal because it can pair with a host of ingredients, but it can use some excitement to perk up its earthiness. In this fiber-packed bowl, it gets upgraded with a super-fragrant green herb paste (featuring Thai basil and cilantro) that clings to every grain of rice. Bright vegetables bring more green and nutrients and a fried egg tops each bowl to marry the components with its decadent runny yolk. You can substitute regular basil for the Thai basil. For an accurate measurement of boiling water, bring a full kettle of water to a boil and then measure out the desired amount. You will need a 12-inch nonstick skillet with a tight-fitting lid.

2⅓ cups boiling water

1½ cups long-grain brown rice, rinsed

5 tablespoons plus 2 teaspoons garlic oil (see page 20), divided

1 teaspoon table salt, divided

1 cup frozen edamame, thawed and patted dry

6 ounces (6 cups) baby spinach, divided

½ cup fresh cilantro leaves

½ cup fresh Thai basil leaves

8 ounces green beans, trimmed and halved

2 teaspoons grated fresh ginger

4 large eggs

⅛ teaspoon pepper

Lime wedges

1 Adjust oven rack to middle position and heat oven to 375 degrees. Combine boiling water, rice, 2 teaspoons oil, and ½ teaspoon salt in 8-inch square baking dish. Cover dish tightly with aluminum foil and bake until rice is tender and no water remains, about 1 hour. Remove rice from oven and fluff with fork, scraping up any rice that has stuck to bottom of dish. Add edamame in even layer over rice. Cover dish with clean dish towel and let sit for 10 minutes.

2 Meanwhile, process 1 cup spinach, cilantro, basil, 3 tablespoons oil, and ¼ teaspoon salt in food processor until smooth, about 1 minute, scraping downs sides of bowl as needed; set herb paste aside.

3 Heat 1 tablespoon oil in 12-inch nonstick skillet over medium-high heat until shimmering. Add green beans and ⅛ teaspoon salt and cook until green beans are spotty brown, 4 to 6 minutes. Add remaining 5 cups spinach and cook, tossing constantly with tongs, until wilted, 1 to 2 minutes. Push vegetables to 1 side of skillet. Add 1 teaspoon oil and ginger to clearing and cook, mashing ginger into skillet, until fragrant, about 30 seconds. Stir ginger mixture into vegetables, then transfer vegetables to bowl and cover with aluminum foil to keep warm; set aside.

4 Heat remaining 2 teaspoons oil in again-empty skillet over medium high heat until shimmering. Crack eggs into 2 small bowls and sprinkle with pepper and remaining ⅛ teaspoon salt. Working quickly, pour eggs into pan. Cover and cook for 1 minute. Remove skillet from heat and let sit, covered, 15 to 45 seconds for runny yolks, 45 to 60 seconds for soft but set yolks, or about 2 minutes for medium-set yolks. Dollop herb paste over rice and edamame, fluff with fork to combine, and season with salt and pepper to taste. Divide rice and edamame among individual serving bowls and top with vegetable mixture and fried eggs. Serve with lime wedges.

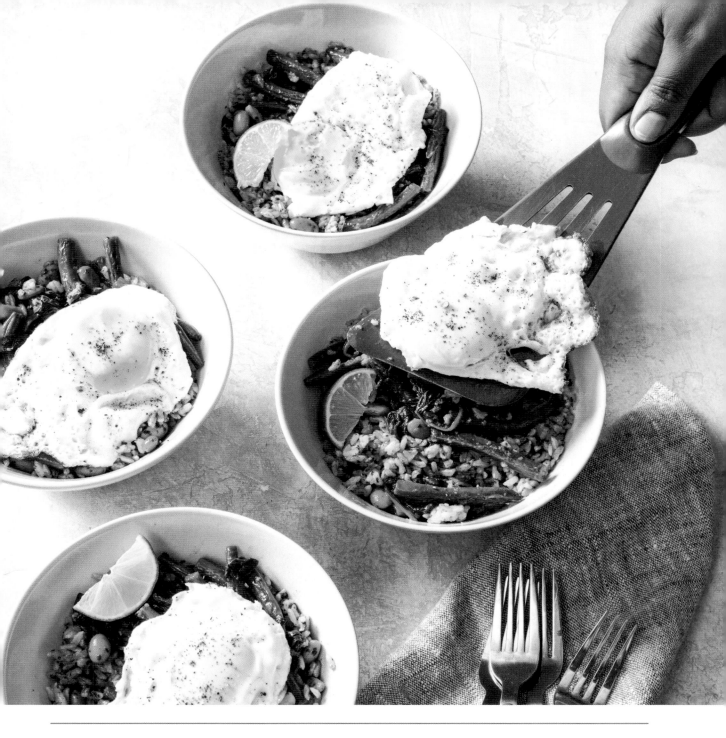

PER SERVING

Dietary Fiber 8g **Cal** 540;
Total Fat 29g, **Sat Fat** 4.5g;
Chol 185mg; **Sodium** 700mg;
Total Carb 61g, **Total Sugars** 3g,
Added Sugars 0g; **Protein** 16g

FARRO BOWLS WITH TOFU, MUSHROOMS, AND SPINACH

SERVES 4

DAIRY FREE

WHY THIS RECIPE WORKS The bowl concept, as illustrated in our Green Rice and Vegetable Bowls with Fried Eggs (page 236), transcends trend; it's an ideal way to layer texturally varied fiberful ingredients in an interesting way. Here nutty farro combines with crispy seared tofu, deeply flavored mushrooms, and wilted spinach. It's all drizzled with a simple creamy miso-ginger sauce, then a fresh finish of scallions adds a touch of aromatic flavor. But the real flavor comes from the sauce that's a gut health winner, with red miso (a fermented powerhouse), sesame oil, sherry vinegar, and ginger (a known digestive aid). We prefer the flavor and texture of whole farro; pearled farro can be used, but the texture may be softer. Do not use quick-cooking or presteamed farro (read the ingredient list on the package to determine this) in this recipe. The cooking time for farro can vary greatly among different brands, so we recommend beginning to check for doneness after 10 minutes.

2 tablespoons mayonnaise

5 teaspoons toasted sesame oil, divided

1 tablespoon red miso

1 tablespoon water

2 teaspoons sherry vinegar, divided

1 teaspoon grated fresh ginger

1 cup whole farro

⅛ teaspoon table salt, plus salt for cooking farro

14 ounces firm tofu

3 tablespoons cornstarch

¼ cup canola oil, divided

10 ounces cremini mushrooms, trimmed and chopped coarse

2 tablespoons dry sherry

10 ounces (10 cups) baby spinach

3 scallions, green parts only, sliced thin

1 Whisk mayonnaise, 1 tablespoon sesame oil, miso, water, 1 teaspoon vinegar, and ginger together in small bowl; set sauce aside for serving.

2 Bring 4 quarts water to boil in large pot. Add farro and 1 teaspoon salt and cook until grains are tender with slight chew, 15 to 30 minutes. Drain farro well and return to now-empty pot. Stir in remaining 2 teaspoons sesame oil and remaining 1 teaspoon vinegar and cover to keep warm.

3 Meanwhile, cut tofu crosswise into 8 equal slabs, arrange over paper towel–lined baking sheet, and let drain for 20 minutes. Gently press dry with paper towels.

4 Spread cornstarch in shallow dish. Coat tofu thoroughly in cornstarch, pressing gently to adhere; transfer to plate. Heat 2 tablespoons canola oil in 12-inch nonstick skillet over medium-high heat until just smoking. Add tofu and cook until crisp and browned, about 4 minutes per side. Transfer to paper towel–lined plate and tent with aluminum foil. Wipe skillet clean with paper towels.

5 Heat 1 tablespoon canola oil in now-empty skillet over medium-high heat until shimmering. Add mushrooms and ⅛ teaspoon salt and cook until beginning to brown, 5 to 8 minutes. Stir in sherry and cook, scraping up any browned bits, until skillet is nearly dry, about 1 minute; transfer to bowl.

6 Heat remaining 1 tablespoon canola oil in again-empty skillet over medium-high heat until shimmering. Add spinach, 1 handful at a time, and cook until just wilted, about 1 minute. Divide farro among individual serving bowls, then top with tofu, mushrooms, and spinach. Drizzle with miso-ginger sauce, sprinkle with scallions, and serve.

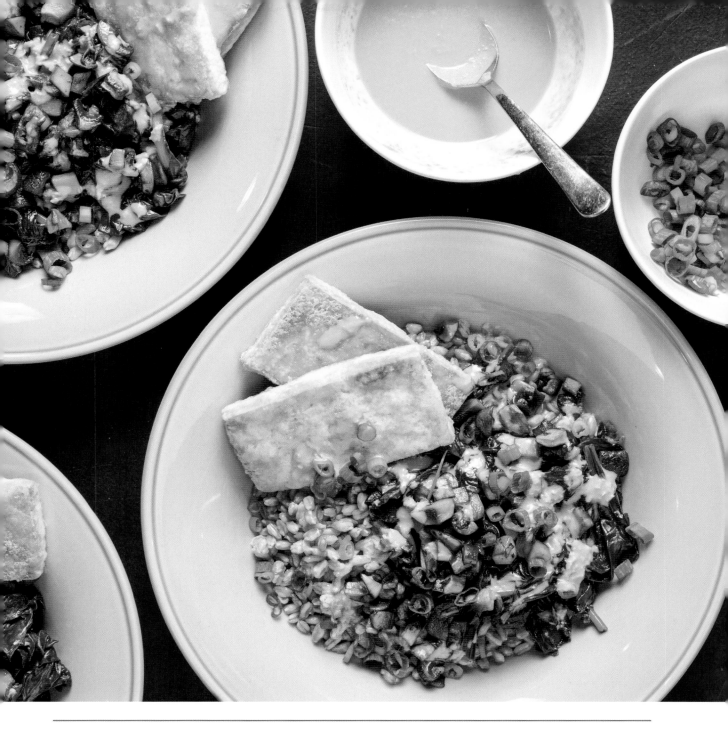

PER SERVING

Dietary Fiber 7g **Cal** 530;
Total Fat 31g, **Sat Fat** 3g;
Chol 5mg; **Sodium** 420mg;
Total Carb 48g, **Total Sugars** 5g,
Added Sugars 0g; **Protein** 18g

LF **MAKE IT LOW FODMAP** Substitute oat berries (groats) (see page 18) for farro and cook for 45 to 50 minutes. Substitute oyster mushrooms for cremini mushrooms.

GF **MAKE IT GLUTEN FREE** Substitute oat berries (groats) (see page 18) for farro and cook for 45 to 50 minutes.

BLACK BEAN CHILAQUILES VERDES

SERVES 4

GLUTEN FREE

WHY THIS RECIPE WORKS Fried tortilla wedges tossed in chile sauce is a dish jam-packed with bright flavor, varying textures, comfort, and, in this case, vegetables. Baking—not frying—tortillas to make our own chips contributes irresistible crunch and chew to our healthful dish. To build a flavorful salsa verde base, we cook mild poblanos and spicier jalapeños in garlic oil with canned tomatillos. To really go green, we add a hefty ½ cup of cilantro leaves. Shredded meat is a common addition, but for a fiber boost we opt for black beans. (You can use whatever beans you have on hand.) We keep texture, aesthetics, and most importantly, vegetables in mind when considering toppings: crispy radishes, creamy avocado, fresh cilantro, and thinly sliced jalapeño. To make this dish less spicy, remove the ribs and seeds from your jalapeños.

¼ cup plain whole-milk yogurt

1 teaspoon grated lime zest plus 1 tablespoon juice

12 (6-inch) corn tortillas (see page 19), each cut into 8 wedges

3 tablespoons garlic oil (see page 20), divided

2 poblano chiles, stemmed, seeded, and chopped coarse

2 jalapeño chiles, stemmed and seeded (1 chopped coarse, 1 sliced thin)

¼ teaspoon table salt

1½ teaspoons ground cumin

1 (26-ounce) can whole tomatillos, drained

1 cup water

¾ cup fresh cilantro leaves, divided

2 (15-ounce) cans black beans, rinsed

1 avocado, halved, pitted, and cut into ½-inch pieces

4 radishes, trimmed and sliced thin

1 Adjust oven racks to upper-middle and lower-middle positions and heat oven to 350 degrees. Combine yogurt and lime zest and juice in small bowl and season with salt and pepper to taste; set yogurt sauce aside until ready to serve.

2 Toss tortillas with 2 tablespoons oil, then spread over 2 rimmed baking sheets. Bake until brown and dried, 16 to 25 minutes, flipping tortillas halfway through baking; set aside to cool.

3 Meanwhile, heat remaining 1 tablespoon oil in Dutch oven over medium heat until shimmering. Add poblanos, coarsely chopped jalapeño, and salt and cook until vegetables are softened and lightly browned, 6 to 8 minutes.

4 Stir in cumin and cook until fragrant, about 30 seconds. Stir in tomatillos and water and simmer until tomatillos are softened, about 10 minutes. Carefully transfer tomatillo mixture to blender, along with ½ cup cilantro, and process until smooth, about 1 minute.

5 Return tomatillo sauce to now-empty pot and bring to simmer over medium heat. Add beans and cook, stirring frequently, until beans are warmed through, about 5 minutes. Stir in cooled tortillas and cook until they begin to soften, about 2 minutes. Season with salt and pepper to taste. Sprinkle with avocado, radishes, thinly sliced jalapeño, and remaining ¼ cup cilantro. Serve with yogurt sauce.

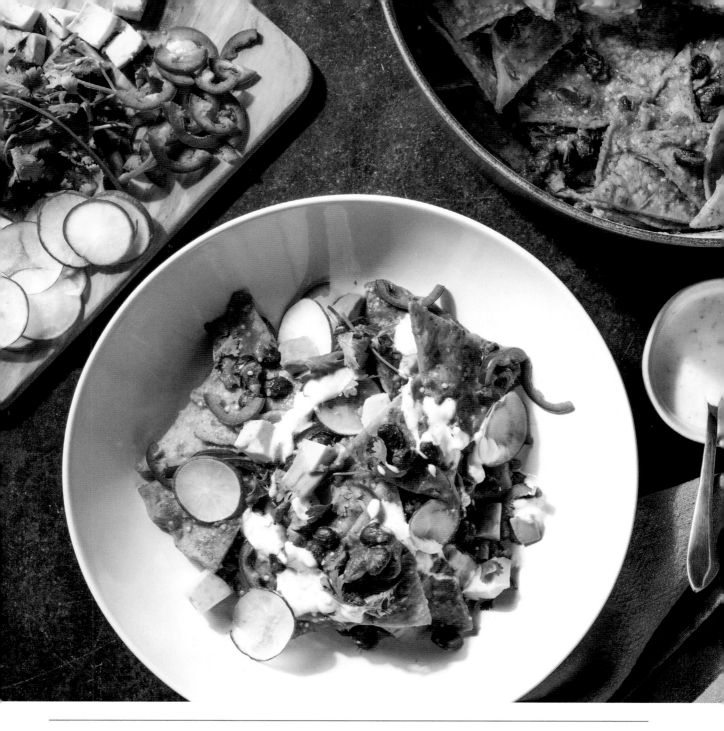

PER SERVING

Dietary Fiber 19g **Cal** 540;
Total Fat 23g, **Sat Fat** 3g;
Chol 0mg; **Sodium** 780mg;
Total Carb 80g, **Total Sugars** 12g,
Added Sugars 0g; **Protein** 15g

DF **MAKE IT DAIRY FREE** Substitute dairy-free yogurt (see page 19) for plain yogurt.

ROASTED CABBAGE WEDGES WITH TOMATOES AND CHICKPEAS

SERVES 4

WHY THIS RECIPE WORKS Think cabbage is humble? Cut it into wedges and roast them to create charred, crispy edges with tender, sweet layers underneath—and upgrade the unassuming vegetable to striking center-of-the-plate status. We first brush the wedges with a curry powder–infused oil, which includes a little sugar to help with browning. Then we cover the cabbage with aluminum foil before putting the baking sheet on the lower rack of a hot oven to steam the wedges and jump-start browning on the undersides. We uncover them for the last part of cooking and add another drizzle of oil to crisp and brown the upper sides while maximizing browning underneath. To complete our meal, while the cabbage roasts we simmer an aromatic chickpea, tomato, and ginger mixture in a skillet on the stovetop to serve as a saucy garnish. When slicing the cabbage into wedges, be sure to slice through the core, leaving it intact so the wedges don't fall apart. A smaller 2-pound cabbage works best here; if you have a larger cabbage, you can remove the outer leaves until it weighs about 2 pounds, though it may not brown as well. Serve with Herbed Yogurt Sauce (page 23), if you like.

7 tablespoons garlic oil (see page 20), divided

1 tablespoon curry powder, divided

1½ teaspoons sugar

½ teaspoon table salt

¼ teaspoon pepper

1 head green cabbage (2 pounds)

2 teaspoons grated fresh ginger

2 (15-ounce) cans chickpeas, undrained

10 ounces grape tomatoes, halved

¼ cup chopped fresh cilantro

1 Adjust oven rack to lowest position and heat oven to 500 degrees. Combine ¼ cup oil, 2 teaspoons curry powder, sugar, salt, and pepper in small bowl. Halve cabbage through core and cut each half into 4 approximately 2-inch-wide wedges, leaving core intact (you will have 8 wedges).

2 Arrange cabbage wedges in even layer on rimmed baking sheet, then brush cabbage all over with oil mixture. Cover tightly with aluminum foil and roast for 10 minutes. Remove foil and drizzle 2 tablespoons oil evenly over wedges. Return cabbage to oven and roast uncovered until cabbage is tender and sides touching sheet are well browned, 12 to 15 minutes.

3 Meanwhile, heat remaining 1 tablespoon oil in 12-inch skillet over medium-high heat until shimmering. Add ginger and remaining 1 teaspoon curry powder and cook, mashing mixture into skillet, until fragrant, about 30 seconds. Add chickpeas and their liquid and tomatoes and bring to simmer. Cook, stirring frequently, until tomatoes begin to break down and mixture has thickened slightly, 7 to 9 minutes. Season with salt and pepper to taste.

4 Divide cabbage among individual plates and spoon chickpea mixture over top. Sprinkle with cilantro and serve.

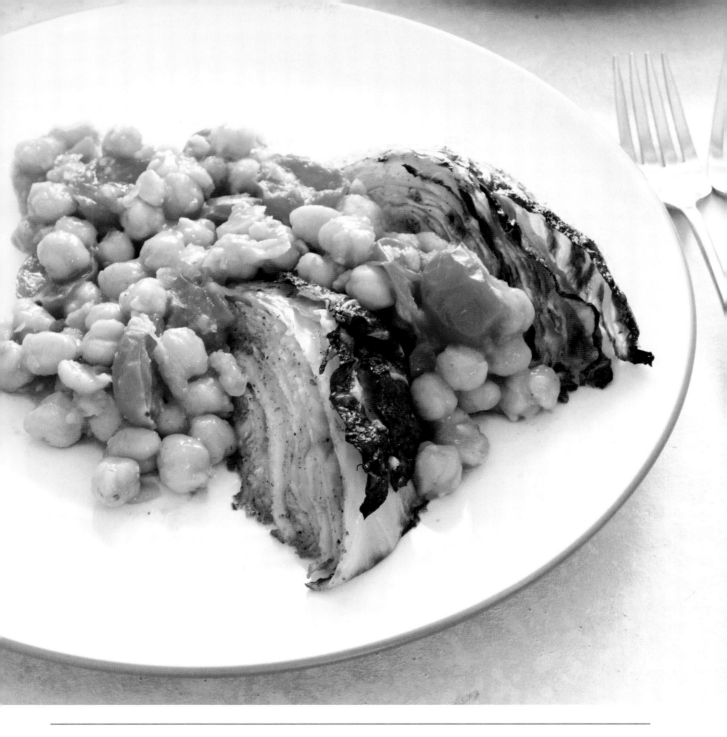

PER SERVING

Dietary Fiber 13g **Cal** 420;
Total Fat 27g, **Sat Fat** 2g;
Chol 0mg; **Sodium** 740mg;
Total Carb 35g, **Total Sugars** 13g,
Added Sugars 2g; **Protein** 10g

STUFFED EGGPLANT WITH BULGUR AND TOMATOES

SERVES 4

WHY THIS RECIPE WORKS Stuffing is a simple way to make vegetables a main meal. Eggplant, with its boat-like shape when halved, is perfect for filling. There are countless variations on stuffed eggplant from around the world, but we found ourselves enamored of a classic Turkish preparation known as imam bayildi and used its flavors as inspiration for the vibrant, warm-spiced tomato-based filling here. We wanted to make sure that the eggplants were rich and creamy and that the filling was hearty and satisfying. Italian eggplants are the perfect size for stuffing, so we started there. Roasting the eggplants prior to stuffing was key to preventing them from turning watery and tasteless. We then let the eggplants drain briefly on paper towels (which got rid of excess liquid) before adding the stuffing. Nutty bulgur made a perfect filling base, plum tomatoes lent bright flavor and a bit of moisture, and Pecorino Romano and pine nuts provided richness and depth. Do not confuse bulgur with cracked wheat, which has a much longer cooking time and will not work in this recipe.

4 (10-ounce) Italian eggplants, halved lengthwise

3 tablespoons extra-virgin olive oil, divided

¾ teaspoon table salt, divided

½ cup medium-grind bulgur, rinsed

¼ cup water

2 teaspoons minced fresh oregano or ½ teaspoon dried

¼ teaspoon ground cinnamon

Pinch cayenne pepper (optional)

1 pound plum tomatoes, cored, seeded, and chopped

2 ounces Pecorino Romano cheese, grated (1 cup), divided

2 tablespoons pine nuts, toasted

2 teaspoons red wine vinegar

2 tablespoons minced fresh parsley

1 Adjust oven racks to upper-middle and lowest positions, place parchment paper–lined rimmed baking sheet on lowest rack, and heat oven to 400 degrees.

2 Score flesh of each eggplant half in 1-inch diamond pattern, about 1 inch deep. Brush scored sides of eggplant with 2 tablespoons oil and sprinkle with ½ teaspoon salt. Lay eggplant cut side down on hot sheet and roast until flesh is tender, 40 to 50 minutes. Transfer eggplant cut side down to paper towel–lined baking sheet and let drain.

3 Toss bulgur with water in bowl and let sit until grains are softened and liquid is fully absorbed, 20 to 40 minutes.

4 Cook remaining 1 tablespoon oil, oregano, cinnamon, and cayenne, if using, in 12-inch skillet until fragrant, about 30 seconds. Off heat, stir in bulgur, tomatoes, ¾ cup Pecorino, pine nuts, vinegar, and remaining ¼ teaspoon salt and let sit until heated through, about 1 minute. Season with salt and pepper to taste.

5 Return eggplant cut side up to rimmed baking sheet. Using 2 forks, gently push eggplant flesh to sides to make room for filling. Mound bulgur mixture into eggplant halves and pack lightly with back of spoon. Sprinkle with remaining ¼ cup Pecorino. Bake on upper rack until cheese is melted, 5 to 10 minutes. Sprinkle with parsley and serve.

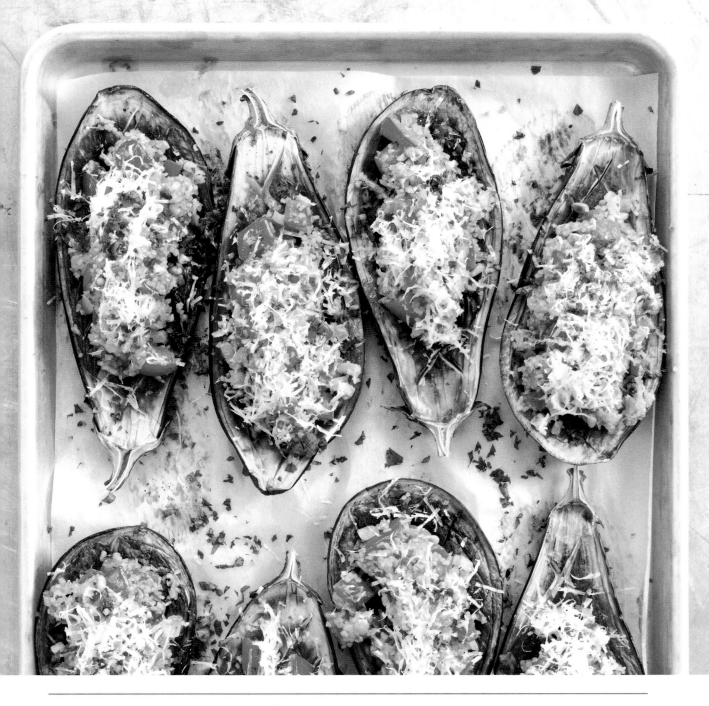

PER SERVING

Dietary Fiber 12g **Cal** 330;
Total Fat 19g, **Sat Fat** 4.5g;
Chol 15mg; **Sodium** 530mg;
Total Carb 36g, **Total Sugars** 13g,
Added Sugars 0g; **Protein** 10g

 MAKE IT DAIRY FREE Omit Pecorino Romano; increase salt
to ½ teaspoon in step 4.

WHOLE POT-ROASTED CAULIFLOWER WITH TOMATOES AND OLIVES

SERVES 4

WHY THIS RECIPE WORKS Diverse vegetable-forward cooking is one of the biggest keys to feeding a good gut. And we think a whole head of cauliflower might be the most impressive, visually striking way to serve a vegetable. This main course cauliflower is hearty and comforting, cloaked in a multidimensional tomato sauce with the flavors of Sicily. The recipes we came across for pot-roasted cauliflower all started by searing the cumbersome whole head first in an attempt to brown the exterior. But we found this task unwieldy, with the cauliflower slipping from our tongs and the hot oil spitting at our forearms. And the browning was spotty at best. Even more, once the cauliflower was coated in our piquant sauce of chunky tomatoes, golden raisins, and briny capers and olives, we couldn't taste or see the difference between browned and unbrowned cauliflower. So we skipped the hassle. To ensure that all of the flavors penetrated the dense vegetable, we started by cooking it upside down in the Dutch oven and spooned some of the sauce over the top so that it seeped into the crevices between the stalk and florets. Then we flipped it right side up, spooned more sauce over the top, and left the pot uncovered to finish cooking. The sauce thickened and the flavors intensified as the cauliflower became fork-tender.

1 **(28-ounce) can whole peeled tomatoes**

¼ **cup garlic oil (see page 20), plus extra for drizzling**

¼ **teaspoon red pepper flakes (optional)**

1 **head cauliflower (2 pounds)**

¼ **cup golden raisins**

¼ **cup pitted kalamata olives, chopped coarse**

3 **tablespoons capers, rinsed**

1 **ounce Parmesan cheese, grated (½ cup)**

¼ **cup minced fresh parsley**

1 Adjust oven rack to middle position and heat oven to 450 degrees. Pulse tomatoes and their juice in food processor until coarsely chopped, 6 to 8 pulses.

2 Cook oil and pepper flakes, if using, in Dutch oven over medium heat, stirring constantly, until fragrant, about 2 minutes. Stir in tomatoes, bring to simmer, and cook until slightly thickened, about 10 minutes.

3 Meanwhile, trim outer leaves of cauliflower and cut stem flush with bottom florets. Stir raisins, olives, and capers into tomatoes in pot, then nestle cauliflower, stem side up, into sauce. Spoon some of sauce over top, cover, transfer pot to oven, and roast until cauliflower is just tender (paring knife slips in and out of core with some resistance), 30 to 35 minutes.

4 Uncover pot and, using tongs, flip cauliflower stem side down. Spoon some of sauce over cauliflower, then scrape down sides of pot. Continue to roast, uncovered, until cauliflower is tender, 10 to 15 minutes.

5 Remove pot from oven. Sprinkle cauliflower with Parmesan and parsley and drizzle with extra oil. Cut cauliflower into wedges and serve, spooning sauce over individual portions.

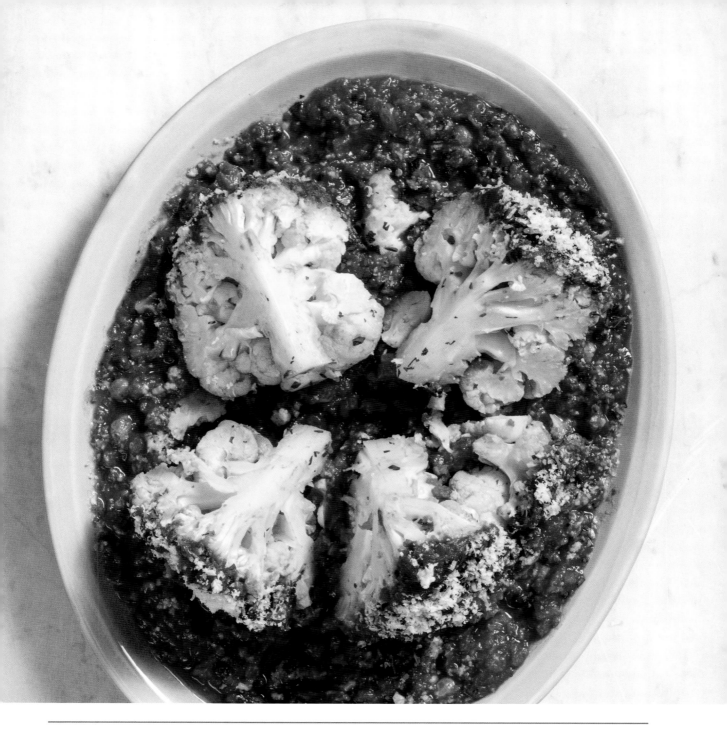

PER SERVING

Dietary Fiber 7g **Cal** 290;
Total Fat 17g, **Sat Fat** 3.5g;
Chol 5mg; **Sodium** 800mg;
Total Carb 28g, **Total Sugars** 17g,
Added Sugars 0g; **Protein** 10g

 MAKE IT DAIRY FREE Omit Parmesan.

PENNE WITH FRESH TOMATO SAUCE, SPINACH, AND FETA

SERVES 4

WHY THIS RECIPE WORKS You may have noticed that many low-FODMAP vegetables are storage vegetables (hearty tubers, squash, carrots), but tomatoes are also a gut-friendly vegetable. Because they have a short seasonal window to shine, we often call for canned, or smaller cherry or grape tomatoes in our recipes. But here we wanted a really stellar, quick but complex tomato sauce that captured the flavor of lightly cooked summer tomatoes. To achieve robust flavors without much cooking, we wilted earthy, fiberful baby spinach into our flavorful tomatoes then added mint and feta. The success of this recipe depends on ripe, in-season tomatoes. The skillet will be quite full when stirring in the spinach in step 1 (stir gently to start), but will become more manageable as the spinach wilts. You can use 12 ounces of any other 100 percent whole-wheat pasta shape instead of the penne, but the cup amount may vary.

2 tablespoons garlic oil (see page 20)

3 pounds ripe tomatoes, cored, peeled, seeded, and cut into ½-inch pieces

5 ounces (5 cups) baby spinach

12 ounces (3½ cups) 100 percent whole-wheat penne

4 ounces feta cheese, crumbled (1 cup), divided

2 tablespoons chopped fresh mint or oregano

1 tablespoon lemon juice

¼ teaspoon table salt, plus salt for cooking pasta

⅛ teaspoon pepper

1 Heat oil in 12-inch skillet over medium heat until shimmering. Add tomatoes and cook until they begin to lose their shape, about 8 minutes. Stir in spinach, 1 handful at a time, and cook until spinach is wilted and tomatoes have made chunky sauce, 2 minutes.

2 Meanwhile, bring 4 quarts water to boil in large pot. Add pasta and 1 tablespoon salt and cook, stirring often, until al dente. Reserve ½ cup cooking water, then drain pasta and return it to pot.

3 Stir ¾ cup feta, mint, lemon juice, salt, and pepper into sauce. Add sauce to pasta and toss to combine. Season with pepper to taste and adjust consistency with reserved cooking water as needed. Sprinkle with remaining ¼ cup feta and serve.

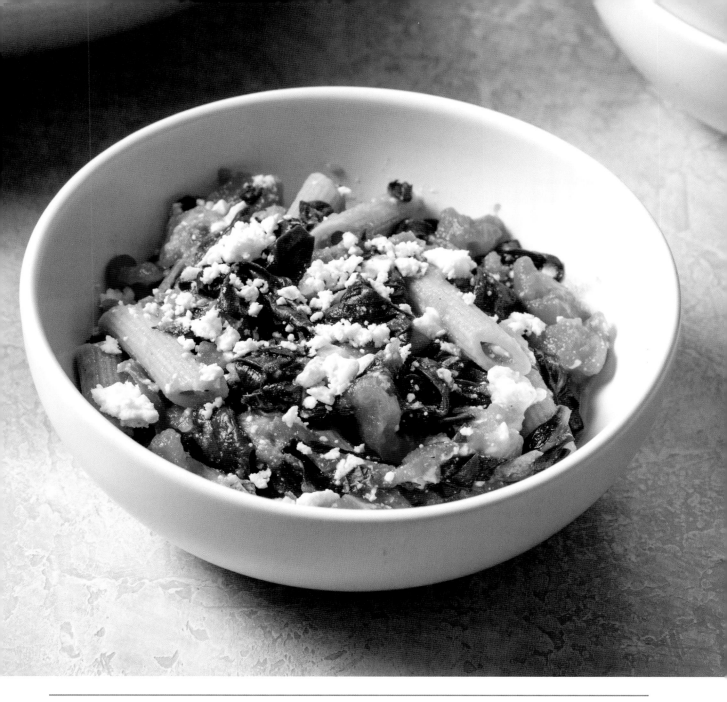

PER SERVING

Dietary Fiber 14g **Cal** 470;
Total Fat 16g, **Sat Fat** 5g;
Chol 25mg; **Sodium** 500mg;
Total Carb 67g, **Total Sugars** 11g,
Added Sugars 0g; **Protein** 18g

LF **MAKE IT LOW FODMAP** Substitute gluten-free pasta
(see page 19) for whole-wheat penne.

DF **MAKE IT DAIRY FREE** Omit feta; increase salt to
½ teaspoon in step 3.

GF **MAKE IT GLUTEN FREE** Substitute gluten-free pasta
(see page 19) for whole-wheat penne.

PEANUT NOODLE BOWLS WITH EDAMAME AND CABBAGE

SERVES 4

WHY THIS RECIPE WORKS Tender-chewy brown rice noodle dishes are a most comforting treat—especially for those with limited noodle options—as they are naturally gluten free and low FODMAP. And that's not where the gut health benefits end for this rich peanut sauce–cloaked noodle bowl. A real stunner, it boasts a colorful medley of vegetables: savory edamame, tangy lightly pickled carrots, and crunchy cabbage. A little curry powder in the sauce adds warmth. There are also plenty of garnishes—fragrant Thai basil, chopped peanuts, and a light pour of additional sauce. If you can't find Thai basil, you can substitute regular basil. To make this dish less spicy, omit or use the lesser amount of chiles. Serve with lime wedges if desired.

1 tablespoon garlic oil (see page 20)

1–2 Thai, serrano, or jalapeño chiles, stemmed, seeded, and minced

1 tablespoon grated fresh ginger

½ teaspoon curry powder

⅓ cup creamy peanut butter

5 tablespoons seasoned rice vinegar, divided

2 tablespoons soy sauce

1 tablespoon sugar

1 cup shredded carrots

12 ounces (¼-inch-wide) flat brown rice noodles

3 tablespoons canola oil, divided

1 cup frozen edamame, thawed

1 cup shredded red cabbage

⅓ cup dry-roasted peanuts, chopped

2 tablespoons torn fresh Thai basil

1 Heat garlic oil in medium saucepan over medium heat until shimmering. Add chiles, ginger, and curry powder and cook until fragrant, about 30 seconds. Stir in ½ cup water, peanut butter, 3 tablespoons vinegar, soy sauce, and sugar and bring to simmer. Cook, stirring occasionally, until thickened slightly and flavors meld, about 2 minutes. Adjust consistency as needed with additional water; set peanut sauce aside.

2 Combine carrots and remaining 2 tablespoons vinegar in small bowl; set aside. Bring 4 quarts water to boil in large pot. Remove from heat, add noodles, and let sit, stirring occasionally, until soft and pliable, but not fully tender. Drain noodles and rinse under cold running water until chilled. Drain noodles well again and toss with 2 teaspoons garlic oil; set aside.

3 Heat 1 tablespoon canola oil in 12-inch nonstick skillet over medium-high heat until just smoking. Add edamame and cook until spotty brown but still bright green, about 2 minutes; transfer to bowl. Heat remaining 4 teaspoons oil in now-empty skillet over medium heat until shimmering. Add noodles, 1¼ cups water, and ½ cup peanut sauce and cook until sauce has thickened slightly and noodles are well coated and tender, about 1 minute.

4 Divide noodles among individual serving bowls, then top with carrots, edamame, and cabbage. Drizzle with remaining peanut sauce, sprinkle with peanuts and basil, and serve.

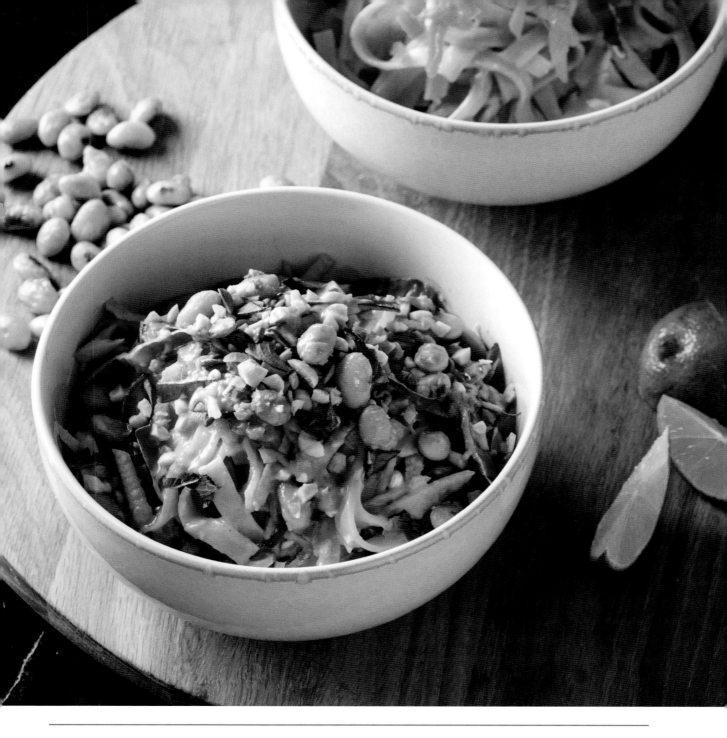

PER SERVING

Dietary Fiber 12g **Cal** 720;
Total Fat 34g, **Sat Fat** 5g;
Chol 0mg; **Sodium** 600mg;
Total Carb 85g, **Total Sugars** 11g,
Added Sugars 3g; **Protein** 20g

SOBA NOODLES WITH ROASTED EGGPLANT AND SESAME

SERVES 4

WHY THIS RECIPE WORKS Soba noodles (when made from 100 percent buckwheat flour) are sneakily gluten- and grain-free, so they're a great noodle choice for many. Hearty eggplant has a satisfyingly meaty texture that stands up quite well to the noodles' rich and nutty flavor and pleasantly chewy texture. To keep preparation straightforward and speedy, we decided that eggplant would be the only vegetable we'd include, so we used a generous amount. Roasting proved an easy, hands-off way to cook the eggplant, concentrate its flavor, and also draw out its moisture, resulting in pieces that were crisped on the outside and creamy on the inside. For the sauce, we started with soy sauce for savory richness. Vegetarian oyster sauce, toasted sesame oil, and some sugar provided a nice balance of spicy and sweet flavors, while a little sake contributed clean, acidic notes that bolstered the complexity of the sauce. A sprinkling of fresh cilantro and sesame seeds brightened up our earthy dish. You may substitute dry vermouth for the sake. Be sure to use 100 percent buckwheat soba noodles and gluten-free soy sauce or tamari if you need this dish to be gluten-free.

3 pounds eggplant, cut into 1-inch pieces

¼ cup canola oil

⅓ cup sugar

3 tablespoons vegetarian oyster sauce

3 tablespoons toasted sesame oil

2 tablespoons water

5 teaspoons sake

1 tablespoon soy sauce (see page 18)

Pinch red pepper flakes (optional)

12 ounces dried soba noodles

¾ cup fresh cilantro leaves

2 teaspoons sesame seeds, toasted

1 Adjust oven racks to upper-middle and lower-middle positions and heat oven to 450 degrees. Line 2 rimmed baking sheets with aluminum foil and spray with canola oil spray. Toss eggplant with canola oil, then spread evenly on prepared baking sheets. Roast until eggplant is well browned and tender, 25 to 30 minutes, stirring and switching sheets halfway through roasting.

2 Combine sugar, oyster sauce, sesame oil, 2 tablespoons water, sake, soy sauce, and pepper flakes, if using, in small saucepan. Cook over medium heat, whisking often, until sugar has dissolved, about 1 minute; cover and set sauce aside.

3 Meanwhile, bring 4 quarts water to boil in large pot. Add noodles and cook, stirring often, until tender. Reserve ½ cup cooking water, then drain noodles and return them to pot. Add sauce and roasted eggplant and toss to combine. Adjust consistency as needed with reserved cooking water. Sprinkle individual portions with cilantro and sesame seeds. Serve.

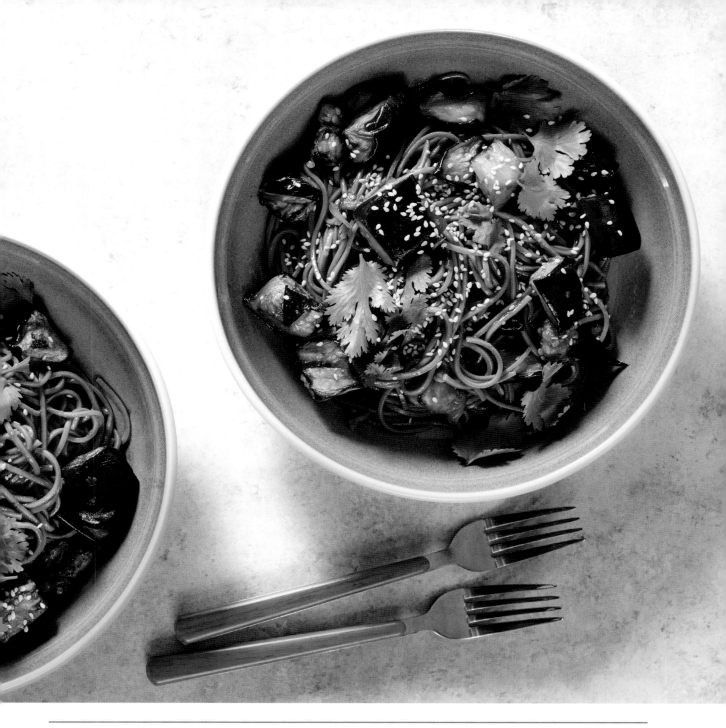

PER SERVING

Dietary Fiber 14g **Cal** 700;
Total Fat 27g, **Sat Fat** 3.5g;
Chol 0mg; **Sodium** 620mg;
Total Carb 105g, **Total Sugars** 33g,
Added Sugars 17g; **Protein** 14g

 MAKE IT GLUTEN FREE Substitute gluten-free soy sauce
or tamari (see page 18) for soy sauce.

BLACK BEAN BURGERS

SERVES 6

WHY THIS RECIPE WORKS Vegetarian burgers are too often weak attempts to replicate meat when what we really want is a satisfying savory patty that packs the qualities ground beef *doesn't*: fiber and gut-supporting nutrition. These hearty burgers are made simply, from mostly black beans. Their flavor profile picks up on elements of Southwestern cuisine thanks to the ground tortilla chips that we use as a binder (so we can include less flour) and the flavor enhancements of cilantro, ground cumin and coriander, and hot sauce. We pulse the tortilla chips with the beans in the food processor, but add the beans near the end of processing so that they maintain some texture. Using some of the liquid from the canned beans helps hold the patties together while boosting the overall flavor of the burgers. To ensure that we retain control over the moisture content of our burgers, we dry the rinsed beans well to remove excess water. When forming the patties, it's important to pack them together firmly.

2 (15-ounce) cans black beans, rinsed, with 6 tablespoons bean liquid reserved

2 tablespoons all-purpose flour

3 tablespoons minced fresh cilantro

1 teaspoon hot sauce (optional)

1 teaspoon ground cumin

½ teaspoon ground coriander

½ teaspoon table salt

¼ teaspoon pepper

1 ounce tortilla chips, crushed (½ cup)

¼ cup canola oil, divided

6 100 percent whole-wheat burger buns, toasted if desired

1 head Bibb lettuce (8 ounces), leaves separated

2 tomatoes, cored and sliced ¼ inch thick

2 avocados, halved, pitted, and sliced ¼ inch thick

1 Line rimmed baking sheet with triple layer of paper towels, spread beans over towels, and let sit for 15 minutes.

2 Whisk reserved bean liquid and flour in large bowl until well combined and smooth. Stir in cilantro, hot sauce, if using, cumin, coriander, salt, and pepper until well combined. Process tortilla chips in food processor until finely ground, about 30 seconds. Add black beans and pulse until beans are coarsely ground, about 5 pulses. Transfer bean mixture to bowl with flour mixture and mix until well combined. (Mixture can be refrigerated for up to 24 hours.)

3 Adjust oven rack to middle position and heat oven to 200 degrees. Divide bean mixture into 6 equal portions. Using your lightly moistened hands, firmly pack each portion into ¾-inch-thick patty. (Patties can be frozen for up to 1 month. Transfer patties to 2 parchment paper–lined rimmed baking sheets and freeze until firm, about 1 hour. Stack patties, separated by parchment paper, wrap in plastic wrap, and place in zipper-lock freezer bag. Thaw completely before cooking.)

4 Heat 1 tablespoon oil in 10-inch nonstick skillet over medium heat until shimmering. Gently lay 3 patties in skillet and cook until crisp and well browned on first side, about 5 minutes. Gently flip patties, add 1 tablespoon oil, and cook until crisp and well browned on second side, 3 to 5 minutes.

5 Transfer burgers to wire rack set in rimmed baking sheet and place in oven to keep warm. Wipe out skillet with paper towels and repeat with remaining 2 tablespoons oil and remaining patties. Transfer to buns and top with lettuce, tomato, and avocado. Serve.

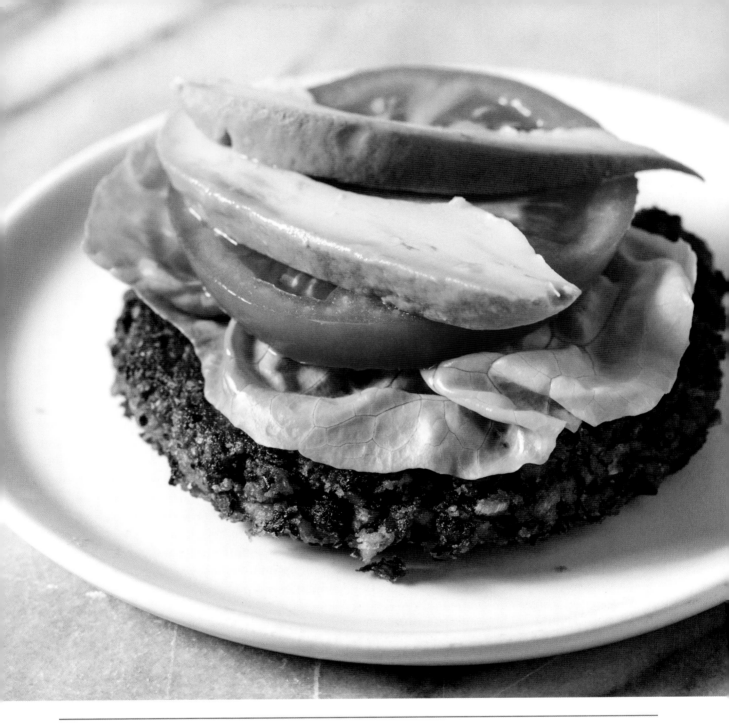

PER SERVING

Dietary Fiber 13g **Cal** 430;
Total Fat 23g, **Sat Fat** 2.5g;
Chol 0mg; **Sodium** 460mg;
Total Carb 48g, **Total Sugars** 6g,
Added Sugars 0g; **Protein** 12g

 MAKE IT GLUTEN FREE Substitute gluten-free flour blend (see page 31) for all-purpose flour. Omit buns or substitute low-FODMAP bread.

SWEET POTATO, POBLANO, AND LENTIL TACOS

SERVES 4

GLUTEN FREE

WHY THIS RECIPE WORKS Combined with spice-roasted cubes of sweet potato and strips of vegetal poblano peppers, earthy lentils make a hearty, almost ground beef–like, filling for tacos with the addition of zero fat and a lot of fiber. In fact, we might be so bold as to suggest that this is the most gut-healthy taco going, with even a unifying crema meeting low-FODMAP serving sizes of avocado and yogurt. Garlic oil, cumin, coriander, and oregano help to give these ingredients taco-Tuesday taste. To top off these robust fillings, we quickly pickle some radishes in lime juice. The bite and acidity freshen everything up and the crunch provides finishing contrast to these complexly flavored vegetarian tacos.

4 radishes, trimmed and sliced thin

¼ cup lime juice (2 limes), divided

1 teaspoon sugar

1¾ teaspoons table salt, divided

3 tablespoons garlic oil (see page 20)

1½ teaspoons ground cumin

1½ teaspoons ground coriander

½ teaspoon dried oregano

½ teaspoon pepper

1 pound sweet potatoes, peeled and cut into ½-inch pieces

4 poblano chiles, stemmed, seeded, and cut into ½-inch-wide strips

½ avocado, halved, pitted, and chopped coarse

½ cup chopped fresh cilantro, divided

¼ cup plain whole-milk yogurt

3 tablespoons water

1 (15-ounce) can lentils, rinsed

12 (6-inch) corn tortillas (see page 19), warmed

1 Combine radishes, 3 tablespoons lime juice, sugar, and 1 teaspoon salt in bowl and let sit at room temperature for 15 minutes. Drain radishes, transfer to bowl, and refrigerate until ready to serve.

2 Adjust oven rack to middle position and heat oven to 450 degrees. Whisk oil, cumin, coriander, oregano, remaining ¾ teaspoon salt, and pepper together in large bowl. Add potatoes and poblanos and toss to coat.

3 Spread vegetable mixture in even layer over aluminum foil–lined rimmed baking sheet. Do not clean bowl. Roast vegetables until tender and golden brown, about 30 minutes, stirring halfway through.

4 Meanwhile, process avocado, ¼ cup cilantro, yogurt, water, and remaining 1 tablespoon lime juice in food processor until smooth, scraping down sides of bowl as needed. Season with salt and pepper to taste. Transfer crema to separate bowl, cover, and refrigerate until ready to serve.

5 Return vegetables to now-empty bowl, add lentils and remaining ¼ cup cilantro, and toss gently to combine. Divide vegetables evenly among warm tortillas and top with avocado crema and pickled radishes. Serve.

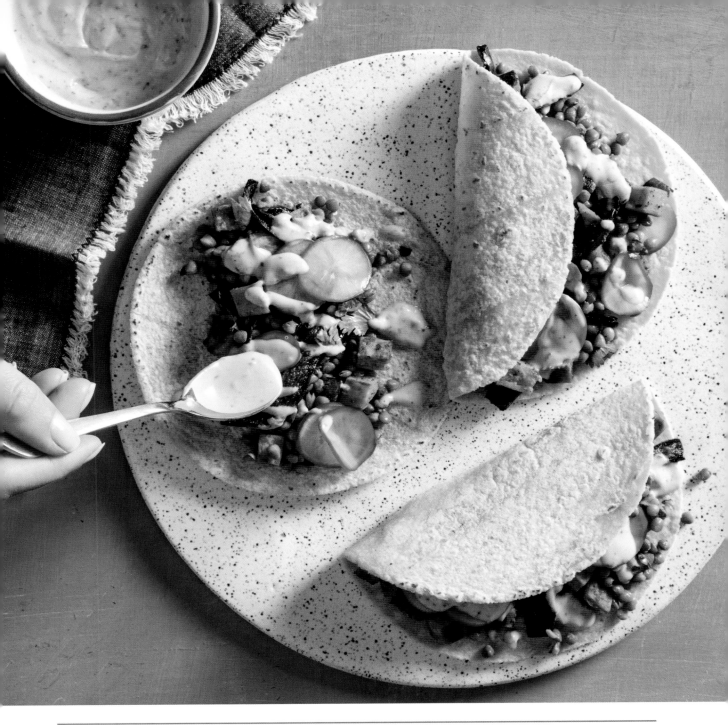

PER SERVING

Dietary Fiber 15g Cal 500;
Total Fat 18g, Sat Fat 2.5g;
Chol 0mg; Sodium 730mg;
Total Carb 75g, Total Sugars 10g,
Added Sugars 0g; Protein 13g

LF **MAKE IT LOW FODMAP** Reduce sweet potato to 10 ounces.

DF **MAKE IT DAIRY FREE** Substitute dairy-free yogurt
(see page 19) for whole-milk yogurt.

SUMMER ROLLS WITH TOFU AND PEANUT DIPPING SAUCE

SERVES 4

WHY THIS RECIPE WORKS Despite their evocative name, many summer rolls contain mostly rice noodles, leaving fresh vegetables as an afterthought. For this version, we skip the noodles altogether and gather up a rainbow of healthful veggies to fill our rice paper wrappers. A mix of red cabbage, red bell pepper, cucumber, and carrots delivers color and crunch. Fresh basil adds herbal notes, and strips of marinated tofu make the rolls hearty enough for lunch. Instead of the typical thin soy dipping sauce, we paired these rolls with a peanut sauce. Be sure to make one roll at a time to keep the wrappers moist and pliable. Brands of rice paper wrappers vary in the time they take to soak and become pliable. You can substitute regular basil for the Thai basil.

6 tablespoons rice wine vinegar, divided

1 tablespoon soy sauce (see page 18)

2 scallions, green parts only, sliced thin on bias

7 ounces extra-firm tofu, cut into 3-inch-long by ½-inch-thick strips

3 cups shredded red cabbage

12 (8-inch) round rice paper wrappers

1 cup fresh Thai basil leaves

1 red bell pepper, stemmed, seeded, and cut into 2-inch-long matchsticks

½ seedless English cucumber, cut into 3-inch-long matchsticks

2 carrots, peeled and shredded

1 recipe Peanut Dipping Sauce (page 23)

1 Whisk 2 tablespoons vinegar, soy sauce, and scallions in small bowl until well combined. Place tofu in shallow dish, then pour soy sauce mixture over top and let sit for 1 hour. Toss cabbage with remaining ¼ cup vinegar and let sit for 1 hour. Drain cabbage in fine mesh strainer, pressing gently with back of spatula to remove as much liquid as possible. Transfer to large plate and pat dry with paper towels.

2 Spread clean, damp dish towel on work surface. Fill 9-inch pie plate with 1 inch room-temperature water. Working with 1 wrapper at a time, submerge in water until just pliable, 10 seconds to 2 minutes; lay softened wrapper on towel. Scatter 3 basil leaves over wrapper. Arrange 5 matchsticks each of bell pepper and cucumber horizontally on wrapper, leaving 2-inch border at bottom. Top with 1 tablespoon carrots, then arrange about 2 tablespoons cabbage on top of carrots. Place 1 strip tofu horizontally on top of vegetables, being sure to shake off excess marinade.

3 Fold bottom of wrapper over filling, pulling back on it firmly to tighten it around filling, then fold sides of wrapper in and continue to roll tightly into summer roll. Transfer to platter and cover with second damp dish towel.

4 Repeat with remaining wrappers and filling. Serve with dipping sauce. (Summer rolls are best eaten immediately but can be covered with a clean, damp dish towel and refrigerated for up to 4 hours.)

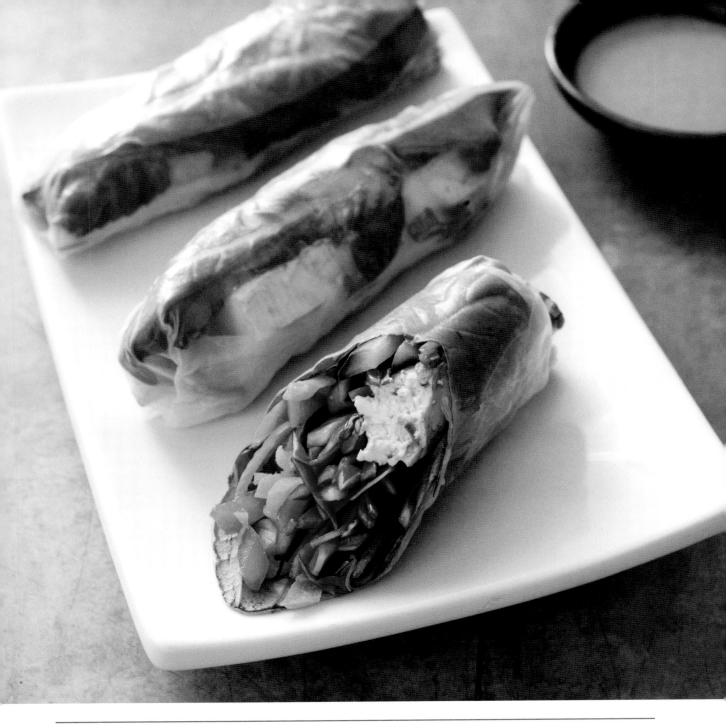

PER SERVING

Dietary Fiber 6g Cal 360;
Total Fat 16g, Sat Fat 3g;
Chol 0mg; Sodium 750mg;
Total Carb 40g, Total Sugars 10g,
Added Sugars 1g; Protein 17g

 MAKE IT GLUTEN FREE Substitute gluten-free soy sauce or
tamari (see page 18) for soy sauce.

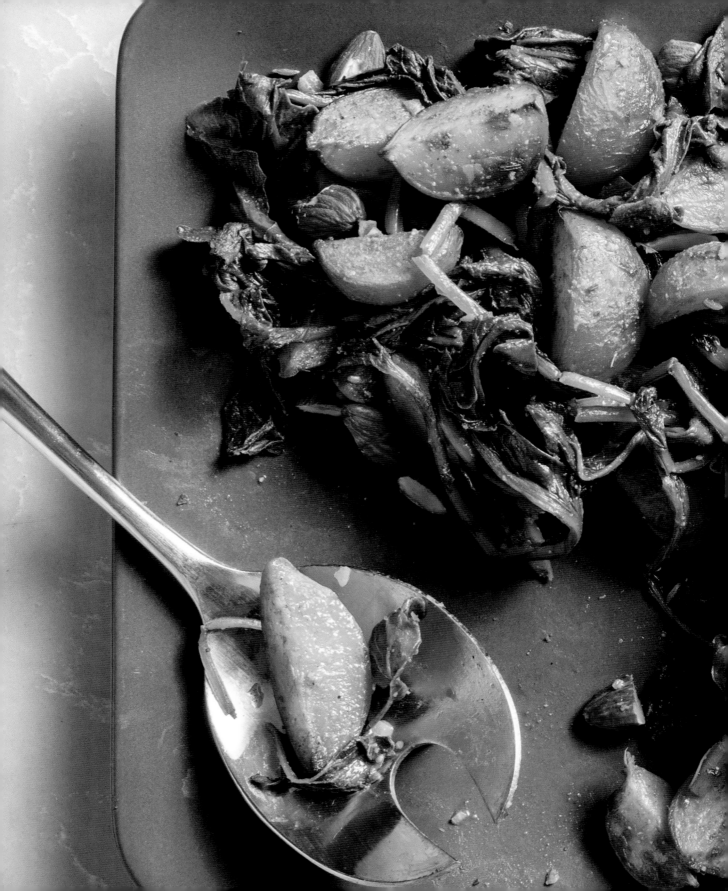

7 Sides

Vegetables

Grains

Beans

PAN-STEAMED KALE

SERVES 4

WHY THIS RECIPE WORKS Kale is a poster child for health, and this should be fact—not trend. The dark leafy greens are fiberful and nutrient dense. Plus, if you're following a low-FODMAP diet it's wise to put kale on your plate—you can eat as much as your appetite tells you to, as it's free from offending carbohydrates. Kale is a hardy green, but it's possible to cook it quickly with both steaming (for tender results) and sautéing (for concentrated flavor and moisture evaporation). We use broth for the steaming medium for deep savor, and we finish the kale with ingredients that don't overpower its natural earthiness, whether that be just a squeeze of bright lemon or delicious bites of pancetta and crunchy toasted pine nuts. It's a perfect accompaniment for dishes like Weeknight Skillet Roast Chicken (page 128).

1 cup chicken or vegetable broth (see page 18)

3 tablespoons garlic oil (see page 20), divided

1¼ pounds curly kale, stemmed and cut into 2-inch pieces (14 cups)

1 teaspoon lemon juice, plus extra for seasoning

1 Bring broth and 2 tablespoons oil to boil in Dutch oven over high heat. Add kale, cover, and reduce heat to medium-high. Cook until kale is tender with some resilience, about 7 minutes, stirring halfway through cooking.

2 Uncover, increase heat to high, and cook, stirring frequently, until liquid has evaporated and kale starts to sizzle, 2 to 3 minutes. Off heat, stir in remaining 1 tablespoon oil and lemon juice. Season with salt and extra lemon juice to taste. Serve.

VARIATION

Pan-Steamed Kale with Pancetta and Pine Nuts
Cook 2 ounces finely chopped pancetta and 1 tablespoon oil in Dutch oven over medium-high heat, stirring frequently, until browned, about 3 minutes. Off heat, using slotted spoon, transfer pancetta to bowl. Substitute fat left in pot for oil in step 1. Substitute balsamic vinegar for lemon juice and sprinkle kale with 2 tablespoons toasted pine nuts and reserved pancetta before serving.

PER SERVING

Dietary Fiber 4g **Cal** 150;
Total Fat 12g, **Sat Fat** 1.5g;
Chol 0mg; **Sodium** 180mg;
Total Carb 9g, **Total Sugars** 3g,
Added Sugars 0g; **Protein** 5g

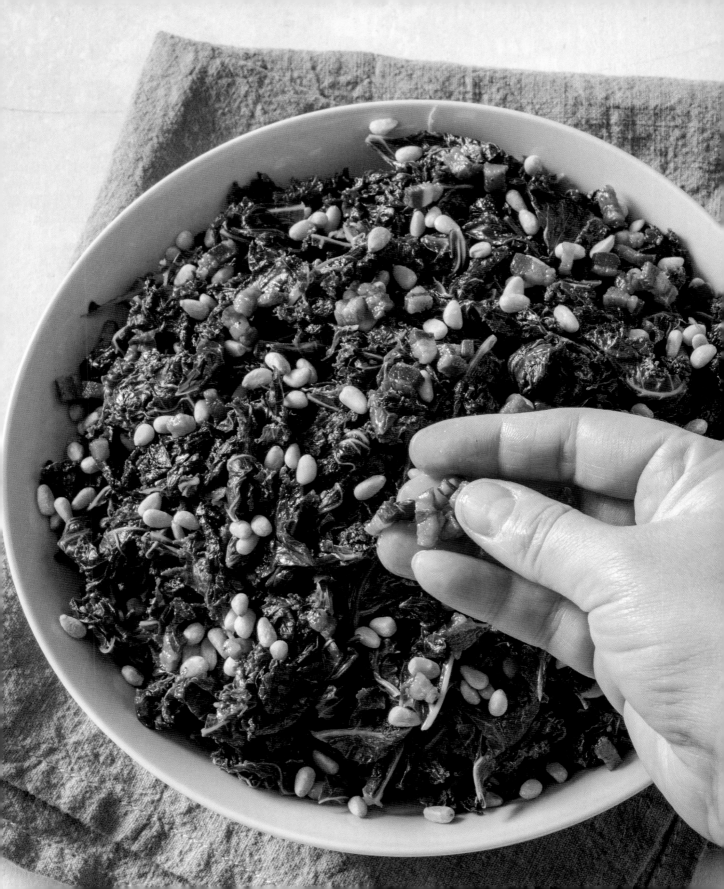

SAUTÉED RADISHES WITH CURRY POWDER AND ALMONDS

SERVES 4

WHY THIS RECIPE WORKS Raw radishes and their uniquely spicy bite grace salads, sandwiches, and crudités plates, but we urge you to try cooking them: They sweeten and gain complexity that gives them a whole new flavor dimension. Since radishes are devoid of FODMAPs, most anyone can eat them to their appetite. To encourage you, we sauté quartered radishes until they're browned and nutty, and then stir in curry powder to release its compounds in the heat and thoroughly coat the quarters. To provide some textural variety, color, and extra nutrition, and to prevent waste, we cook the radish greens at the end. The greens retain a slight crispness that complements the meatier radish pieces. If you can't find radishes with their greens, skip cooking them in step 2.

3 tablespoons garlic oil (see page 20), divided

1½ pounds radishes with their greens, radishes trimmed and quartered, 8 cups greens reserved

¼ teaspoon plus ⅛ teaspoon table salt, divided

1½ teaspoons curry powder

2 tablespoons whole almonds, toasted and coarsely chopped

1 Heat 2 tablespoons oil in 12-inch skillet over medium-high heat until shimmering. Add quartered radishes and ¼ teaspoon salt and cook, stirring occasionally, until radishes are lightly browned and crisp-tender, 10 to 12 minutes. Stir in curry powder and cook until fragrant, about 30 seconds; transfer to bowl.

2 Heat remaining 1 tablespoon oil in now-empty skillet over medium heat. Add radish greens and remaining ⅛ teaspoon salt and cook, stirring frequently, until wilted, about 1 minute. Off heat, stir in radishes and season with salt to taste. Sprinkle with almonds and serve.

PER SERVING
Dietary Fiber 4g **Cal** 160;
Total Fat 13g, **Sat Fat** 1.5g;
Chol 0mg; **Sodium** 290mg;
Total Carb 9g, **Total Sugars** 4g,
Added Sugars 0g; **Protein** 4g

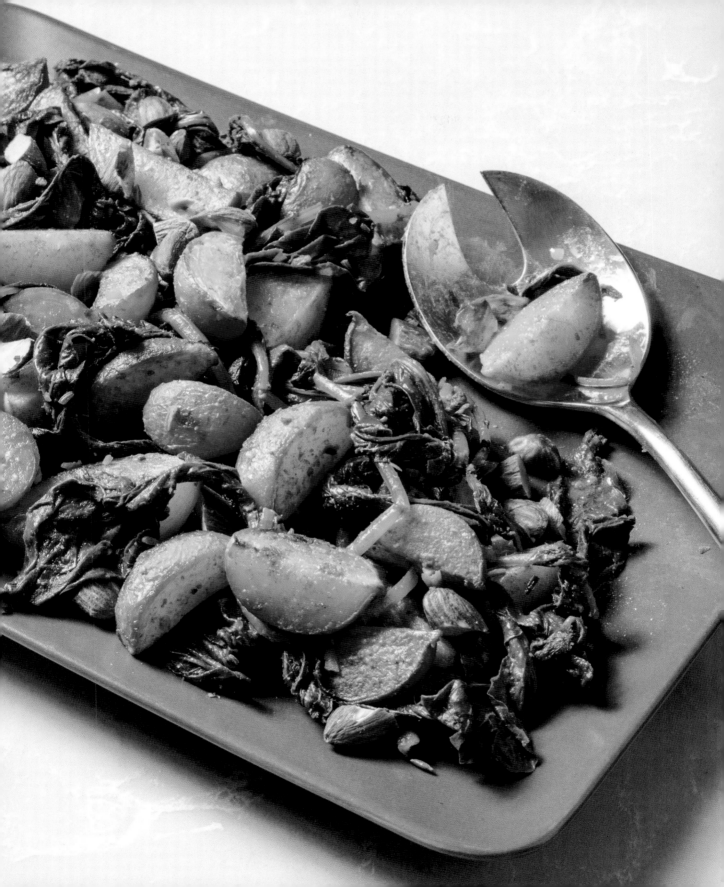

SAUTÉED GREEN BEANS WITH FRESH HERBS

SERVES 4

WHY THIS RECIPE WORKS There might not be a green food that's unhealthful, and green beans live up to the color in their name, with a boastworthy amount of fiber. (Not to mention that the fiber content comes at a very low calorie cost.) String beans play equally well first-string next to an elegant roast (see page 182) as they do with a weeknight fish dish (see page 212) since they're quick to cook. But quick means the line between raw and crunchy and muddy-colored and mushy is thin. We like ours crisp-tender with appealing browning, which we achieve with a three-part sauté: We sauté the beans until spotty brown; add water to the pan, cover, and cook the beans through; and then lift the lid to evaporate the water and promote more browning. Finishing with some bright lemon juice and parsley contrasts the more woodsy flavor of the thyme in the recipe. If you prefer beans that are softer or if you are using large, tough beans, increase the amount of water by 1 tablespoon and cook, covered, for 1 minute longer.

4 teaspoons garlic oil (see page 20), divided

1 teaspoon minced fresh thyme

1 pound green beans, trimmed and cut into 2-inch lengths

¼ teaspoon table salt

⅛ teaspoon pepper

¼ cup water

2 teaspoons lemon juice

1 tablespoon minced fresh parsley, basil, and/or mint

1 Combine 1 tablespoon oil and thyme in bowl. Heat remaining 1 teaspoon oil in 12-inch nonstick skillet over medium heat until just smoking. Add green beans, salt, and pepper and cook, stirring occasionally, until spotty brown, 4 to 6 minutes. Add water, cover, and cook until beans are bright green and still crisp, about 2 minutes.

2 Uncover, increase heat to high, and cook until water evaporates, 30 to 60 seconds. Add oil mixture and cook, stirring often, until green beans are crisp-tender, lightly browned, and beginning to wrinkle, 1 to 3 minutes. Off heat, stir in lemon juice and parsley and season with pepper to taste. Serve.

VARIATION

Sautéed Green Beans with Thyme, Coriander, and Sesame Seeds
Add ¼ teaspoon ground coriander and ¼ teaspoon ground cumin to oil with thyme. Substitute 1 tablespoon toasted sesame seeds for parsley.

PER SERVING

Dietary Fiber 3g **Cal** 70;
Total Fat 5g, **Sat Fat** 0.5g;
Chol 0mg; **Sodium** 150mg;
Total Carb 7g, **Total Sugars** 3g,
Added Sugars 0g; **Protein** 2g

 MAKE IT LOW FODMAP Reduce green beans to 10 ounces. Add 8 ounces grape tomatoes, halved, to skillet with oil mixture and cook until green beans are crisp-tender and tomatoes begin to break down, 1 to 3 minutes.

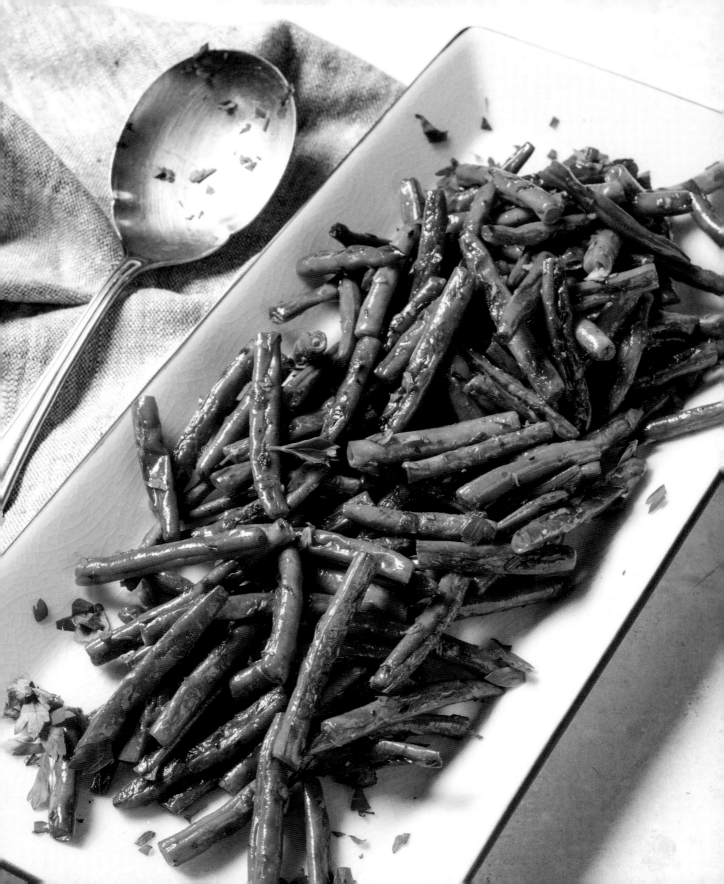

PAN-ROASTED PARSNIPS

SERVES 4

WHY THIS RECIPE WORKS Uniquely floral, candy-sweet, fully filling, superlatively high in fiber, and FODMAP-free, parsnips may seem too good (for you) to be true. But they're not, and that's why we love them. In this convenient recipe, we replicate the sweet caramelized flavor of oven-roasted parsnips on the stovetop. After browning the parsnips in oil, we add water to the pan before covering— this creates a gentle steaming effect that guarantees perfectly cooked interiors every time. Cutting the parsnips into ½-inch-thick pieces on the bias assures even and plentiful browning as well as an attractive presentation. A sprinkling of fresh herbs and a squeeze of citrus may seem simple but their brightness does a delicious job of balancing the earthy vegetable and cutting through its sweetness. Look for parsnips no wider than 1 inch at their base, or you may need to discard their fibrous cores. Poultry is a favorite parsnip pairing.

1 tablespoon extra-virgin olive oil

1¼ pounds parsnips, peeled and cut ½ inch thick on bias

½ cup water

¼ teaspoon table salt

1 teaspoon minced fresh parsley

Lemon wedges

1 Heat oil in 12-inch skillet over medium-high heat until shimmering. Add parsnips and cook, stirring occasionally, until golden, 8 to 10 minutes.

2 Add water and salt and bring to simmer. Cover, reduce heat to medium-low, and cook, stirring occasionally, until parsnips are tender and liquid has evaporated, 8 to 10 minutes. Off heat, stir in parsley and season with salt and pepper to taste. Serve with lemon wedges.

VARIATION

Pan-Roasted Parsnips with Cilantro and Lime
Add ½ teaspoon chipotle chile powder to skillet with parsnips in step 1. Substitute cilantro for parsley. Add ¼ teaspoon lime zest plus 1½ teaspoons lime juice to parsnips with cilantro. Serve with lime wedges.

PER SERVING
Dietary Fiber 6g **Cal** 120;
Total Fat 4g, **Sat Fat** 0.5g;
Chol 0mg; **Sodium** 160mg;
Total Carb 22g, **Total Sugars** 6g,
Added Sugars 0g; **Protein** 1g

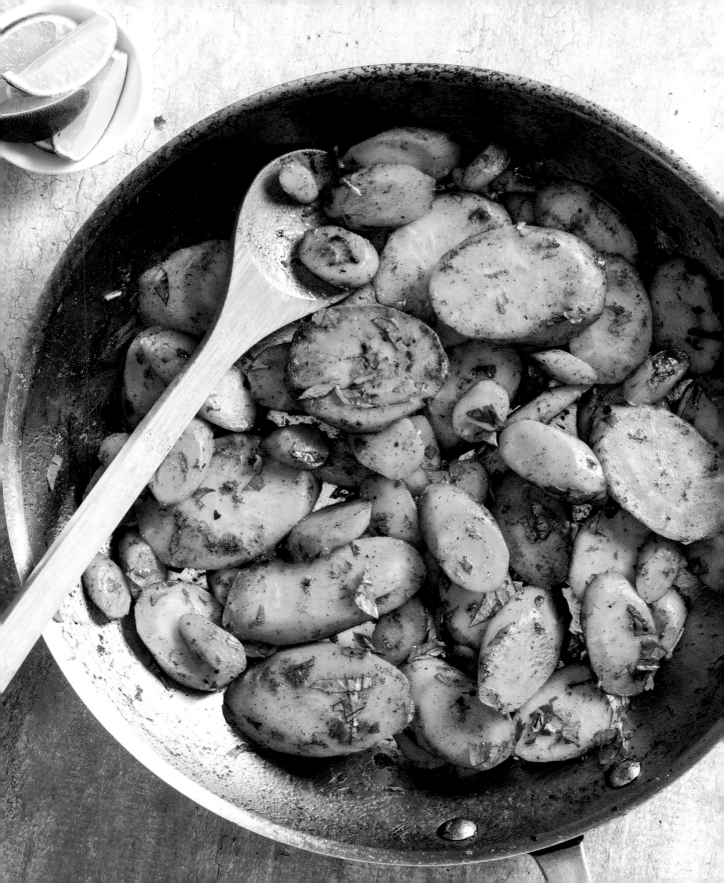

SKILLET-ROASTED BROCCOLI

SERVES 4

WHY THIS RECIPE WORKS Eating your broccoli is easy if it's deeply browned and nutty and cooked evenly from stem to floret. Steaming won't get you there; roasting will, but it's a nonstarter if you have your main dish in the oven. Luckily, we've found a way to achieve the impressive browning of roasting quickly on the stovetop. We cut broccoli crowns into wedges to create large flat sides that sit flush with the surface of a generously oiled skillet, and we steam the broccoli initially to soften it. When the water evaporates, the oil fills any gaps between the broccoli and the skillet for optimal heat transfer and browning. Pressing the wedges against the skillet with a spatula between cooking stages creates even deeper browning, yielding generously sized crisp wedges—with meaty stems and delicate florets—that go with anything. Or, make the variation with a crunchy umami-rich topping for broccoli that steals the show.

1¼ **pounds broccoli crowns**

¼ **cup extra-virgin olive oil**

¾ **teaspoon kosher salt**

2 **tablespoons water**

1 Cut broccoli crowns into 4 wedges (if 3 to 4 inches in diameter) or 6 wedges (if 4 to 5 inches in diameter). Add oil to 12-inch non-stick skillet and tilt skillet until oil covers surface. Add broccoli, cut side down (pieces will fit snugly; if a few pieces don't fit in bottom layer, place on top). Sprinkle evenly with salt and drizzle with water. Cover and cook over high heat, without moving broccoli, until broccoli is bright green, about 4 minutes.

2 Uncover and press gently on broccoli with back of spatula. Cover and cook until undersides of broccoli are deeply browned and stems are crisp-tender, 4 to 6 minutes. Off heat, uncover and turn broccoli so second cut side is touching skillet. Move any pieces that were on top so they are flush with skillet surface. Continue to cook, uncovered, pressing gently on broccoli with back of spatula, until second cut side is deeply browned, 3 to 5 minutes longer. Serve.

VARIATION

Skillet-Roasted Broccoli with Smoky Sunflower Seed Topping
Nutritional yeast is a flaky, golden, nonleavening form of yeast with a nutty, tangy flavor; look for it in natural foods stores.

Using spice grinder or mortar and pestle, grind 2 tablespoons toasted sunflower seeds, 1 tablespoon nutritional yeast, ½ teaspoon grated lemon zest, ¼ teaspoon smoked paprika, and ¼ teaspoon kosher salt to coarse powder. Sprinkle one-third mixture onto platter, top with cooked broccoli, and sprinkle with remaining topping.

PER SERVING

Dietary Fiber 3g **Cal** 170;
Total Fat 14g, **Sat Fat** 2g;
Chol 0mg; **Sodium** 250mg;
Total Carb 7g, **Total Sugars** 2g,
Added Sugars 0g; **Protein** 4g

 MAKE IT LOW FODMAP Reduce broccoli to 10 ounces. After uncovering skillet in step 2, add 2 red bell peppers, stemmed, seeded, and sliced thin, and cook, tossing occasionally, until softened, 3 to 5 minutes.

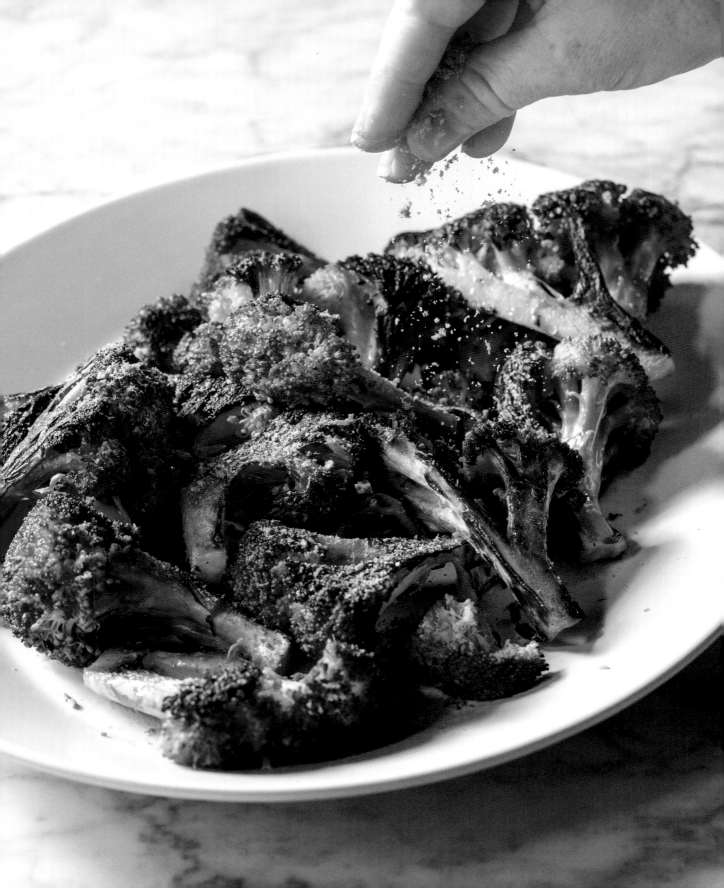

SAUTÉED CABBAGE

SERVES 4

WHY THIS RECIPE WORKS If you think cooked cabbage dishes are heavy and maybe a little smelly, poor preparation has misled you; this simple recipe brings out the vegetable's natural sweetness while maintaining its crisp-tender texture. A precooking step of soaking the cabbage reduces any bitterness (and smelliness) while providing extra moisture to help the cabbage steam. We then pan-steam and sauté the cabbage over relatively high heat to cook it quickly and add an extra layer of flavor from browning. The garlic cooking oil provides depth, and fresh parsley offers a bright finish. Finally, a bacony caraway variation makes things a little extra rich—if you're inclined. Skip the slaw; make this and instantly up the fiber content of your dinner. We particularly like cabbage with pork chops (see page 174), but we think you'll be incorporating it into many meals.

1 small head green cabbage (1¼ pounds), cored and sliced thin

2 tablespoons garlic oil (see page 20)

½ teaspoon table salt

¼ teaspoon pepper

¼ cup chopped fresh parsley

1½ teaspoons lemon juice

1 Place cabbage in large bowl and cover with cold water; let stand for 3 minutes. Drain well.

2 Heat oil in 12-inch nonstick skillet over medium-high heat until shimmering. Add cabbage and sprinkle with salt and pepper. Cover and cook, without stirring, until cabbage is wilted and lightly browned on bottom, about 3 minutes. Stir and continue to cook, uncovered, until cabbage is crisp-tender and lightly browned in places, about 4 minutes, stirring once halfway through cooking. Off heat, stir in parsley and lemon juice and season with salt and pepper to taste. Serve.

VARIATION

Sautéed Cabbage with Bacon and Caraway Seeds
Omit oil, parsley, and lemon juice. Substitute red cabbage for green. Whisk 1 tablespoon cider vinegar, 2 teaspoons packed brown sugar, and 1 teaspoon toasted caraway seeds together in medium bowl. Cook 4 slices chopped bacon in skillet over medium-high heat until rendered and crispy, 5 to 7 minutes. Transfer bacon to paper towel–lined plate and pour off all but 1 tablespoon fat. Cook drained cabbage in fat left in skillet. Stir bacon and vinegar mixture into cabbage before serving.

PER SERVING

Dietary Fiber 4g **Cal** 110;
Total Fat 7g, **Sat Fat** 1g;
Chol 0mg; **Sodium** 330mg;
Total Carb 9g, **Total Sugars** 5g,
Added Sugars 0g; **Protein** 2g

 MAKE IT LOW FODMAP Reduce cabbage to ½ small cabbage. Add cabbage and 8 ounces kale, stemmed and sliced thin, to skillet, one handful at a time, and cook until slightly wilted. Sprinkle with salt and pepper, cover, and continue to cook as directed.

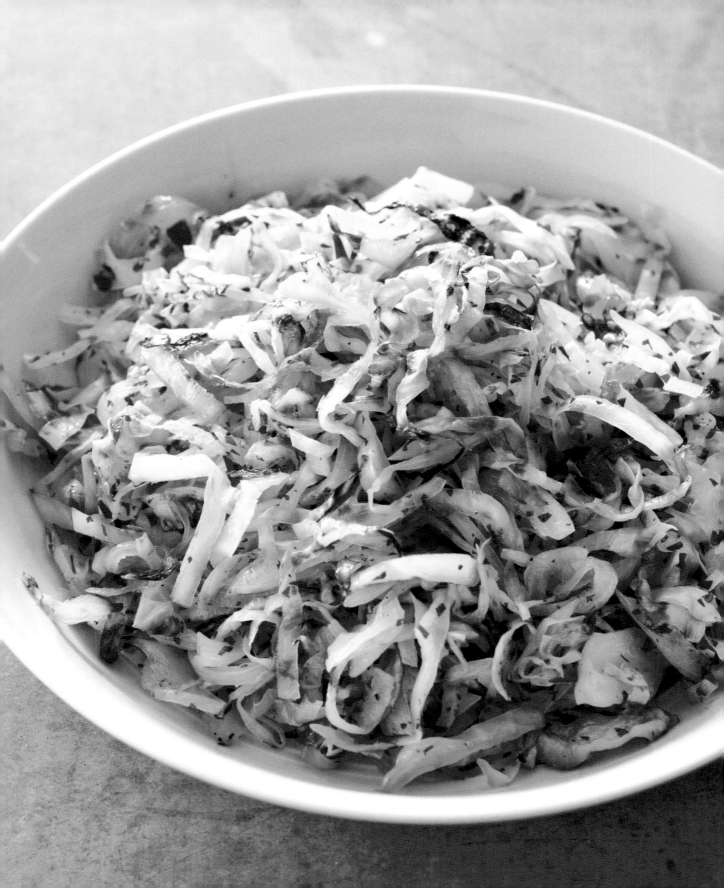

ESCAROLE AND ORANGE SALAD WITH GREEN OLIVES

SERVES 4

WHY THIS RECIPE WORKS Leafy, produce-packed salads are an excellent way to both display seasonal veggies in their purest forms and add fiber to your meal. We encourage you to move beyond more delicate baby spinach and arugula and fill your bowl with escarole. Of course we love that it's packed with fiber and that you can have a more generous portion if you're following a low-FODMAP diet. But a real draw is how much more character it has than many other salad greens; not as hardy as kale, not as leafy as lettuce, this chicory has an appealing bite but isn't bracingly bitter. Two whole oranges brighten up the greens and provide fruitiness (and extra nutrition); green olives add a briny, meaty element to pierce through it all; and slivered almonds offset these ingredients with richness. We use the orange's zest to boost the vinaigrette and we cut the oranges into sections instead of larger rounds, so they are evenly distributed throughout the salad. When arranging the orange segments on the escarole, leave behind any juice that is released; it will dilute the dressing.

2 oranges

3 tablespoons garlic oil
(see page 20)

2 tablespoons sherry vinegar

1 head escarole (1 pound),
trimmed and chopped

½ cup chopped brine-cured
green olives

¼ cup slivered almonds,
toasted

1 Grate 1 teaspoon zest from orange; set zest aside. Cut away peel and pith from oranges. Holding fruit over second bowl, use paring knife to slice between membranes to release segments; set aside.

2 Whisk oil, vinegar, and orange zest in large bowl until combined. Add escarole and olives and toss to coat. Season with salt and pepper to taste. Divide dressed greens among individual serving plates, top with orange segments, and sprinkle with almonds. Serve.

PER SERVING

Dietary Fiber 5g **Cal** 200;
Total Fat 16g, **Sat Fat** 2g;
Chol 0mg; **Sodium** 260mg;
Total Carb 14g, **Total Sugars** 7g,
Added Sugars 0g; **Protein** 3g

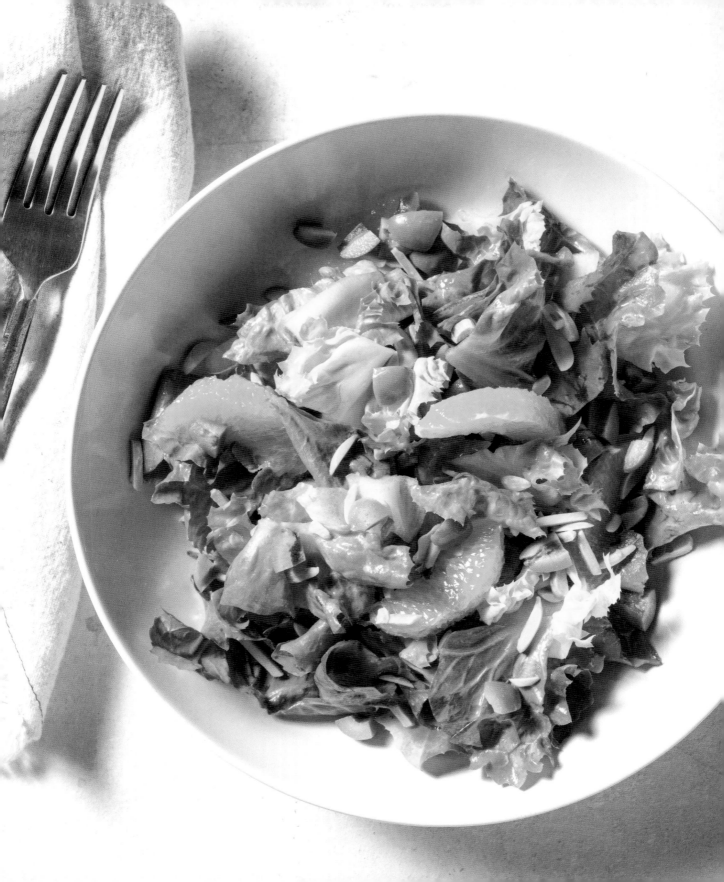

ROASTED RED POTATOES

SERVES 4

WHY THIS RECIPE WORKS Roasted potatoes feel like comfort food, so it can be hard to remember you're getting your vegetables when you're eating them. But potatoes are plenty good for you: They're gentle on the gut, moderate in fiber, and do not contain FODMAPs. To arrive at our ideal—potatoes with deep golden, crisp crusts and creamy, soft interiors—we take advantage of the high moisture content of red potatoes. We arrange them cut side down on a foil-lined rimmed baking sheet and also cover them with foil; they turn tender as they steam in their own moisture. Finishing the potatoes uncovered crisps the outsides. Contact with the baking sheet is important for browning, so we flip the potatoes partway through for crispness on every side. If using very small potatoes, cut them in half instead of into wedges and flip them cut side up during the final 10 minutes of roasting.

1½ pounds red potatoes, unpeeled, cut into ¾-inch wedges

2 tablespoons extra-virgin olive oil

¼ teaspoon table salt

⅛ teaspoon pepper

1 Adjust oven rack to middle position and heat oven to 425 degrees. Line rimmed baking sheet with aluminum foil. Toss potatoes with oil, salt, and pepper in bowl. Arrange potatoes cut side down on prepared sheet. Cover with foil and roast for 20 minutes.

2 Remove foil and roast until sides of potatoes touching pan are crusty and golden, about 15 minutes. Flip potatoes over and roast until crusty and golden on second side, about 8 minutes. Season with salt and pepper to taste, and serve.

VARIATION
Roasted Red Potatoes with Rosemary
Substitute garlic oil (see page 20) for olive oil. During final 3 minutes of roasting, sprinkle 1 tablespoon minced fresh rosemary over potatoes.

PER SERVING

Dietary Fiber 3g **Cal** 180;
Total Fat 7g, **Sat Fat** 1g;
Chol 0mg; **Sodium** 180mg;
Total Carb 27g, **Total Sugars** 2g,
Added Sugars 0g; **Protein** 3g

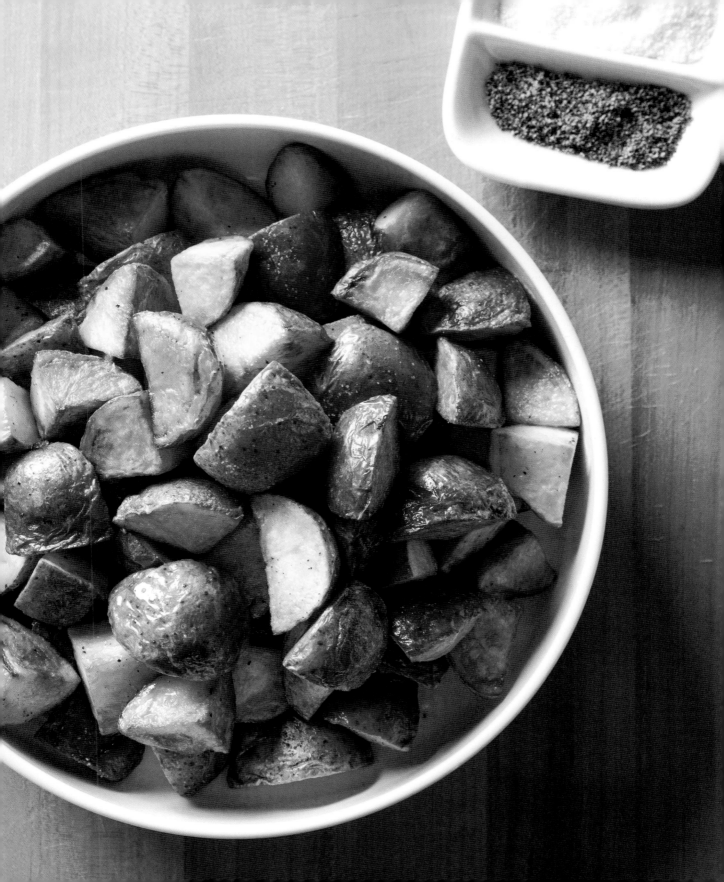

MASHED POTATOES AND ROOT VEGETABLES

SERVES 4

WHY THIS RECIPE WORKS Mashed potatoes, with their generous butter and cream, are a luxury, often a special-occasion side; we made a mashed vegetable side with double the fiber and nutrition and none of the dairy—but all of the luxury. Carrots or parsnips add earthy flavor and sweetness to potatoes, but because they have different starch levels and water content, treating them the same as the potatoes creates a bad mash. We found that a 1:3 ratio of root vegetables to potatoes gave us an optimal creamy consistency, and caramelizing the root vegetables in oil before simmering helped bring out their sweetness. Vegetable broth was the perfect cooking medium; we didn't want this mash so rich that the root vegetables didn't shine. Russet potatoes will yield a slightly fluffier, less creamy mash, but they can be used in place of the Yukon Gold potatoes if desired. It is important to cut the potatoes and root vegetables into evenly sized pieces so that they cook at the same rate. This recipe can be doubled; use a large Dutch oven and increase the simmering time in step 2 to 40 minutes.

1½ pounds Yukon Gold potatoes, peeled, quartered lengthwise, and cut crosswise into ¼-inch-thick slices

3 tablespoons extra-virgin olive oil

8 ounces carrots or parsnips, peeled, halved lengthwise and sliced ¼ inch thick

1 cup vegetable broth (see page 20), plus extra as needed

¼ teaspoon table salt

3 tablespoons minced fresh chives

1 Rinse potatoes using 3 or 4 changes of cold water, then drain well. Heat oil in large saucepan over medium heat until shimmering. Add carrots and cook, stirring occasionally, until dark brown and caramelized, 10 to 12 minutes. (If after 4 minutes carrots have not started to brown, increase heat to medium-high.)

2 Stir in potatoes, broth, and salt; cover; and reduce heat to low. Simmer gently, stirring occasionally and adjusting heat as needed, until potatoes fall apart easily when poked with fork and all liquid has been absorbed, 25 to 30 minutes. Remove pan from heat, remove lid, and allow steam to escape for 2 minutes.

3 Gently mash potatoes and carrots in saucepan with potato masher (do not mash vigorously). Adjust consistency with extra warm broth as needed. Fold in chives and season with salt and pepper to taste. Serve.

VARIATION

Mashed Potatoes and Root Vegetables with Paprika and Parsley
Toast 1½ teaspoons smoked or sweet paprika in 8-inch skillet over medium heat until fragrant, about 30 seconds. Substitute parsley for chives and fold toasted paprika into potatoes with parsley.

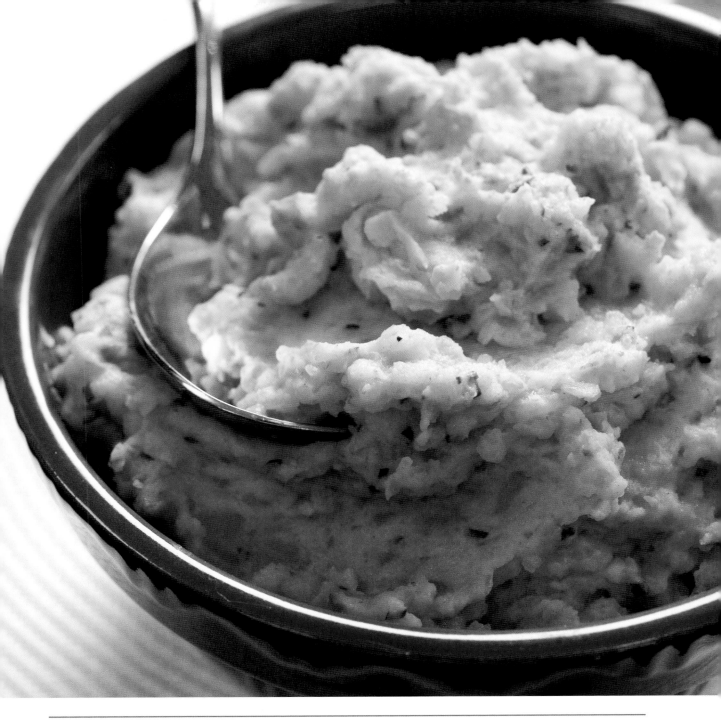

PER SERVING

Dietary Fiber 6g **Cal** 290;
Total Fat 12g, **Sat Fat** 4g;
Chol 15mg; **Sodium** 300mg;
Total Carb 44g, **Total Sugars** 6g,
Added Sugars 0g; **Protein** 5g

ROASTED KABOCHA SQUASH WITH MAPLE AND SAGE

SERVES 4

WHY THIS RECIPE WORKS You might be used to roasting butternut squash when fall arrives; if so, we'll introduce you to kabocha squash. Kabocha looks like a squat, green pumpkin and is a wise (and incredibly delicious) way to meet your daily fiber minimum because, unlike other winter squashes, it's low FODMAP. Why else? When roasted, its flesh becomes rich and creamy, and its skin tender to eat, so this recipe gives us more fiber than many other winter squash recipes. The flesh is close in flavor to a sweet potato, with a hint of sweet heat. We build on that heat, coating squash wedges in paprika as well as coriander, which provide a hint of complementary warmth. The spice-roasted squash becomes something truly special when adorned with a simple vinaigrette that we whisk together from garlic oil, maple syrup, cider vinegar, and sage. The warm squash drinks up the dressing to achieve the perfect sweet-savory balance.

1 kabocha squash (3 pounds), halved lengthwise and seeded

¼ cup garlic oil (see page 20), divided

2 teaspoons ground paprika

1 teaspoon ground coriander

½ teaspoon table salt

½ teaspoon pepper

1 tablespoon cider vinegar

1 tablespoon maple syrup

2 teaspoons minced fresh sage

1 Adjust oven rack to middle position and heat oven to 475 degrees. Line rimmed baking sheet with parchment paper.

2 Cut each squash half into 2½- to 3-inch pieces. Whisk 2 tablespoons oil, paprika, coriander, salt, and pepper together in large bowl. Add squash and toss until evenly coated. Arrange squash cut side down in single layer on prepared sheet. Roast until bottoms of most pieces are deep golden brown, 15 to 20 minutes.

3 Remove sheet from oven. Gently flip squash and switch outer pieces with inner pieces on sheet. Continue to roast until squash is tender and most pieces are deep golden brown on second side, 15 to 20 minutes.

4 Whisk vinegar, maple syrup, sage, and remaining 2 tablespoons oil together in small bowl. Transfer squash to serving platter and drizzle with vinaigrette. Serve.

VARIATION
Roasted Kabocha Squash with Honey and Five-Spice Powder
Omit pepper. Substitute 2 teaspoons five-spice powder for paprika and coriander, honey for maple syrup, white wine vinegar for cider vinegar, and minced chives for sage.

PER SERVING
Dietary Fiber 5g **Cal** 200;
Total Fat 14g, **Sat Fat** 1g;
Chol 0mg; **Sodium** 290mg;
Total Carb 32g, **Total Sugars** 15g,
Added Sugars 3g; **Protein** 4g

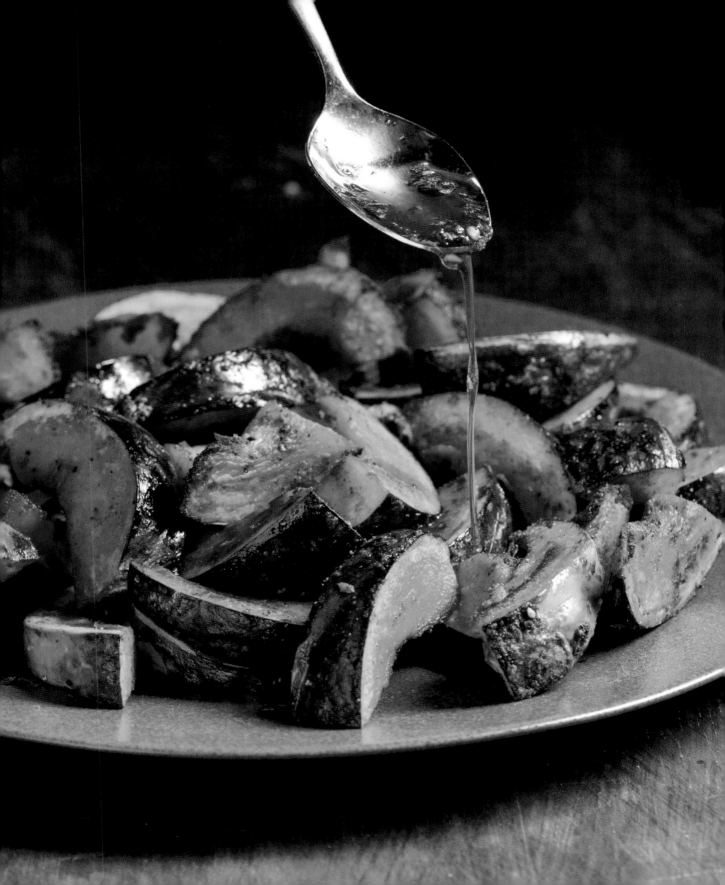

BAKED WILD RICE

SERVES 6

WHY THIS RECIPE WORKS Wild rice isn't actually rice, but a grass with more fiber than regular rice. Beyond its fiber boost, we love its nuttiness in a savory side dish, but its chewy outer husk means it can take nearly an hour to become tender on the stovetop. We turn to the oven to make wild rice a hands-off affair. We spread the rice in a baking dish, pour boiling water over top, and bake until it's tender. After a little more than an hour, you have evenly cooked, tender grains with great chew that are good for all guts and perfect with fish, chicken, turkey, beef, or pork. The recipe can be doubled easily using a 13 by 9-inch baking dish. Be sure to cover the pot when bringing the water to a boil in step 2; any water loss due to evaporation will affect how the rice cooks. Do not use quick-cooking or presteamed wild rice in this recipe; you may need to read the ingredient list on the package carefully to determine if the wild rice is presteamed.

1½ cups wild rice, rinsed

3 cups water

2 teaspoons extra-virgin olive oil

¾ teaspoon table salt

1 Adjust oven rack to middle position and heat oven to 375 degrees. Spread rice in 8-inch square baking dish.

2 Bring water, oil, and salt to boil in covered medium saucepan over high heat. Once boiling, stir to combine, then immediately pour over rice. Cover dish tightly with double layer of aluminum foil and bake until liquid is absorbed and rice is tender, 1 hour 10 minutes to 1 hour 20 minutes.

3 Remove dish from oven, uncover, and fluff rice with fork. Re-cover dish with foil and let rice sit for 10 minutes before serving.

PER ¾-CUP SERVING

Dietary Fiber 3g **Cal** 210;
Total Fat 2.5g, **Sat Fat** 0g;
Chol 0mg; **Sodium** 290mg;
Total Carb 40g, **Total Sugars** 1g,
Added Sugars 0g; **Protein** 7g

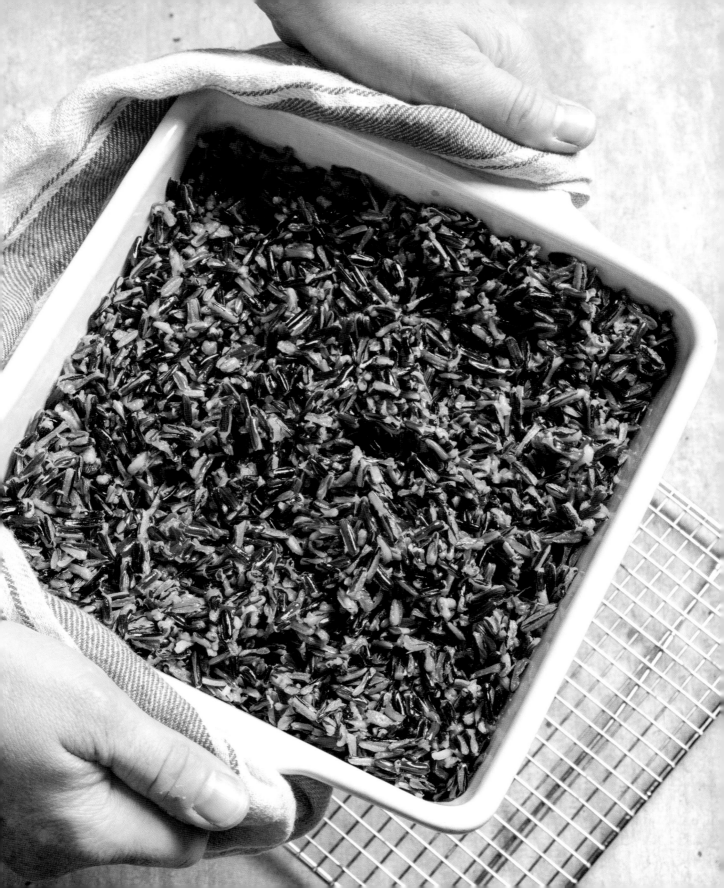

TOMATO RICE WITH LENTILS

SERVES 6

WHY THIS RECIPE WORKS Cooking rice with tomatoes, as in the Mexican dish arroz rojo, makes a flavorful, rich side dish from low-FODMAP white rice. But while white rice is friendly to the gut, it doesn't contain much fiber, so we stir canned lentils into the rice after cooking. To keep the tender grains of rice distinct, we rinse the rice first to remove excess starch and then pan-fry it in garlic oil before adding the liquid to create a satisfying texture and mild toasted flavor. For the rice cooking liquid, we puree fresh tomatoes and combine with vegetable broth for a savory backbone. Cilantro, jalapeño, and lime juice complement the richer tones of the cooked tomatoes and the allium flavor from the garlic oil. Use an ovensafe pot about 12 inches in diameter so that the rice cooks evenly and in the time indicated. We've successfully used both a straight-sided sauté pan and a Dutch oven. Whichever type of pot you use, it should have a tight-fitting, ovensafe lid. The dish is hearty on its own but also an exciting side for meat dishes like Grilled Chicken Fajitas (page 126).

2 ripe tomatoes, cored and quartered

3 tablespoons garlic oil (see page 20)

1 cup long-grain brown rice

2 jalapeño chiles, stemmed, seeded, and minced (optional), divided

1¼ cups chicken or vegetable broth (see page 18), plus extra as needed

2 teaspoons tomato paste

⅛ teaspoon table salt

1 (15-ounce) can lentils, rinsed

¼ cup minced fresh cilantro

Lime wedges

1 Adjust oven rack to middle position and heat oven to 350 degrees. Process tomatoes in food processor until smooth, about 15 seconds. Transfer to liquid measuring cup and spoon off excess to measure 1 cup (or, if necessary, add extra broth to equal 1 cup).

2 Heat oil in Dutch oven over medium-high heat for 1 to 2 minutes. Drop 3 or 4 grains rice in oil; if grains sizzle, oil is ready. Add rice and cook, stirring often, until rice is light golden and translucent, 2 to 4 minutes.

3 Reduce heat to medium. Stir in two-thirds of jalapeños, if using, and cook until fragrant, about 1½ minutes. Stir in tomatoes, broth, tomato paste, and salt. Increase heat to medium-high and bring to boil.

4 Cover pot, transfer to oven, and cook until liquid is absorbed and rice is tender, 45 minutes to 1 hour, stirring after 30 minutes.

5 Remove pot from oven. Fold in lentils and let sit, covered, until heated through, about 5 minutes. Stir in cilantro and remaining jalapeño, if using. Serve with lime wedges.

PER ¾-CUP SERVING

Dietary Fiber 4g **Cal** 220;
Total Fat 7g, **Sat Fat** 0.5g;
Chol 0mg; **Sodium** 230mg;
Total Carb 33g, **Total Sugars** 2g,
Added Sugars 0g; **Protein** 6g

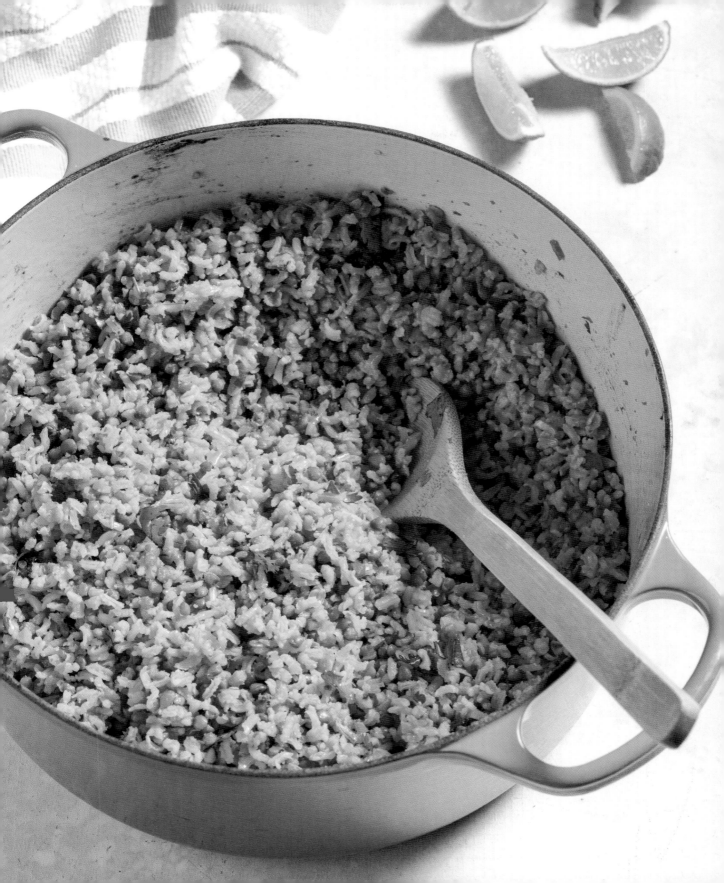

CREAMY PARMESAN POLENTA

SERVES 6

WHY THIS RECIPE WORKS With deep corn flavor and a creamy, porridge-like texture, a warm bowl of polenta is a classic pairing for stews, ragus, or vegetable toppings (which you can even make from the sides in this chapter). It is also a comfort food that will make your gut feel good. But we didn't want to work too hard for our comforts, and polenta has a reputation for requiring almost constant stirring to avoid forming intractable lumps. Instead, we found a way to achieve smooth polenta without exercise. Coarse-ground cornmeal gave us a soft but hearty texture and nutty flavor. Adding a pinch of baking soda to the pot helped soften the cornmeal's endosperm, which cut down on the cooking time. The baking soda also encouraged the granules to break down and release their starch, creating a silky consistency with minimal stirring. Naturally low-lactose Parmesan cheese, plus a tablespoon of olive oil, stirred in at the last minute gave the polenta a satisfying, rich flavor. If the polenta bubbles or sputters even slightly after the first 10 minutes, the heat is too high and you may need to move the saucepan to a smaller burner.

5 cups water

½ teaspoon table salt

Pinch baking soda

1 cup coarse-ground cornmeal

1 ounce Parmesan cheese, grated (½ cup), plus extra for serving

1 tablespoon extra-virgin olive oil

2 tablespoons minced fresh chives

1 Bring water to boil in large saucepan over medium-high heat. Stir in salt and baking soda. Slowly pour cornmeal into water in steady stream while stirring back and forth with wooden spoon or silicone spatula. Bring mixture to boil, stirring constantly, about 1 minute. Reduce heat to lowest setting and cover.

2 After 5 minutes, whisk polenta to smooth out any lumps that may have formed and scrape down sides and bottom of pot. Cover and continue to cook, without stirring, until polenta grains are tender but slightly al dente, about 25 minutes. (Polenta should be loose and barely hold its shape; it will continue to thicken as it cools.)

3 Remove from heat, stir in Parmesan and oil, and season with pepper to taste. Let sit, covered, for 5 minutes. Serve, sprinkling individual portions with chives and passing extra Parmesan separately.

PER ¾-CUP SERVING

Dietary Fiber 3g **Cal** 110;
Total Fat 4.5g, **Sat Fat** 1g;
Chol 5mg; **Sodium** 300mg;
Total Carb 15g, **Total Sugars** 0g,
Added Sugars 0g; **Protein** 3g

 MAKE IT DAIRY FREE Omit Parmesan cheese. Season to taste with nutritional yeast, if desired.

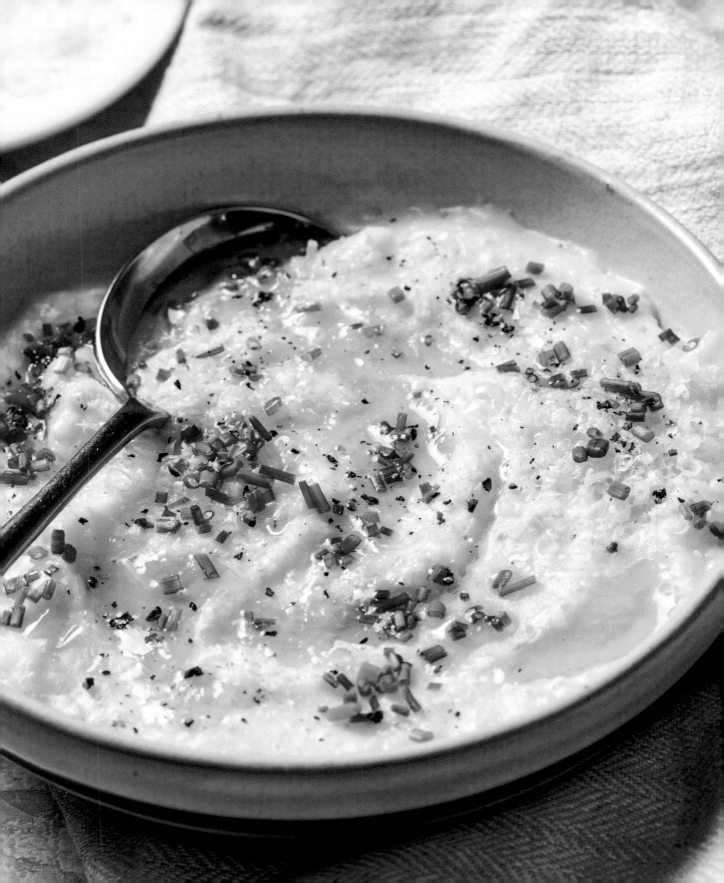

BAKED QUINOA WITH LEMON AND PARSLEY

SERVES 6

WHY THIS RECIPE WORKS Quinoa, the ancient seed that you may know is packed with protein and gluten-free, is also low in FODMAPs, so we think it deserves to be a staple for anyone. There are many ways to prepare quinoa, but this hands-off method delivers perfectly cooked "grains" every time. For the cooking liquid, we turn to chicken broth (vegetable broth works well, too), which we microwave with lemon zest, so the dish has citrus flavor throughout. We pour the hot liquid over the quinoa in a baking dish, cover it with foil, and bake. Lemon juice and parsley stirred in before serving lend bright notes to this pilaf to go alongside a delicate protein like Pan-Roasted Cod (page 202), or with a hearty side like Sautéed Radishes with Curry Powder and Almonds (page 264). We like the convenience of prewashed quinoa. If you buy unwashed quinoa (or if you are unsure whether it's washed), rinse it before cooking to remove its bitter protective coating (called saponin).

1½ cups prewashed white quinoa

2 tablespoons extra-virgin olive oil

1½ cups chicken or vegetable broth (see page 18)

1 teaspoon grated lemon zest plus 1 teaspoon juice

¼ teaspoon table salt

2 tablespoons minced fresh parsley

1 Adjust oven rack to middle position and heat oven to 450 degrees. Combine quinoa and oil in 8-inch square baking dish.

2 Bring broth, lemon zest, and salt to boil in covered medium saucepan over high heat. Pour hot broth over quinoa mixture and cover dish tightly with double layer of aluminum foil. Bake quinoa until tender and no liquid remains, about 25 minutes.

3 Remove dish from oven, uncover, and fluff quinoa with fork, scraping up any quinoa that has stuck to bottom. Re-cover dish with foil and let sit for 10 minutes. Fold in lemon juice and parsley, and season with salt and pepper to taste. Serve.

VARIATION

Baked Quinoa with Tomatoes, Parmesan, and Basil
Omit lemon zest, lemon juice, and parsley. Fold 1 finely chopped tomato, ½ cup grated Parmesan, and 2 tablespoons chopped fresh basil into quinoa before serving.

PER ½-CUP SERVING
Dietary Fiber 3g **Cal** 200;
Total Fat 7g, **Sat Fat** 1g;
Chol 0mg; **Sodium** 230mg;
Total Carb 28g, **Total Sugars** 1g,
Added Sugars 0g; **Protein** 7g

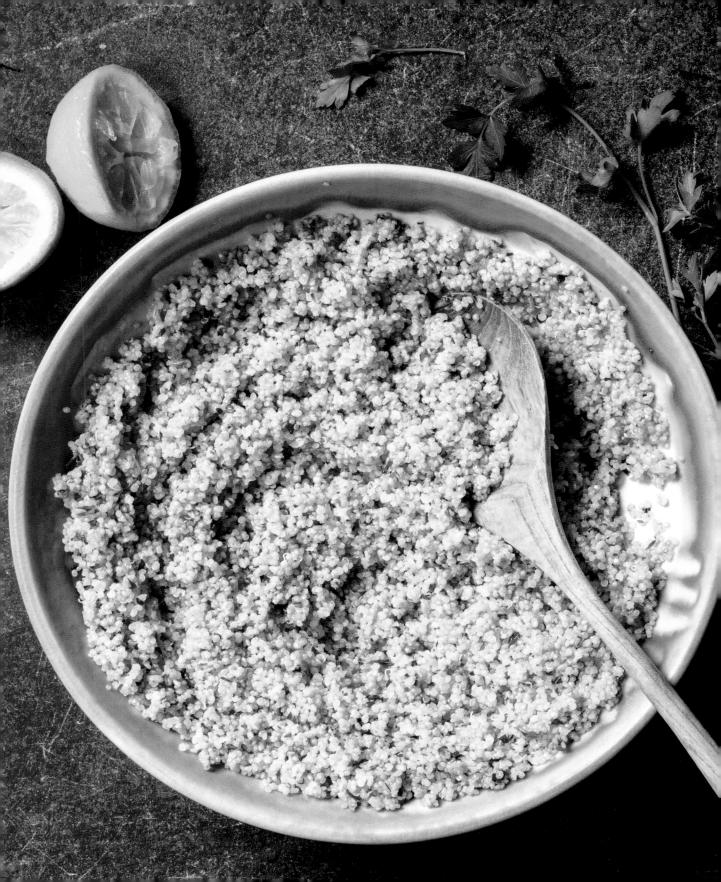

CURRIED MILLET PILAF WITH ALMONDS AND RAISINS

SERVES 6

WHY THIS RECIPE WORKS Millet, a tiny cereal grass seed that has a mellow corn flavor and is gluten-free and low-FODMAP at a reasonable serving size, packs a whopping amount of good-for-you fiber: This dish clocks in at 10 grams per serving. It can be flavored with interest just like any other rice or grain dish. For our pilaf, first things in the pan are some garlic oil and curry powder; cooking the spice before incorporating the millet blooms its flavor. Then we toast rinsed and dried millet in the oil for a spell before simmering to give the seeds nutty depth. After some testing, we landed on a 2:1 ratio of liquid to millet, which ensured evenly cooked, fluffy seeds. Plentiful fresh herbs, sweet raisins, and crunchy sliced almonds are lively stir-ins. We dollop the pilaf with yogurt for richness and an appealing cooling counterpoint to the warmth of the curry. We have found that, unlike other grains, millet can become gluey if allowed to steam off the heat. Once all the liquid has been absorbed, use a gentle hand to stir in the herbs, raisins, almonds, and scallion greens and serve immediately, alone or next to dishes like Grilled Beef Kebabs (page 166).

1 tablespoon garlic oil (see page 20)

1 teaspoon curry powder

1½ cups millet, rinsed and dried on dish towel

3 cups water

¾ teaspoon table salt

½ cup chopped fresh mint

¼ cup raisins

¼ cup sliced almonds, toasted

3 scallions, green parts only, sliced thin

¼ cup plain yogurt

1 Cook oil and curry powder in large saucepan over medium heat until fragrant, about 1 minute. Add millet and cook, stirring often, until lightly browned, about 2 minutes. Stir in water and salt and bring to boil. Reduce heat to low, cover, and simmer until liquid is absorbed, 15 to 20 minutes.

2 Off heat, fluff millet with fork and gently stir in basil, raisins, almonds, and scallion greens. Season with salt and pepper to taste. Serve, dolloping individual portions with yogurt.

PER ⅔-CUP SERVING

Dietary Fiber 10g **Cal** 280;
Total Fat 7g, **Sat Fat** 1g;
Chol 5mg; **Sodium** 310mg;
Total Carb 48g, **Total Sugars** 6g,
Added Sugars 0g; **Protein** 9g

 MAKE IT DAIRY FREE Omit yogurt or substitute dairy-free yogurt (see page 19).

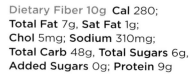

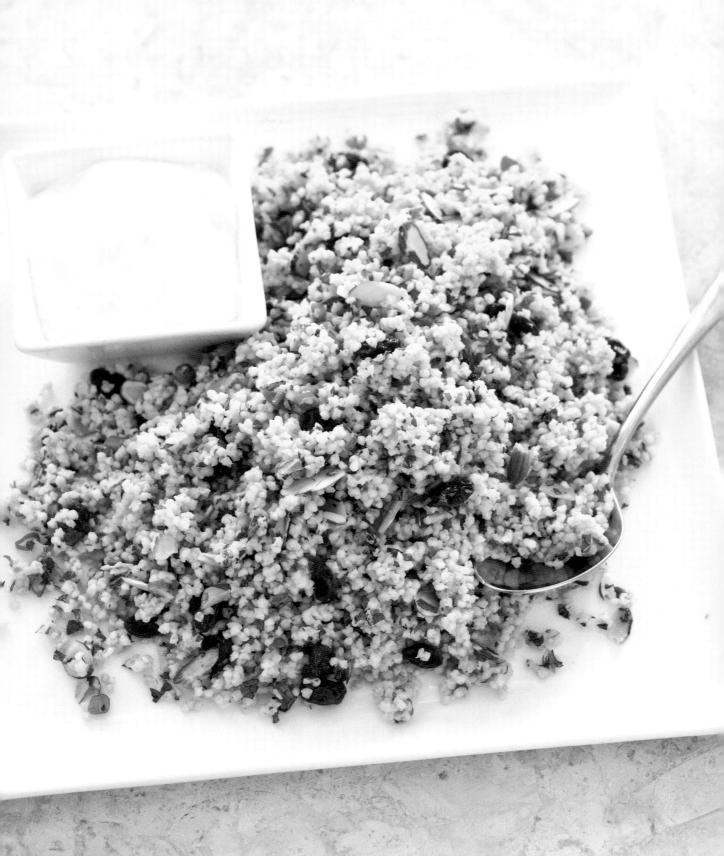

OAT BERRY, CHICKPEA, AND ARUGULA SALAD

SERVES 6

WHY THIS RECIPE WORKS Every grain has unique qualities that make it an interesting side served plain, enhanced with just some acid and herbs, or made into a pilaf. Here, an ingredient-packed cold salad is a great way to highlight the versatility of grains and stretch their use. Nutty oat berries are a suitably substantial grain salad base. To ensure that the oat berries retain their chewy, tender texture when cooled, we cook them in a large amount of water, pasta style, and then drain and rinse them under cold water to stop the cooking so that the grains don't end up mushy. For the leafy component of our salad, assertive, peppery arugula pairs well with the oat berries, and we add chickpeas for a little more heft and complementary buttery flavor and creamy texture. Roasted red peppers contribute a lively sweetness and feta lends creaminess and salty bite. A simple lemon and cilantro dressing spiked with cumin, paprika, and cayenne infuse the oat berries with brightness and spice.

¾ cup oat berries (groats) (see page 18), rinsed

¼ teaspoon table salt, plus salt for cooking oat berries

3 tablespoons extra-virgin olive oil

2 tablespoons lemon juice

2 tablespoons minced fresh cilantro

1 teaspoon honey

¼ teaspoon ground cumin

⅛ teaspoon paprika

Pinch cayenne pepper (optional)

1 (15-ounce) can chickpeas, rinsed

6 ounces (6 cups) baby arugula

½ cup jarred roasted red peppers, drained, patted dry, and chopped

2 ounces feta cheese, crumbled (½ cup)

1 Bring 2 quarts water to boil in large saucepan. Add oat berries and 1½ teaspoons salt, partially cover, and cook, stirring often, until tender but still chewy, 45 to 50 minutes. Drain oat berries, spread over large plate, and let cool completely, about 15 minutes; transfer to large bowl.

2 Whisk oil, lemon juice, cilantro, honey, cumin, paprika, cayenne, if using, and ¼ teaspoon salt together in small bowl, then drizzle over oat berries. Stir in chickpeas, arugula, roasted red peppers, and feta. Season with salt and pepper to taste, and serve.

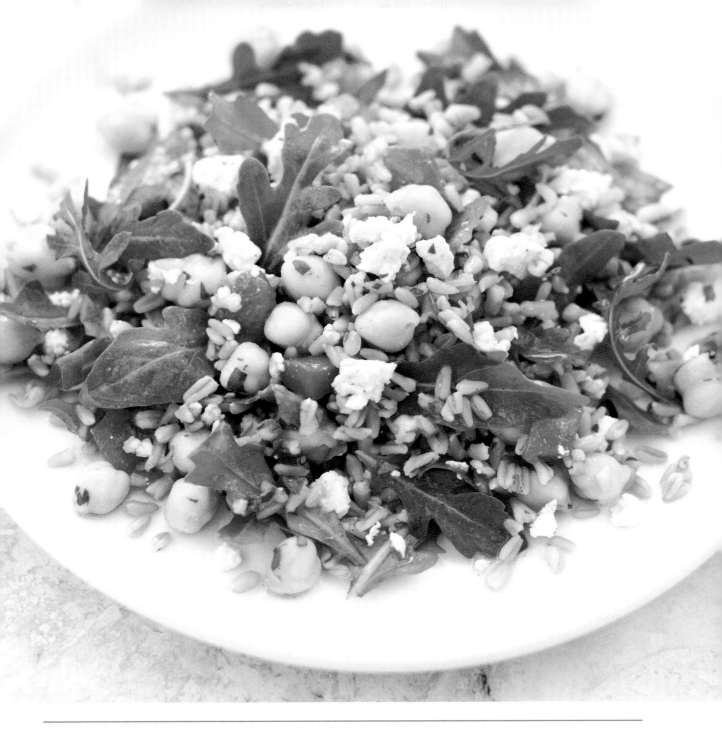

PER 1¼-CUP SERVING

Dietary Fiber 5g **Cal** 260;
Total Fat 12g, **Sat Fat** 3g;
Chol 10mg; **Sodium** 380mg;
Total Carb 30g, **Total Sugars** 4g,
Added Sugars 1g; **Protein** 9g

DF **MAKE IT DAIRY FREE** Omit feta cheese.

SKILLET CANNELLINI BEANS

SERVES 6

WHY THIS RECIPE WORKS Beans like creamy cannellini help you reach your fiber goals fast with their high amount per serving—and they can be on the table fast, too, when you start with a can. There's no need to soak or simmer; canned cannellini beans are perfectly tender and need just to be heated and flavored. To easily transform our beans, we simmer them in broth, which imparts a savory backbone to the dish without overpowering it and then reduces to a bean-coating glaze. Garlic oil, parsley, and lemon juice are final touches that round out the flavors of this satisfying dish.

- 2 (15-ounce) cans cannellini beans, rinsed
- 1 cup chicken or vegetable broth
- 2 tablespoons garlic oil (see page 20)
- 2 tablespoons minced fresh parsley
- 2 teaspoons lemon juice

Bring beans and broth to simmer in 12-inch nonstick skillet over medium-high heat. Reduce heat to low, cover, and cook until beans are heated through, about 5 minutes. Uncover, increase heat to medium-high, and simmer until liquid has reduced to light glaze, about 3 minutes. Off heat, stir in oil, parsley, and lemon juice. Season with salt and pepper to taste. Serve.

PER ½-CUP SERVING

Dietary Fiber 4g **Cal** 130;
Total Fat 7g, **Sat Fat** 1g;
Chol 0mg; **Sodium** 350mg;
Total Carb 13g, **Total Sugars** 0g,
Added Sugars 0g; **Protein** 5g

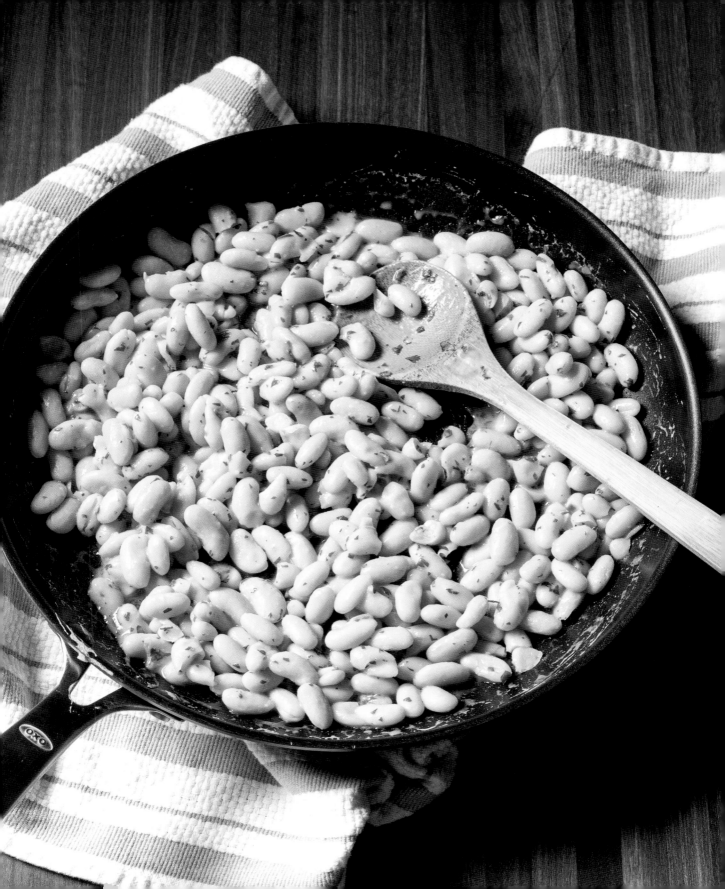

LENTIL SALAD WITH POMEGRANATE AND WALNUTS

SERVES 6

WHY THIS RECIPE WORKS If you're used to dried lentils, we want you to get to know the canned variety. High-fiber lentils are easy to transform into something special—they're a great stir-in but also make a standout salad or side dish on their own. And, through the canning process, lentils are the only legume that lose their oligosaccharides, so you don't need to bid every bean goodbye on a low-FODMAP diet. This impressive side pairs the firm-on-the-outside, creamy-on-the-inside canned legume with a tart vinaigrette, pomegranate seeds for juicy pops of sweetness, and some crunchy walnuts. Sliced radishes and liberal chopped parsley bring welcome freshness to a complexly flavored, beautifully textured, good-for-you salad that's not much more difficult than opening a can.

3 tablespoons extra-virgin olive oil

1½ tablespoons lemon juice

¼ teaspoon table salt

¼ teaspoon pepper

2 (15-ounce) cans lentils, rinsed

¼ cup chopped fresh parsley

6 radishes, trimmed, halved, and sliced thin

¼ cup walnuts, toasted and chopped coarse, divided

½ cup pomegranate seeds, divided

Whisk oil, lemon juice, salt, and pepper together in large bowl. Add lentils, parsley, radishes, half of walnuts, and half of pomegranate seeds to dressing and toss to combine. Season with salt and pepper to taste. Transfer to serving dish and sprinkle with remaining walnuts and pomegranate seeds. Serve.

VARIATION

Lentil Salad with Spiced Carrots and Cilantro
Combine 3 carrots, peeled and cut into 2-inch-long matchsticks, 1 teaspoon cumin, ½ teaspoon cinnamon, and ⅛ teaspoon cayenne pepper (optional) in bowl. Cover and microwave until carrots are crisp-tender, 2 to 4 minutes. Substitute cilantro for parsley and carrot mixture for radishes, walnuts, and pomegranate seeds.

PER ⅔-CUP SERVING
Dietary Fiber 9g **Cal** 210g;
Total Fat 10g, **Sat Fat** 1.5g;
Chol 0mg; **Sodium** 290mg;
Total Carb 23g, **Total Sugars** 4g,
Added Sugars 0g; **Protein** 9g

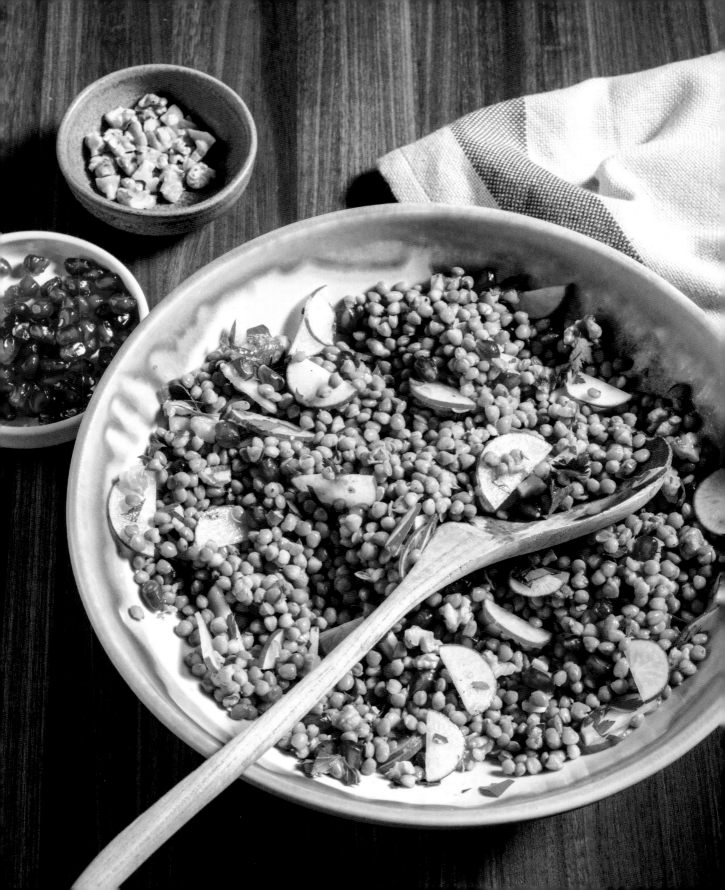

SPICED CRANBERRY BEANS

SERVES 8

WHY THIS RECIPE WORKS Pretty-pink and nutrient-dense cranberry beans have a more delicate flavor than pinto beans and are as creamy as cannellini beans; we wanted to highlight these special beans in a spiced side dish. Eating more fiber can mean eating more beans for many, so it's nice to embrace canned beans. But it's also nice to take the time and care to perfect cooking dried beans. To help our cranberry beans cook up creamy and tender, we soak them overnight in salt water before thoroughly rinsing them to remove any excess salt. We sauté carrots in aromatic garlic oil, along with tomato paste for depth of flavor; just a touch of cinnamon imparts a subtle sweet, warm spice. In addition to broth, we cook the beans in white wine for acidity, and letting them cook through in the gentle heat of the oven ensures that they are perfectly cooked without constant monitoring. We complete our dish with lemon juice and mint, which nicely balance the warm, rich flavors of the beans. If cranberry beans are not available, you can substitute pinto beans.

3 tablespoons table salt for brining

1 pound (2½ cups) dried cranberry beans, picked over and rinsed

¼ cup garlic oil (see page 20)

2 carrots, peeled and chopped fine

1 tablespoon tomato paste

½ teaspoon ground cinnamon

¼ teaspoon pepper

½ cup dry white wine

4 cups chicken or vegetable broth (see page 18)

2 tablespoons lemon juice, plus extra for seasoning

2 tablespoons minced fresh mint

1 Dissolve salt in 4 quarts cold water in large container. Add beans and soak at room temperature for at least 8 hours or up to 24 hours. Drain and rinse well.

2 Adjust oven rack to lower-middle position and heat oven to 350 degrees. Heat oil in Dutch oven over medium heat until shimmering. Add carrots and cook until softened, about 5 minutes. Stir in tomato paste, cinnamon, and pepper and cook until fragrant, about 1 minute. Stir in wine, scraping up any browned bits. Stir in broth, ½ cup water, and beans and bring to boil. Cover, transfer pot to oven, and cook until beans are tender, about 1½ hours, stirring every 30 minutes.

3 Stir in lemon juice and mint. Season with salt, pepper, and extra lemon juice to taste. Adjust consistency with extra hot water as needed. Serve.

PER ¾-CUP SERVING
Dietary Fiber 15g **Cal** 280;
Total Fat 8g, **Sat Fat** 1g;
Chol 0mg; **Sodium** 390mg;
Total Carb 38g, **Total Sugars** 2g,
Added Sugars 0g; **Protein** 14g

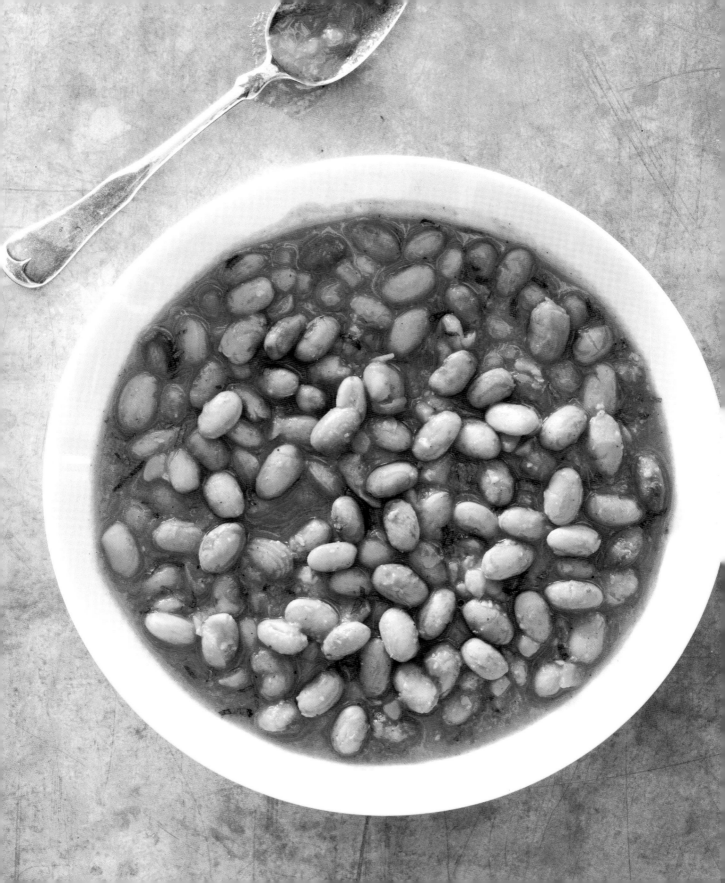

REFRIED BEANS

SERVES 6

WHY THIS RECIPE WORKS With their rich flavor and creamy texture, these refried beans resemble those made with pinto beans in northern parts of Mexico and might just be the most satisfying high-fiber side dish there is. Dried beans are typically cooked in lard and mashed. Canned pinto beans worked fine for us and kept our cooking time short. Instead of using lard, we reached for salt pork, which we sautéed to render its fat to use to cook chiles (two types for complexity) and deepen the flavor of the beans. Usually the beans are hand mashed, but processing a portion in the food processor with broth before frying created the creamy texture we were after, and pulsing the remaining beans ensured some chunky bites. Make sure you rinse the beans thoroughly before cooking to get rid of excess salt. For a less spicy dish, reduce the chiles.

2 (15-ounce) cans pinto beans, rinsed, divided

½ cup chicken broth (see page 18), plus extra as needed

1 tablespoon garlic oil (see page 20)

3 ounces salt pork, rind removed, chopped fine

1 poblano chile, stemmed, seeded, and chopped fine

1 jalapeño chile, stemmed, seeded, and minced

½ teaspoon ground cumin

1 tablespoon minced fresh cilantro

2 teaspoons lime juice

1 Process all but 1 cup beans with broth in food processor until smooth, about 30 seconds, scraping down sides of bowl as needed. Add remaining beans and pulse until coarsely ground, about 5 pulses.

2 Heat oil in 12-inch nonstick skillet over medium heat until shimmering. Add salt pork and cook, stirring occasionally, until rendered and well browned, 10 to 15 minutes; discard pork, leaving fat behind in skillet.

3 Add poblano and jalapeño to fat left in skillet and cook over medium heat until vegetables are softened and beginning to brown, about 8 minutes. Stir in cumin and cook until fragrant, about 30 seconds. Stir in processed beans and cook, stirring often, until well combined and thickened slightly, about 5 minutes. Off heat, stir in cilantro and lime juice and season with salt and pepper to taste. Adjust consistency with extra hot broth as needed. Serve.

PER ½-CUP SERVING
Dietary Fiber 6g **Cal** 160;
Total Fat 6g, **Sat Fat** 0.5g;
Chol 0mg; **Sodium** 370mg;
Total Carb 21g, **Total Sugars** 1g,
Added Sugars 0g; **Protein** 7g

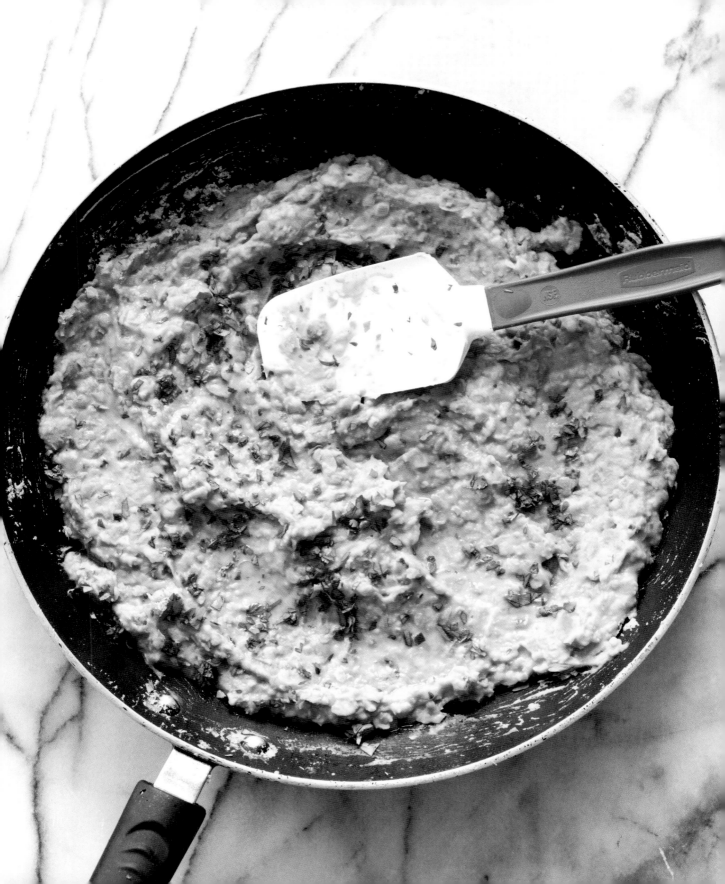

CHICKPEA SALAD WITH ORANGE AND CELERY

SERVES 6

WHY THIS RECIPE WORKS Chickpeas are a popular salad bean for good reason: They have a firm texture and nutty flavor, and they add fiber and protein to any meal. Canned chickpeas work perfectly in salads, and we pair them with juicy, crisp feel-good ingredients—oranges and sliced celery. With a garlic-sherry vinaigrette to bring everything together, our simple salad requires little more than a toss and yet has surprisingly complex flavor.

2 oranges

2 (15-ounce) cans chickpeas, rinsed

3 celery ribs, sliced thin on bias

¼ cup chopped fresh parsley

2 tablespoons garlic oil (see page 20)

2 teaspoons sherry vinegar

¼ teaspoon table salt

Cut away peel and pith from oranges. Quarter oranges, then slice crosswise into ½-inch-thick pieces. Combine oranges, chickpeas, celery, parsley, oil, vinegar, and salt in bowl and let sit for 20 minutes. Season with salt and pepper to taste. Serve.

VARIATION

Chickpea Salad with Cucumber and Olives
Omit oranges. Substitute ½ English cucumber, quartered lengthwise and sliced ½ inch thick, for celery, and mint for parsley. Add ¼ cup chopped pitted kalamata olives with beans.

PER ½-CUP SERVING

Dietary Fiber 6g **Cal** 150;
Total Fat 7g, **Sat Fat** 1g;
Chol 0mg; **Sodium** 380mg;
Total Carb 19g, **Total Sugars** 4g,
Added Sugars 0g; **Protein** 5g

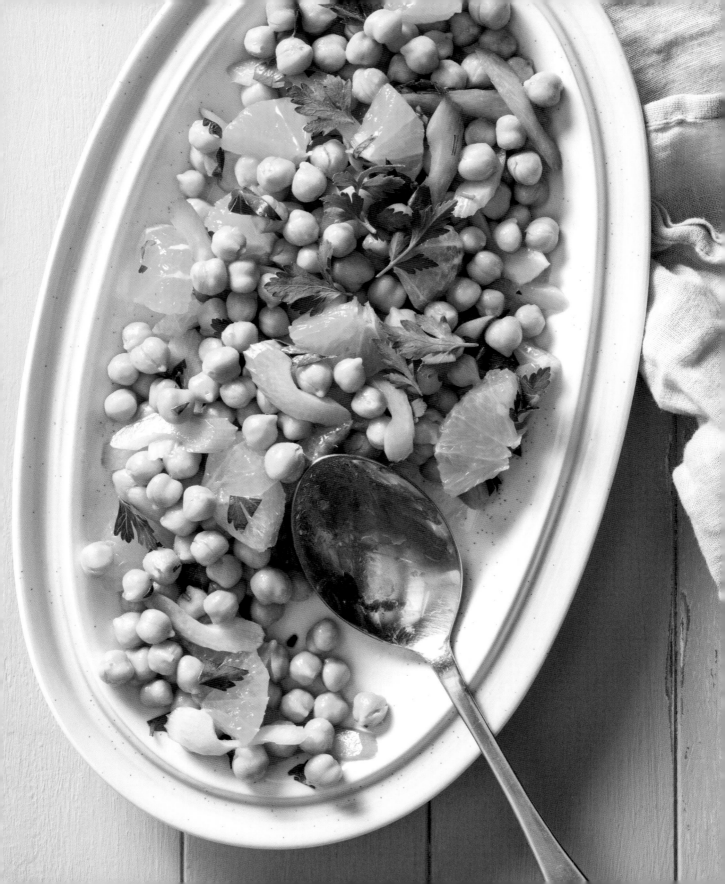

NUTRITIONAL INFORMATION FOR OUR RECIPES

To calculate the nutritional values of our recipes per serving, we used The Food Processor SQL by ESHA research. When using this program, we entered all the ingredients, using weights for important ingredients such as most vegetables. We also used our preferred brands in these analyses. Any ingredient listed as "optional" was excluded from the analyses. We did not include salt or pepper for food that's "seasoned to taste." If there is a range in the serving size, we used the highest number of servings to calculate the nutritional values.

	Calories	Total Fat (g)	Sat Fat (g)	Chol (mg)	Sodium (mg)	Total Carb (g)	Dietary Fiber (g)	Total Sugars (g)	Added Sugar (g)	Protein (g)
Gut-Friendly Meal Builders										
Garlic Oil	120	14	1	0	0	0	0	0	0	0
Make-Ahead Vinaigrette	100	11	1.5	0	100	1	0	1	1	0
Basil Pesto	70	7	1	0	30	0	0	0	0	1
Chimichurri	70	7	1	0	75	0	0	0	0	0
Chermoula	70	7	1	0	35	0	0	0	0	0
Fresh Tomato Salsa	20	1.5	0	0	0	2	1	1	0	0
Orange-Basil Relish	70	2.5	0	0	0	12	2	9	0	1
Herbed Yogurt Sauce	15	0	0	0	5	1	0	0	0	1
Tzatziki	20	1.5	1	0	40	0	0	0	0	1
Peanut Dipping Sauce	40	3	0.5	0	150	1	0	1	0	2
Fresh Tomato Salsa	70	5	1	0	220	4	1	3	0	1
Chicken Broth	20	0	0	0	276	0	0	0	0	4
Beef Broth	53	0	0	0	248	0	0	0	0	13
Vegetable Broth	9	0	0	0	288	0	0	0	0	1
Cucumber-Lemon Water	0	0	0	0	0	0	0	0	0	0
Cantaloupe-Mint Iced Green Tea	25	0	0	0	15	7	0	6	6	0
Raspberry-Basil Iced Black Tea	30	0	0	0	5	7	0	6	6	0
Switchel	60	0	0	0	75	14	0	12	12	0
Sourdough Bread	30	0	0	0	65	6	0	0	0	1
Gluten-Free Whole-Grain Sandwich Bread	180	5	1	40	290	28	6	3	3	6
Sauerkraut	15	0	0	0	200	3	1	2	0	1
Kimchi	30	0	0	0	190	1	3	2	2	1

	Calories	Total Fat (g)	Sat Fat (g)	Chol (mg)	Sodium (mg)	Total Carb (g)	Dietary Fiber (g)	Total Sugars (g)	Added Sugar (g)	Protein (g)
Gut-Friendly Meal Builders *(cont.)*										
Homemade Yogurt	40	2	1	5	50	3	3	0	0	2
Homemade Greek-Style Almond Milk Yogurt	40	2	1	5	50	3	3	0	0	2
Homemade Almond Milk Yogurt	10	0.5	0	0	45	0	0	0	0	0
Homemade Greek-Style Almond Milk Yogurt	10	0.5	0	0	45	0	0	0	0	0
Breakfast										
Avocado and Bean Toast	340	14	2	0	600	48	13	6	0	11
Eggs with Swiss Chard Hash and Sweet Potato Hash	440	24	5	370	670	39	6	6	0	18
Chickpea Shakshuka	350	18	6	380	720	23	7	9	0	22
Ratatouille with Poached Eggs	280	18	4	190	650	18	7	11	0	14
Pea and Feta Frittata	420	25	8	575	730	19	6	9	0	28
Kale and Black Bean Breakfast Burritos	320	15	4	250	750	31	8	2	0	16
Mushroom and Artichoke Hash with Parmesan Croutons	440	29	7	10	650	33	7	6	0	13
Steel-Cut Oatmeal with Blueberries and Almonds	230	5	0.5	0	150	39	6	6	3	7
Steel-Cut Oatmeal with Raspberries, Orange, and Pecans	220	6	0.5	0	150	37	6	5	3	6
Maple-Vanilla Granola	380	26	11	0	120	35	6	14	6	7
Chia Pudding with Fresh Fruit and Coconut	260	14	6	10	200	27	10	14	6	8
Hazelnut and Coconut Muesli	300	13	5	10	40	43	6	16	0	8
Yogurt Parfaits	390	26	4.5	15	60	30	10	16	0	14
Whole-Wheat Pancakes with Raspberry-Chia Compote	470	19	2.5	80	670	63	9	15	8	15
Blueberry Oat Pancakes	350	13	2	65	390	49	6	14	6	13
Pumpkin Spice Waffles	580	24	4	105	630	74	10	21	12	19
Power Smoothies	270	12	1.5	0	160	40	7	16	0	6
Berry Smoothies	250	9	3	15	210	38	8	21	0	9

	Calories	Total Fat (g)	Sat Fat (g)	Chol (mg)	Sodium (mg)	Total Carb (g)	Dietary Fiber (g)	Total Sugars (g)	Added Sugar (g)	Protein (g)
Soups & Stews										
Chicken and Vegetable Soup	220	6	1	65	860	18	6	7	0	25
Smoky Chicken and Lentil Soup with Swiss Chard	360	15	2	65	810	27	8	5	0	30
Beef and Oat Berry Soup	520	25	5	75	750	37	7	4	0	35
Beef, Cabbage, and Tofu Soup with Gochugaru	400	22	3.5	40	710	24	6	5	0	29
Miso-Ginger Soup with Halibut and Zucchini Noodles	320	14	1.5	55	750	21	6	10	0	29
New England-Style Fish and Vegetable Chowder	400	13	4	75	720	42	7	6	0	32
Mushroom and Wheat Berry Soup	310	8	0.5	0	710	44	7	6	0	11
Chickpea and Escarole Soup with Fennel and Orange	280	7	0	0	520	45	15	10	0	14
Chicken Stew with Collard Greens and Black-Eyed Peas	340	16	4	120	680	19	7	4	0	32
Vegetable and Beef Stew	430	10	2.5	100	790	34	8	9	0	41
Fish Tagine	310	11	1	55	800	26	9	8	0	27
Okra Pepper Pot	200	9	4	0	750	27	9	7	0	6
Tuscan Bean Stew	290	6	1.5	10	700	43	22	4	0	17
Pumpkin Turkey Chili	290	8	2	30	700	30	11	6	0	27
White Chicken Chili	450	19	2.5	90	790	36	12	6	0	38
Poultry										
Poached Chicken Breasts with Warm Tomato-Ginger Vinaigrette	280	12	2	125	310	2	1	1	0	39
Parmesan Chicken with Bitter Greens and Fennel	560	27	4	220	490	29	7	9	0	51
Pan-Seared Chicken Breasts with Artichoke, Tomato, and Bulgur Pilaf	610	25	6	145	700	48	9	4	0	50
One-Pot Chicken with Braised Spring Vegetables	430	15	2	125	680	27	7	6	0	46
Pan-Roasted Chicken Breasts with Vermouth Pan Sauce	380	24	9	110	530	2	0	2	0	29
Roasted Chicken Breasts with Kabocha Squash and Kale	510	28	6	90	560	29	6	12	0	38

	Calories	Total Fat (g)	Sat Fat (g)	Chol (mg)	Sodium (mg)	Total Carb (g)	Dietary Fiber (g)	Total Sugars (g)	Added Sugar (g)	Protein (g)
Poultry (cont.)										
Braised Chicken Breasts with Chickpeas, Fennel, and Chermoula	540	26	4	100	480	34	10	6	0	41
Grilled Yogurt Chicken and Warm Oat Berry Salad	570	26	3.5	130	770	35	7	9	0	48
Roasted Chicken Thighs with Root Vegetables	520	35	8	120	620	29	7	7	1	25
Chicken Mole with Cilantro-Lime Rice and Beans	520	15	2	105	700	72	9	7	0	32
Stir-Fried Ginger-Orange Chicken and Long Beans	340	18	2	85	790	15	6	7	0	31
Grilled Chicken Fajitas	690	24	5	125	810	66	11	12	1	49
Weeknight Skillet Roast Chicken	300	17	5	110	660	0	0	0	0	34
Roast Chicken with Ras el Hanout and Carrots	430	22	6	110	620	20	6	10	0	36
Super Cobb Salad	490	29	6	210	670	25	11	8	0	34
Chopped Salad with Chicken and Jícama	280	10	3.5	70	570	23	9	11	0	24
Black Rice and Chicken Salad with Snap Peas and Ginger-Sesame Vinaigrette	500	20	2.5	60	370	58	6	6	3	27
Pasta with Kale Pesto, Tomatoes, and Chicken	700	28	4.5	125	540	58	11	4	0	53
Chicken Enchiladas	380	21	5	90	570	29	6	4	0	24
Turkey Meatballs with Lemony Wild Rice and Artichokes	480	12	3	90	720	56	9	4	0	41
Turkey Burgers	590	28	14	115	720	30	7	4	0	51
Easy Roast Turkey Breast	260	10	3	100	230	0	0	0	0	39
Turkey Shepherd's Pie	370	14	4	90	730	29	8	11	0	35
Farfalle with Broccoli and Turkey Sausage	600	24	4	30	690	71	12	6	0	32
Beef & Pork										
Flank Steak with Parsnips and Baby Kale	470	23	7	80	780	38	10	10	0	28
Pan-Seared Sirloin Steak with Mushroom Pan Sauce	320	16	6	85	320	4	0	3	0	26
Steak Tips with Spiced Millet and Spinach	490	17	4.5	75	720	49	12	7	0	33

	Calories	Total Fat (g)	Sat Fat (g)	Chol (mg)	Sodium (mg)	Total Carb (g)	Dietary Fiber (g)	Total Sugars (g)	Added Sugar (g)	Protein (g)
Beef & Pork (cont.)										
Stir-Fried Beef with Gai Lan and Oyster Sauce	390	23	4.5	80	750	17	6	6	3	28
Steak Tacos with Napa Cabbage Slaw	470	19	4.5	75	410	52	3	12	4	30
Sirloin Steak with Wilted Escarole and Chickpea Salad	480	28	5	80	670	22	9	5	1	34
Grilled Beef Kebabs	410	25	4	55	670	17	6	7	2	30
Spaghetti and Meatballs	530	14	4	105	790	65	12	9	0	39
Meaty Lasagna	370	17	9	75	480	32	6	6	0	27
Meatloaf with Roasted Potatoes and Green Beans	460	19	4.5	100	750	40	6	6	0	34
Roasted Pork Chops and Vegetables with Parsley Vinaigrette	450	17	3.5	55	730	47	10	11	0	26
Grilled Pork Chops with Sweet Potato Salad	470	22	5	65	670	40	6	7	0	28
Chipotle-Braised Pork and Rice	390	12	3.5	75	720	39	7	5	0	30
Maple-Ginger Roasted Pork Tenderloin with Swiss Chard and Carrots	350	16	2	75	790	25	6	15	9	29
Caraway-Crusted Pork Tenderloin with Sauerkraut and Apples	380	11	2	105	820	34	7	24	7	35
Grilled Pork Tenderloin with Pineapple-Lentil Salad	350	14	2	70	430	28	8	14	1	30
Roasted Pork Loin with Butternut and Brussels	480	21	4	90	710	39	9	9	2	38
Seafood										
Oven-Roasted Salmon with Tangerine-Ginger Relish	330	20	4	60	360	12	2	9	0	24
Sesame Salmon with Snap Pea Slaw	540	34	6	65	570	22	9	8	0	39
Pomegranate-Roasted Salmon with Lentils and Swiss Chard	450	24	4.5	60	680	26	8	9	0	32
Salmon, Avocado, Orange and Watercress Salad	280	18	2.5	30	650	17	9	10	0	14
Salmon Tacos	480	28	5	60	490	31	8	1	0	27

	Calories	Total Fat (g)	Sat Fat (g)	Chol (mg)	Sodium (mg)	Total Carb (g)	Dietary Fiber (g)	Total Sugars (g)	Added Sugar (g)	Protein (g)
Seafood *(cont.)*										
Salmon Cakes with Sautéed Beet Greens and Lemon-Parsley Sauce	400	27	5	65	710	12	6	2	0	28
Pan-Roasted Cod	130	4.5	0	50	350	1	0	1	1	20
Sautéed Halibut with Succotash	480	17	4.5	70	580	51	10	6	0	35
Crispy Snapper with Charred Okra and Tomatoes	310	16	1.5	40	600	15	6	7	0	28
Roasted Halibut, Broccolini, and Potatoes with Mustard Sauce	450	22	3	55	610	35	6	8	4	28
Blackened Red Snapper with Sautéed Spinach and Black Rice	480	16	2.5	45	710	57	8	2	0	33
Roasted Trout with White Bean and Tomato Salad	470	25	4	65	680	27	8	5	0	33
Coconut-Ginger Swordfish Packets with Couscous, Snow Peas, and Bell Pepper	530	18	7	75	630	57	10	8	0	34
Grilled Tuna Steaks with Cucumber-Mint Farro Salad	620	25	4	45	790	63	8	9	3	39
Seared Shrimp with Fresh Tomato Sauce and Cilantro-Lime Quinoa	560	27	3.5	145	770	55	13	5	0	27
Linguini with Shrimp, Peas, and Preserved Lemon	480	16	4.5	120	670	61	12	4	0	25
Shrimp with White Beans and Arugula	370	19	3	145	690	26	7	4	0	21
Seared Scallops with Barley and Beet Risotto	520	10	1	30	760	73	14	6	0	24
Vegetable Mains										
Rainbow Salad with Crispy Tempeh	390	24	3	0	480	34	10	15	0	13
Fattoush with Escarole	360	26	3.5	0	710	30	8	5	0	6
Quinoa Taco Salad	350	21	3	5	710	34	10	3	0	9
Freekeh Salad with Sweet Potato, Walnuts, and Raisins	570	26	3	0	520	72	14	10	0	13
Green Rice and Vegetable Bowls with Fried Eggs	540	29	4.5	185	700	61	8	3	0	16

	Calories	Total Fat (g)	Sat Fat (g)	Chol (mg)	Sodium (mg)	Total Carb (g)	Dietary Fiber (g)	Total Sugars (g)	Added Sugar (g)	Protein (g)
Vegetable Mains *(cont.)*										
Farro Bowls with Tofu, Mushrooms, and Spinach	530	31	3	5	420	48	7	5	0	18
Black Bean Chilaquiles Verdes	540	23	3	0	780	80	19	12	0	15
Roasted Cabbage Wedges with Tomatoes and Chickpeas	420	27	2	0	740	35	13	10	2	10
Stuffed Eggplant with Bulgur and Tomatoes	330	19	4.5	15	530	36	12	13	0	10
Whole Pot-Roasted Cauliflower with Tomatoes and Olives	290	17	3.5	5	800	28	7	17	0	10
Penne with Fresh Tomato Sauce, Spinach, and Feta	470	16	5	25	500	67	14	11	0	18
Peanut Noodle Bowls with Edamame and Cabbage	400	18	3	0	490	47	9	7	1	15
Soba Noodles with Roasted Eggplant and Sesame	700	27	3.5	0	620	105	14	33	17	14
Black Bean Burgers	430	23	2.5	0	460	48	13	6	0	12
Sweet Potato, Poblano, and Chickpea Tacos	500	18	2.5	0	730	75	15	10	0	13
Summer Rolls with Tofu and Peanut Dipping Sauce	360	16	3	0	750	40	6	10	1	17
Sides										
Pan-Steamed Kale	150	12	1.5	0	180	9	4	3	0	5
Pan-Steamed Kale with Pancetta and Pine Nuts	140	9	1.5	5	260	10	4	3	0	7
Sautéed Radishes with Curry Powder and Almonds	160	13	1.5	0	290	9	4	4	0	4
Sautéed Green Beans with Fresh Herbs	70	5	0.5	0	150	7	3	3	0	2
Sautéed Green Beans with Thyme, Coriander, and Sesame Seeds	90	6	1	0	150	8	3	3	0	2
Pan-Roasted Parsnips	120	4	0.5	0	160	22	6	6	0	1
Pan-Roasted Parsnips with Cilantro and Lime	120	4	0.5	0	160	22	6	6	0	2
Skillet-Roasted Broccoli	170	14	2	0	250	7	3	2	0	4
Skillet-Roasted Broccoli with Smoky Sunflower Seed Topping	190	17	2.5	0	320	8	4	2	0	5

	Calories	Total Fat (g)	Sat Fat (g)	Chol (mg)	Sodium (mg)	Total Carb (g)	Dietary Fiber (g)	Total Sugars (g)	Added Sugar (g)	Protein (g)
Sides *(cont.)*										
Sautéed Cabbage	110	7	1	0	330	40	9	5	0	2
Sautéed Cabbage with Bacon and Caraway Seeds	130	8	2	10	480	10	3	2	0	5
Escarole and Orange Salad with Green Olives	200	16	2	0	260	14	5	7	0	3
Roasted Red Potatoes	180	7	1	0	180	27	3	2	0	3
Roasted Red Potatoes with Rosemary	180	7	1	0	180	27	3	2	0	3
Mashed Potatoes and Root Vegetables	290	12	4	15	300	44	6	6	0	5
Mashed Potatoes and Root Vegetables with Paprika and Parsley	290	12	4	15	300	44	6	6	0	5
Roasted Kabocha Squash with Maple and Sage	200	14	1	0	290	32	5	15	3	4
Roasted Kabocha Squash with Honey and Five-Spice	200	14	1	0	290	33	5	16	4	4
Baked Wild Rice	210	2.5	0	0	290	40	3	1	0	7
Tomato Rice with Lentils	210	2.5	0	0	290	40	3	1	0	7
Creamy Parmesan Polenta	110	4.5	1	5	300	15	3	0	0	3
Baked Quinoa with Lemon and Parsley	200	7	1	0	230	28	3	1	0	7
Baked Quinoa with Tomatoes, Parmesan, and Basil	250	10	2.5	5	390	28	3	2	0	11
Curried Millet with Almonds and Raisins	280	7	1	5	310	48	10	6	0	9
Oat Berry, Chickpea, and Arugula Salad	260	12	3	10	380	30	5	4	1	9
Skillet Cannellini Beans	130	4.5	0.5	0	350	13	4	0	0	5
Lentil Salad with Pomegranate and Walnuts	210	10	1.5	0	290	23	9	4	0	9
Lentil Salad with Spiced Carrots and Cilantro	190	8	1	0	310	23	9	4	0	9
Spiced Cranberry Beans	280	8	1	0	390	38	15	2	0	14
Refried Beans	160	6	0.5	0	370	21	6	1	0	7
Chickpea Salad with Orange and Celery	150	7	1	0	380	19	6	4	0	5
Chickpea Salad with Cucumber and Olives	130	7	0.5	0	380	13	5	0	0	5

CONVERSIONS AND EQUIVALENTS

Some say cooking is a science and an art. We would say that geography has a hand in it, too. Flours and sugars manufactured in the United Kingdom and elsewhere will feel and taste different from those manufactured in the United States. So we cannot promise that the loaf of bread you bake in Canada or England will taste the same as a loaf baked in the States, but we can offer guidelines for converting weights and measures. We also recommend that you rely on your instincts when making our recipes. Refer to the visual cues provided. If the dough hasn't "come together in a ball" as described, you may need to add more flour—even if the recipe doesn't tell you to. You be the judge.

The recipes in this book were developed using standard U.S. measures following U.S. government guidelines. The charts below offer equivalents for U.S. and metric measures. All conversions are approximate and have been rounded up or down to the nearest whole number.

EXAMPLE

1 teaspoon	=	4.9292 milliliters, rounded up to 5 milliliters
1 ounce	=	28.3495 grams, rounded down to 28 grams

VOLUME CONVERSIONS

U.S.	METRIC
1 teaspoon	5 milliliters
2 teaspoons	10 milliliters
1 tablespoon	15 milliliters
2 tablespoons	30 milliliters
¼ cup	59 milliliters
⅓ cup	79 milliliters
½ cup	118 milliliters
¾ cup	177 milliliters
1 cup	237 milliliters
1¼ cups	296 milliliters
1½ cups	355 milliliters
2 cups (1 pint)	473 milliliters
2½ cups	591 milliliters
3 cups	710 milliliters
4 cups (1 quart)	0.946 liter
1.06 quarts	1 liter
4 quarts (1 gallon)	3.8 liters

WEIGHT CONVERSIONS

OUNCES	GRAMS
½	14
¾	21
1	28
1½	43
2	57
2½	71
3	85
3½	99
4	113
4½	128
5	142
6	170
7	198
8	227
9	255
10	283
12	340
16 (1 pound)	454

CONVERSIONS FOR COMMON BAKING INGREDIENTS

Baking is an exacting science. Because measuring by weight is far more accurate than measuring by volume, and thus more likely to produce reliable results, in our recipes we provide ounce measures in addition to cup measures for many ingredients. Refer to the chart below to convert these measures into grams.

INGREDIENT	OUNCES	GRAMS
Flour		
1 cup all-purpose flour*	5	142
1 cup cake flour	4	113
1 cup whole-wheat flour	5½	156
Sugar		
1 cup granulated (white) sugar	7	198
1 cup packed brown sugar (light or dark)	7	198
1 cup confectioners' sugar	4	113
Cocoa Powder		
1 cup cocoa powder	3	85
Butter†		
4 tablespoons (½ stick or ¼ cup)	2	57
8 tablespoons (1 stick or ½ cup)	4	113
16 tablespoons (2 sticks or 1 cup)	8	227

* U.S. all-purpose flour, the most frequently used flour in this book, does not contain leaveners, as some European flours do. These leavened flours are called self-rising or self-raising. If you are using self-rising flour, take this into consideration before adding leaveners to a recipe.

† In the United States, butter is sold both salted and unsalted. We generally recommend unsalted butter. If you are using salted butter, take this into consideration before adding salt to a recipe.

OVEN TEMPERATURES

FAHRENHEIT	CELSIUS	GAS MARK
225	105	¼
250	120	½
275	135	1
300	150	2
325	165	3
350	180	4
375	190	5
400	200	6
425	220	7
450	230	8
475	245	9

CONVERTING TEMPERATURES FROM AN INSTANT-READ THERMOMETER

We include doneness temperatures in many of the recipes in this book. We recommend an instant-read thermometer for the job. Use this simple formula to convert Fahrenheit degrees to Celsius:

Subtract 32 degrees from the Fahrenheit reading, then divide the result by 1.8 to find the Celsius reading.

EXAMPLE
"Roast chicken until thighs register 175 degrees."

To convert:
175°F − 32 = 143°
143° ÷ 1.8 = 79.44°C, rounded down to 79°C

INDEX

Note: Page references in *italics* indicate photographs.

C

E

Edamame

and Cabbage, Peanut Noodle Bowls with, 250–51, *251*

Green Rice and Vegetable Bowls with Fried Eggs, 236–37, *237*

Miso-Ginger Soup with Halibut and Zucchini Noodles, 80–81, *81*

Sesame Salmon with Snap Pea Slaw, 192–93, *193*

Eggplant

Grilled Beef Kebabs, 166–67, *167*

Ratatouille with Poached Eggs, 42–43, *43*

Roasted, and Sesame, Soba Noodles with, 252–53, *253*

Stuffed, with Bulgur and Tomatoes, 244–45, *245*

Eggs

Chickpea Shakshuka, 40, *41*

Fried, Green Rice and Vegetable Bowls with, 236–37, *237*

Kale and Black Bean Breakfast Burritos, 46–47, *47*

Pea and Feta Frittata, 44–45, *45*

Poached, Ratatouille with, 42–43, *43*

Super Cobb Salad, 132–33, *133*

with Swiss Chard and Sweet Potato Hash, 38–39, *39*

Enchiladas, Chicken, 140–41, *141*

Escarole

and Chickpea Soup with Fennel and Orange, 86–87, *87*

Chopped Salad with Chicken and Jícama, 134, *135*

Fattoush with, 230–31, *231*

and Orange Salad with Green Olives, 274, *275*

Quinoa Taco Salad, 232–33, *233*

Wilted, and Chickpea Salad, Sirloin Steak with, 164–65, *165*

F

Fajitas, Grilled Chicken, 126–27, *127*

Farfalle with Broccoli and Turkey Sausage, 150–51, *151*

Farro

Bowls with Tofu, Mushrooms, and Spinach, 238–39, *239*

Salad, Cucumber-Mint, Grilled Tuna Steaks with, 216–17, *217*

Fats, healthful, 7, 17

Fattoush with Escarole, 230–31, *231*

Fennel

and Bitter Greens, Parmesan Chicken with, 106–7, *107*

Chickpeas, and Chermoula, Braised Chicken Breasts with, 116–17, *117*

and Orange, Chickpea and Escarole Soup with, 86–87, *87*

Pea and Feta Frittata, 44–45, *45*

Fermentable carbohydrates, 13

Fiber, 6, 8, 9, 17

Fish

Blackened Red Snapper with Sautéed Spinach and Black Rice, 210–11, *211*

Coconut-Ginger Swordfish Packets with Couscous, Snow Peas, and Bell Pepper, 214–15, *215*

Crispy Snapper with Charred Okra and Tomatoes, 206–7, *207*

Grilled Tuna Steaks with Cucumber-Mint Farro Salad, 216–17, *217*

Miso-Ginger Soup with Halibut and Zucchini Noodles, 80–81, *81*

Oven-Roasted Salmon with Tangerine-Ginger Relish, 190–91, *191*

Pan-Roasted Cod, 202, *203*

Fish *(cont.)*

Pomegranate-Roasted Salmon with Lentils and Swiss Chard, 194–95, *195*

Roasted Halibut with Broccolini, and Potatoes with Mustard Sauce, 208–9, *209*

Roasted Trout with White Bean and Tomato Salad, 212, *213*

Salmon, Avocado, Orange, and Watercress Salad, 196–97, *197*

Salmon Cakes with Sautéed Beet Greens and Lemon-Parsley Sauce, 200–201, *201*

Salmon Tacos, 198–99, *199*

Sautéed Halibut with Succotash, 204–5, *205*

Sesame Salmon with Snap Pea Slaw, 192–93, *193*

Tagine, 92–93, *93*

and Vegetable Chowder, New England–Style, 82–83, *83*

Flavor boosters, 19

Flour Blends

ATK All-Purpose Gluten-Free, 31

ATK Whole-Grain Gluten-Free, 31

FODMAPs

defined, 12, 13

high FODMAP foods, 14

low FODMAP foods, 14

FODMAP stacking, 16

Freekeh Salad with Sweet Potatoes, Walnuts, and Raisins, 234–35, *235*

Frittata, Pea and Feta, 44–45, *45*

Fructans, 13, 15–16, 20

Fructose, 13

Fruits

high and low FODMAP, 14

low-fructose, stocking up on, 19

see also Berry(ies); *specific fruits*

Functional GI disorders (FGID), 10–11

K

Kale

Baby, and Parsnips, Flank Steak with, 154–55, *155*

and Black Bean Breakfast Burritos, 46–47, *47*

Chicken and Vegetable Soup, 72–73, *73*

and Kabocha Squash, Roasted Chicken Breasts with, 114–15, *115*

Pan-Steamed, 262

Pan-Steamed, with Pancetta and Pine Nuts, 262, *263*

Pesto, Tomatoes, and Chicken, Pasta with, 138–39, *139*

Power Smoothies, 66, *67*

Super Cobb Salad, 132–33, *133*

Tuscan Bean Stew, 96–97, *97*

Vegetable and Beef Stew, 90–91, *91*

Kimchi, 32

L

Lactose, 13

Lactose-free products, 19

Lactose intolerance, 13

Lasagna, Beef and Spinach, 170–71, *171*

Leaky gut syndrome, 6

Legumes

high and low FODMAP, 14

see also Bean(s); Lentil(s)

Lemon

-Cucumber Water, 26

and Parsley, Baked Quinoa with, 288, *289*

-Parsley Sauce and Sautéed Beet Greens, Salmon Cakes with, 200–201, *201*

Lemon *(cont.)*

Preserved, Shrimp, and Peas, Linguine with, 220–21, *221*

Lentil(s)

and Chicken Soup, Smoky, with Swiss Chard, 74–75, *75*

Chipotle-Braised Pork and Rice, 178–79, *179*

-Pineapple Salad, Grilled Pork Tenderloin with, 184–85, *185*

Salad with Pomegranate and Walnuts, 296, *297*

Salad with Spiced Carrots and Cilantro, 296

Sweet Potato, and Poblano Tacos, 256–57, *257*

and Swiss Chard, Pomegranate-Roasted Salmon with, 194–95, *195*

Tomato Rice with, 284, *285*

Lime and Cilantro, Pan-Roasted Parsnips with, 268, *269*

Linguine with Shrimp, Peas, and Preserved Lemon, 220–21, *221*

Long Beans and Ginger-Orange Chicken, Stir-Fried, 124–25, *125*

Low FODMAP Diet

allium alternatives for, 15, 20

breads for, 27–31

broths for, 24–25

choosing ingredients for, 18

dairy and lactose in, 13

dairy products for, 19

dairy-free products for, 19

flavor boosters for, 19

flavorful beverages for, 26–27

foundational sauces for, 21–23

fruits for, 19

gluten-free flour blends for, 31

grains and grain alternatives for, 19

greens for, 19

herbs for, 19

high-fiber foods for, 17

lactose-free products for, 19

Low FODMAP Diet *(cont.)*

limiting or eliminating fructans, 15–16

Monash app for, 16

overview of, 12–13

phased dietary approach, 12

probiotic partners for, 31–33

vegetables for, 19

wheat for, 15–16

Low-lactose diet, 13

M

Mannitol, 13

Maple (syrup)

-Ginger Roasted Pork Tenderloin with Swiss Chard and Carrots, 180–81, *181*

and Sage, Roasted Kabocha Squash with, 280

Switchel, *26, 27*

-Vanilla Granola, 52, *53*

Meatballs

Spaghetti and, 168–69, *169*

Turkey, with Lemony Wild Rice and Artichokes, 142–43, *143*

Meatloaf with Roasted Potatoes and Green Beans, 172–73, *173*

Meaty Lasagna, 170–171, *171*

Microbes, 5

Microbiome, 5

Millet

Pilaf, Curried, with Almonds and Raisins, 290, *291*

Spiced, and Spinach, Steak Tips with, 158, *159*

Mint

-Cantaloupe Iced Green Tea, 26

-Cucumber Farro Salad, Grilled Tuna Steaks with, 216–17, *217*

Fattoush with Escarole, 230–31, *231*

Herbed Yogurt Sauce, 23